Disease and the Environment in the Medieval and Early Modern Worlds

This volume brings together environmental and human perspectives, engages with both historians and scientists, and, being mindful that environments and disease recognize no boundaries, includes studies that touch on Europe, the wider Mediterranean world, Asia, Africa, and the Americas.

Disease and the Environment in the Medieval and Early Modern Worlds explores the intertwined relationships between humans, the natural and manmade environments, and disease. Urgency gives us a sense that we need a longer view of human responses and interactions with the airs, waters, and places in which we live, and a greater understanding of the activities and attitudes that have led us to the present. Through a series of new research studies, two salient questions are explored: What are the deeper patterns in thinking about disease and the environment? What can we know about the environmental and ecological parameters of emergent human diseases over a longer period – aspects of disease that contemporary persons were not able to know or understand in the way that we do today?

The broad chronological and geographical approach makes this volume perfect for students and scholars interested in the history of disease, environment, and landscape in the medieval and early modern worlds.

Lori Jones is a medical historian at Carleton University and the University of Ottawa, Canada. Her research focuses primarily on plague texts and images. She is the author of *Patterns of Plague* (2022) and co-editor of *Death and Disease in the Medieval and Early Modern World* (2022) with Nükhet Varlık.

Themes in Environmental History

Themes in Environmental History is a series of books aimed at 2nd and 3rd year undergraduate students and postgraduate students in the fields of history and environmental studies. The collection covers key areas of environmental history from across the globe, running from 500 CE to the present day. These books bring together chapters on the historiography of the field and the new research that is being done to move the field forward, making engaging reading for students. Topics covered are varied and expansive and emphasize the importance of looking back at environmental history to date to understand where we are today.

Water in North American Environmental History
Martin V. Melosi

Disease and the Environment in the Medieval and Early Modern Worlds
Edited by Lori Jones

For more information about this series, please visit: https://www.routledge.com/Themes-in-Environmental-History/book-series/TIEH

Disease and the Environment in the Medieval and Early Modern Worlds

Edited by
Lori Jones

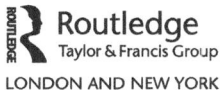
Routledge
Taylor & Francis Group

LONDON AND NEW YORK

Cover image: Tacuinum Sanitatis. 14th century. Medieval handbook of health. A man drinks water from a river. Folio 90v © PRISMA ARCHIVO/Alamy Stock Photo

First published 2022
by Routledge
4 Park Square, Milton Park, Abingdon, Oxon OX14 4RN

and by Routledge
605 Third Avenue, New York, NY 10158

Routledge is an imprint of the Taylor & Francis Group, an informa business

British Library Cataloguing-in-Publication Data
A catalogue record for this book is available from the British Library

Library of Congress Cataloging-in-Publication Data
Names: Jones, Lori (Medical historian), editor.
Title: Disease and the environment in the medieval and early modern worlds / edited by Lori Jones.
Description: Abingdon, Oxon ; New York, NY : Routledge, 2022. | Series: Themes in environmental history | Includes bibliographical references and index.
Identifiers: LCCN 2021060024 (print) | LCCN 2021060025 (ebook) | ISBN 9780367151737 (hardback) | ISBN 9780367151720 (paperback) | ISBN 9780429055478 (ebook)
Subjects: LCSH: Environmentally induced diseases—History. | Environmental health—History. | Medical climatology—History. | Public health—History. | Medicine, Medieval.
Classification: LCC RB152.5 .D573 2022 (print) | LCC RB152.5 (ebook) | DDC 616.9/8—dc23/eng/20220324
LC record available at https://lccn.loc.gov/2021060024
LC ebook record available at https://lccn.loc.gov/2021060025

ISBN: 978-0-367-15173-7 (hbk)
ISBN: 978-0-367-15172-0 (pbk)
ISBN: 978-0-429-05547-8 (ebk)

DOI: 10.4324/9780429055478

Typeset in Bembo
by codeMantra

Contents

Figures

Maps

Tables

Contributors

Abigail Agresta is Assistant Professor of History at George Washington University. She specializes in medieval European and Mediterranean history, with an emphasis on environmental history, urban history, and history of public health. Her book *The Keys to Bread and Wine: Faith, Nature, and Infrastructure in Late Medieval Valencia* will be published by Cornell University Press in 2022.

Lucy C. Barnhouse has been Assistant Professor of History at Arkansas State University since autumn 2020, having previously held visiting positions at the College of Wooster and Wartburg College. Her forthcoming monograph, *Houses of God, Places for the Sick*, examines hospitals in the religious and social networks of late medieval cities. She has edited and translated leprosy examination letters for punctum's *Medieval Disability Sourcebook: Western Europe* and contributed to the collection *Leprosy and Identity in the Middle Ages: From England to the Mediterranean*. She teaches courses in premodern and medical history and is a founding member of the Footnoting History podcast.

Gérard L. Chouin is an Associate Professor of African History in the Harrison Ruffin Tyler Department of History at William & Mary, which he joined in 2014 after spending twenty years in Ghana, Nigeria, and The Gambia. His research interests include medieval to modern African history and archaeology, landscape, urbanization and environmental studies, global health, and the social and natural histories of diseases. He is currently the co-director of the Ife-Sungbo Archaeological Project that focuses on social, political, and environmental change in southwestern Nigeria, before and after the opening of the Atlantic trade.

Sharon N. DeWitte is a Professor of Anthropology at the University of South Carolina, Columbia. Her research specialties are bioarchaeology, palaeoepidemiology, and palaeodemography. She engages in the reconstruction of life, health, disease, and demography in the past using data from human skeletal remains, and is ultimately interested in the ways in which research on past populations informs our understanding of and promotes health among living people. For the last fifteen years, her research has primarily centred around the Black Death (*c.* 1346–53), one of the most devastating and influential pandemics in human history.

Cindy Ermus is Assistant Professor of History at the University of Texas at San Antonio. She has published on catastrophe and crisis management in eighteenth-century Europe and the Atlantic, as well as on digital history and the future of the historical profession. She is also the editor of a volume entitled *Environmental Disaster in the Gulf South: Two Centuries of Catastrophe, Risk and Resilience* (Baton Rouge, 2018). Her current book project is a transnational study of the Plague of Provence of 1720 ("Great Plague of Marseille"), one of the last outbreaks of plague in Western Europe. Beyond the classroom, she is a co-founder, executive editor, and contributor for the digital academic publication, *Age of Revolutions* (www. ageofrevolutions.com).

Lori Jones is a historian of medieval and early modern medicine at Carleton University and the University of Ottawa. After receiving her PhD in history at the University of Ottawa, she held consecutive post-doctoral fellowships at Carleton University funded by the Associated Medical Services and Nova Scotia Health Research Foundation and by the Social Sciences and Humanities Research Council of Canada. Her research focuses on plague texts and images and on early modern medical manuscripts. She is the author of *Patterns of Plague: Changing Ideas about Plague in England and France, 1348–1750* (Montreal, 2022) and co-editor of *Death and Disease in the Medieval and Early Modern World: Perspectives From Across the Mediterranean and Beyond* (York, 2022) with Nükhet Varlık. She has also published several book chapters and journal articles on plague treatises and images.

Courtney Krolikowski is a PhD candidate in the Department of History and Classical Studies at McGill University in Montreal, Quebec, working under the supervision of Dr. Faith Wallis. Her current research explores the status of lepers in Bologna, Italy, in the High Middle Ages with a focus on the interaction of the social, religious, and medical aspects of the disease as well as arguing for the inclusion of leprosy in the cadre of medieval disabilities. She co-organized the "Leprosy and the 'Leper' Reconsidered" Conference in 2018 at McGill University with Anna Peterson.

Guillaume Linte has a PhD in history from the University of Paris-Est. His thesis focused on naval medicine and health issues related to transoceanic travel in France during the early modern period. He is currently a Swiss National Science Foundation Postdoctoral Researcher at the Institute for Ethics, History, and the Humanities (iEH2) at the University of Geneva. His research interests include the history of health, science, and colonization. He is the author of several articles and book chapters dealing with the history of medicine in France and its Empire during the early modern period, and the Portuguese expeditions to Africa in the fifteenth century.

Anna M. Peterson earned her PhD in medieval history from the University of St Andrews in 2017, was awarded a Mellon Fellowship at the Pontifical Institute of Mediaeval Studies (Toronto) from 2018 to 2019, and is currently an adjunct at the Universidad Europea Miguel de Cervantes. Her research has focused on assistive institutions in France and Italy, especially on their relationship with religious and secular bodies as well as responses to corruption. She is the co-founder of "Leprosy and the 'Leper' Reconsidered" along with Courtney Krolikoski. Currently, she is a member of the project *Hermenéutica del Cuerpo Visible: Conceptualizaciones y Prácticas en la Medicina Medieval de Tradición Latina/Hermeneutics of the Visible Body: Conceptualisations and Practices in Medieval Medicine in the Latin Tradition* (PID2019–107671GB-I00).

Nükhet Varlık is Associate Professor of History at Rutgers University – Newark. She is a historian of the Ottoman Empire interested in disease, medicine, and public health. She is the author of *Plague and Empire in the Early Modern Mediterranean World: The Ottoman Experience, 1347–1600* (Cambridge, 2015), editor of *Plague and Contagion in the Islamic Mediterranean* (Kalamazoo, 2017), and co-editor of *Death and Disease in the Medieval and Early Modern World: Perspectives From Across the Mediterranean and Beyond* (York, 2022) with Lori Jones. Her new book project, *Empire, Ecology, and Plague: Rethinking the Second Pandemic (ca.1340s–ca. 1940s)*, examines the 600-year-old Ottoman plague experience in a global ecological context. She is involved in the Black Death Digital Archive and contributes to multidisciplinary research projects that incorporate perspectives from palaeogenetics, bioarchaeology, disease ecology, and climate science into historical inquiry.

Acknowledgements

I thank Laura Pilsworth at Taylor and Francis for approaching me in the first instance to put this volume together and Monica H. Green for recommending me. Steering a volume about environment and disease during a pandemic has been both a challenge and an opportunity. A challenge, of course, because my and everyone else's attention and energy had to pivot over the past two years to more immediate concerns, notably staying healthy. I am grateful to each contributor in this volume for staying the course and for submitting such insightful, new research with only relatively minor delays. I am also appreciative of those authors who fully intended to participate in the volume but who, for pandemic-related reasons, were not able to do so in the end. I trust and hope that their valuable work will be forthcoming in another format sometime soon. Producing this volume during a pandemic has also been an opportunity of sorts, as living in an era marked by a worldwide disease outbreak that emerged from some as-yet unconfirmed environment has made the topics addressed in this book's chapters all the more relevant.

I acknowledge the scholars who reviewed individual chapters in this volume and provided thoughtful and valuable feedback: Ellen Arnold, Hannah Barker, Hugh Cagle, Ann G. Carmichael, Sasha Pfau, Junko Takeda, Paul-Arthur Tortosa, Wendy J. Turner, and Brittany S. Walter. Their time and effort has made the work presented here that much better.

The publication team at Routledge has been both helpful and supportive, and I would especially like to note the pleasure of working with Isabel Voice, whose constant (and very friendly) check-ins helped keep the project on track.

Introduction

Diseases in Historical Environments

Lori Jones

This volume offers an interdisciplinary examination of the intertwined relationships between humans, the natural and manmade environments, and
disease in the medieval and early modern worlds. Recognizing the inherent
value of studies that offer a more holistic view of the past and that generate
new insights, it brings together environmental and human perspectives and
engages with both historians and scientists. Being mindful that pre-modern
environments and disease clearly recognized no boundaries – just as they
do not today – the volume includes studies that touch on Europe, the wider
Mediterranean world, Asia, Africa, and the Americas. People throughout
western Eurasia, North Africa, and around the Mediterranean basin lived in
similar disease and mortality environments and imposed their thinking about
what constituted a healthy environment onto regions further away; what we
thus learn by stepping beyond Europe's borders helps us to better understand
that "European" history of disease and the environment cannot be understood in a vacuum. The volume's *longue durée* time frame, stretching from the
High Middle Ages to the dawn of the modern era, also bypasses traditional
periodization, since environmental challenges and peoples' responses to them
did not suddenly shift gears once an imaginary timeline was crossed.

In the twenty-first century, we are facing and attempting to manage accelerating climate change, environmental encroachment and degradation, and
unprecedented extinction of species and loss of biodiversity – together with
what sometimes seems to be a growing flood of emerging and re-emerging
diseases. More than fifty serious outbreaks of emerging (i.e., newly recognized) or re-emerging (i.e., resurging after a period of quiet, appearing in
new locations, or of drug-resistant variants) infectious diseases have been
recorded since 1998 (Public Health England 2019). Urgency gives us a new
sense that we need a longer view of human responses and interactions with
the airs, waters, and places in which we live, and a greater understanding of
the activities and attitudes that have led us to today. The salient questions
explored in the volume are, what are the deeper patterns in thinking about
disease and the environment? What can we know about the environmental
and ecological parameters of emergent human diseases over a longer period

DOI: 10.4324/9780429055478-1

of time – aspects of disease that persons at the time were not in a position to know or understand in the way that we do today?

Interactions between humans and their environments in the past have affected the environment that we now live in; indeed, many of our current challenges can be better understood through a thorough knowledge and understanding of what transpired in the past. At the same time, we must recognize that humans and human societies have never stood apart from the environments in which they existed. Humans have significantly altered disparate landscapes – and to an extent the entire planet – for more than 40,000 years, likely over 100,000. We are patch disturbers. And human decisions and human actions have contributed to today's global climate crisis, of that there is no doubt. Yet it is not solely human agency that drives environmental change over time, and stepping beyond the anthropocentric gaze that has so long dominated our thinking allows us to see humans as actors in an environment over which they do not always have control.

Environmental history scholarship in the French tradition – notably the *Annales* school with its emphasis on the *longue durée* – paid significant attention to geography, the environment, and the climate as historical influencers. Pioneering work by Fernand Braudel (1972–73, 1949) focused explicitly on how slow, at times imperceptible, changes in the environment impacted social organization and culture. Braudel's *Annales* successor, Emmanuel Le Roy Ladurie, also explored in some detail the impact of long-term shifts in the environment on the human condition, intertwining them with political, cultural, economic, and social change (Le Roy Ladurie 2004–2009, 1967); he was also among the first to specifically explore the environmental globalization of disease (Le Roy Ladurie 1981). The early Anglo-American tradition – led in the 1960s and 1970s by Hubert H. Lamb (1977, 1966) and Clarence Glacken (1967), among others – tended instead to look at humans and their interactions with the environment, exploring climatic and landscape change over time within familiar European historical temporal and spatial frameworks (McNeill, 2010a, 2003). Despite Le Roy Ladurie's earlier broaching of the topic, it wasn't really until Alfred W. Crosby's works appeared – *The Columbian Exchange: Biological and Cultural Consequences of 1492* (1972) and *Ecological Imperialism: The Biological Expansion of Europe, 900–1900* (1986) – that diseases of plants, animals, and humans were systematically pulled into the broader temporal/spatial narratives of human and environmental history. Crosby examined the ecological underpinnings and impacts of a European expansion and colonialism endeavour that substantially altered environmental and disease landscapes along with their human populations in Europe, Asia, and the Americas. Subsequent scholars adapted the scope of Crosby's take on history-through-ecology and disease to explore Africa (Curtin 1998), China (Elvin and Ts'ui-jung 1998; Marks 1998), the Indian Ocean (Arnold 1991), and England (Dobson 1997), among other places.

Over the past twenty years, much additional scholarship has followed, as historians and other scholars have explored environment–disease links in specific pre-modern geographical regions, including China (Marks 2017), Egypt (Borsch 2005; Derr 2019; Mikhail 2012), the Mediterranean littoral (Davis 2007; Gratien 2017; Tabak 2009), Africa (Akyeampong 2006), Eurasia (Campbell 2016; Green 2018), and the American and Indian colonies (Sivaramakrishnan 2011; Wear 2011). Cross-cultural approaches to the topic have also appeared recently (Bretelle-Establet et al. 2019). The impact of disease on entire ancient civilizations, such as Neolithic societies or the Roman Empire, has likewise received attention (Harper 2016; 2017; Little 2007; Rascovan et al. 2019; Selassie 2011). Others have examined how, in the very act of creating civilization – which inherently required environmental transformation – and then revising, expanding, and transferring that civilization to new regions of the globe, human beings have constantly altered their surroundings and created conditions suitable for the emergence and spread of disease (Barrett and Armelagos 2013; Kenny 2021; King et al. 2017). Further studies have explored the role of climate change(s), natural disasters, as well as human intervention in the environment, among other factors, on the creation, evolution, and maintenance of actual or perceived pre-modern disease ecologies or regimes around the globe (Cagle 2015; Campbell 2016; Dey 2018; McCandless 2011; McNeill 2010b; Sallares 2002; 2006; Varlık 2015; Warren 2020; Webster 2021; White 2010; Ziegler 2016b). Recent work has, moreover, taken Crosby and Le Roy Ladurie's ideas even further back in time to explore the deep-in-time historical globalization of infectious disease (Green 2017).

Humans have not, however, always behaved or thought themselves at the mercy of *unmanageable* environmental threats, including diseases. Instead, they have actively sought to manage them. By identifying and distinguishing between healthy and unhealthy landscapes and climates, the original Hippocratic *Airs, Waters, and Places* (fifth century BCE) instructed itinerant healers how to deflect dis-ease onto the local environment and underlay medieval and early modern understanding of the relationship between environments and the generation of disease (Wear 2008). The resultant attempts to manage potentially diseased environments – what we might consider to be the origins of public health – have become another rich field of study in recent years (Ciecieznski 2013; Coomans 2021; Fay 2015; Geltner 2013; 2019; Jørgensen 2013; Rawcliffe 2013; Rawcliffe and Weeda 2019; Zaneri and Geltner 2020). Victorian portrayals of medieval and early modern cities and towns as rubbish-strewn dung heaps inhabited by mangy dogs, poxy livestock, and humans too ignorant and apathetic to improve them have largely been dispelled. Indeed, it has been established beyond doubt that medieval and early modern city governments and their inhabitants were concerned about hygiene and managing the spread of disease. Many pre-modern cities left much to be desired when judged by modern sensitivities, yet by taking account of contemporary worldviews to understand the impetuses that lay behind the broad range of public works, regulations, and policies enacted to improve local environments, we can better piece together how pre-modern peoples perceived the relationship between their environments and disease.

Human agency cannot explain everything in the environment, just as historical studies alone cannot answer all the questions that new analytical technologies are bringing to the study of the environment proper: the determinants of a plague outbreak, for example, or the causes of the Little Ice Age. We thus see scholarly advances on multiple fronts. Recognition of the innate relationship between environment and disease, for example, led to the development of landscape epidemiology, a methodology that uses the "landscape as a frame for understanding" the emergence, persistence, and transmission of disease in the environment (Ziegler 2016a, 99; see also Lambin et al. 2010 and Reisen 2010). Those diseases that have been transmitted to humans from animals, that require an insect or other living creature for their transmission, or that arise from contaminated water or food are best understood as diseases of the environment. In each case, a microbe that lives naturally in a specific environment – whether a bacterium, a virus, a fungus, or a protozoa – enters the bodies of people and causes disease. The transmission of disease is thus linked to particular landscapes, and often to human encroachment into them, disruption of them, or, in some cases, the very creation of them (think of mosquito-borne diseases increasing in areas where humans have created ideal conditions for mosquitoes: standing pools of water in discarded tires, for example).

While descriptive studies of premodern landscapes, including changes to human-dominated spaces, have much explanatory value, it has increasingly been recognized that studying, and attempting to understand, interrelationships between the environment and disease in the past requires information far beyond that left behind by human activities and studied by historians. Scientific fields, such as archaeology, palaeogenetics, bio- and medical anthropology, climatology, and more, have much to offer and allow us to think much more broadly, forcing us, in some cases, to revisit our texts and documentary evidence with new questions. Advances in the palaeosciences, for example, have allowed the legacy of Crosby's scope to be narrowed to the level of microscopic pathogens, showing how (or at least, asking how) the environment enabled the emergence, spread, and, eventually, "settling in" of longstanding sylvatic – or wild animal – diseases into new hosts, humans. Plague is at the forefront of these new studies, and efforts to reconstruct an environmental history of the pathogen itself, rather than simply its appearance in human populations, is well underway (Eroshenko et al. 2017; Kausrud et al. 2010). So too are explorations into whether (and again how) plague, initially a rodent disease of Central Asia, became endemic in parts of Europe for centuries before mysteriously disappearing once again (Bos et al. 2016; Carmichael 2014; Morozova et al. 2020; Siefert et al. 2016; Spyrou et al. 2019). Studies of other pathogens are following suit to show how, for example, diseases changed genetically as they spread across and through different environments (Green 2017; Green and Jones 2020).

Bioarchaeologists too are uncovering the health impacts of climatic and environmental change on skeletal remains. Their work not only highlights how changes in the environment affected disease patterns but also demonstrates the increased risk that the urban environment posed to the health of humans in the past, regardless of where in the world they lived (Betsinger and DeWitte 2020; Robbins Schug 2020; Walter and DeWitte 2017). The role played by historical climates and climate change in disease generation, spread, and persistence in the past are likewise gaining attention among historians and other scholars, not only for creating the environments that are conducive to human-to-human transmission and the survival and replication of disease vectors such as insects but also for upending those environments and creating the conditions that lead to the spill over of zoonotic (animal) diseases into human populations (Ben Ari et al. 2011; Brooke 2014; Campbell and Ludlow 2020; Green 2018; Luterbacher et al. 2020; McMichael 2017; Newfield 2016; Webb 2018).

This volume was conceived with all of this fast-moving scholarship in mind, and each chapter highlights some of the critical changes that have subtly (or not so subtly) been taking place in the history of pre-modern disease and the environment in recent years. Taken together, they address themes that resonate strongly today, including tensions between competing interests in how the environment is to be shaped or utilized (and, thus, its tendency towards healthiness or unhealthiness), synergies between distantly located environments, and changing ideas about what "the environment" itself entails.

The volume is organized into three overlapping sections. Section 1, "Cleansing and Managing Local *Airs, Waters, and Places*," includes three chapters that explore how pre-modern people in different regions of medieval Europe perceived and responded to local threats of disease by attempting to manage their surroundings. In a sense, these chapters follow the traditional approach to humans as directors and managers who tamed and governed their environments. Yet each offers a novel approach to the documentary evidence, showing that a distinctive pre-modern environmentalism was informed by medical notions of healthscaping: policy decisions and infrastructure projects undertaken by municipal governments to create and maintain healthy environments, or alternatively to mitigate the environments that they considered to be health-harming, throughout and beyond their cities (Geltner 2013; 2020). More than economic development or environmentalism in the modern sense, these chapters reveal wider meanings of health, environment, and civic responsibility than we see today. Taken together, they demonstrate how a shared culture of healthscaping was adapted to meet locally specific environmental challenges.

In Chapter 1, Anna M. Peterson and Courtney Krolikowski take us to the pre-Black Death northern Italian cities of Bologna and Siena. Each city was both a powerful commercial hub and an important religious centre, in addition to developing strong municipal legislative bodies governed by comprehensive law codes. Here, we can see medieval urban environmental policy management at work. Yet, we also see here that health, disease, and even the environment in this context had much wider meanings than they do today: morally and spiritually clean environments were as important in the urban context as was one clear of detritus and foul-smelling industrial by-products. By diving into the cities' respective archival records to see how healthscaping policies and practices were conceived and enacted, and focusing, in particular, on the management of food, water, and assistive (i.e., charitable) institutions in the built environment, Peterson and Krolikowski demonstrate how various aspects of civic life were impacted by a desire to keep the urban environment clean, disease-free, and respectable.

In Chapter 2, Abigail Agresta turns our attention to late medieval Valencia, in south-eastern Spain. While urban environmental health threats in Valencia largely mirrored those faced in other medieval cities, here we find one additional key issue: water management. While a network of canals irrigated the land surrounding the city and made it one of the richest agricultural areas around the Mediterranean, not all water was created equal. Clean running water was vital to the city's population – for drinking, turning the mill wheels that ground the city's flour, and irrigating the crops that fed and enriched the city; but stagnant water, such as that used to flood rice fields or that settled in poorly managed canals, was believed to cause infections, illness, and death. Managing health and keeping the urban environment disease-free therefore required city officials to constantly calibrate and oversee the city's waterways. And, as Agresta demonstrates, these very actions sometimes led to conflict between local residents when their personal interests were affected.

In contrast to northern Italy and southeastern Iberia, Lucy C. Barnhouse's Chapter 3 on cities in the Upper Rhineland's prosperous trading zone showcases how the promotion of moral and physical well-being in medieval towns did not necessarily require centralized governance and infrastructure or top-down control. Mainz, Worms, and Speyer each had their own set of customs and laws determining how matters of public health were negotiated. By examining each city's legal codes, penitentiary records, business agreements, and, most interestingly, records of disputes, Barnhouse reveals that despite their lack of centralized government, municipal authorities were neither indifferent to concerns with healthful environmental management nor powerless to enact relevant legislation when necessary. Instead, public health regulation and environmental management were incorporated into each city's customs and adapted as needed to accommodate the rights of individual citizens. Barnhouse gives us insight into the types of unhealthy or potentially diseased environments that gave rise to disputes between neighbours, including blocked wastewater channels, undesirable clientele in bathhouses, bad or offensive behaviour, and conflict over access to and proper management of wells and public latrines. Here, as in the previous chapters, we see that medieval ideas of health and disease in the urban environment were broadly conceived.

The thinking behind, and actions associated with, medieval healthscaping and managing the environment continued well into the early modern era. Especially during recurrent outbreaks of plague and, later, other diseases, municipal authorities across Europe stepped up their efforts to keep their streets clean of foul-smelling, disease-inducing waste and to control the movement of people assumed to generate or carry disease, notably the poor, the criminal, and the immoral. However, these longstanding efforts also failed to control plague, and gradually eroded Europeans' commitment to the shared cultural and religious bases of environmental responsibility that had marked the medieval era. An accumulation of disruptions to their shared sense of purpose and meaning in local healthscaping coincided with an age of exploration and colonialism that took Europeans farther afield into new, unfamiliar environments seemingly full of novel disease threats. And, as new medical and scientific thinking took hold, old ways of thinking about disease and its place in the environment started to crumble, giving rise to vigorous debate and new approaches to disease containment and management.

Three chapters in Section 2, "Recalibrating *Airs, Waters, and Places*: New Environments, New Mentalities," explore how early modern Europeans began to reconsider the environmental causes of disease. Here, we see writers attempting to understand and explain the unusual environments, unfamiliar climates, and novel diseases that they faced in Africa, Asia, and the Americas. They did so, in part, by comparing them with what was familiar, ultimately deeming foreign landscapes to be unhealthy and disease-ridden in contrast to their own purportedly healthy homelands. Here, too, we see Europeans gradually shifting the geographical and environmental origins of plague to foreign sources and foreign environments. The Plague of Provence (1720–22), in some ways, marks the culmination of these attempts: in that epidemic it is possible to trace a significant change in mentality about contagion, environment, and disease management.

As Lori Jones discusses in Chapter 4, when the Black Death struck medieval Eurasia, the Hippocratic *Airs, Waters, and Places* tradition was easily incorporated into medical writers' attempts to explain the origin and cause of plague. Plague tract authors pointed to domestic environments, including ubiquitous swamps, marshes, and foul-smelling urban industries, to explain local outbreaks. Mitigation efforts, in turn, focused on cleaning up these local sites of disease. Yet, as Jones's analysis of English and French plague treatises reveals, although the overall environment–disease relationship remained largely intact in these texts across the centuries, changing medical norms and contemporary socio-cultural and political considerations ultimately shifted the location of places that tract writers associated with plague. Before the early eighteenth century and the great outbreak in southern France, plagued environments were re-located from localized European spaces to definitively foreign sites. The Ottoman Empire – long stereotyped as a despotic, violent, terror-inducing regime, and its people as immoral and religiously suspect – became the plaguescape *par excellence*, its crowded streets and stagnant swamps blamed for outbreaks that reached European cities. As outbreaks continued there with force after they appeared to have declined in the West, the assumption that plague had always come from the diseased environments of the eastern Mediterranean became entrenched in modern historiography.

Cindy Ermus maintains our focus on the Plague of Provence (1720–22) in Chapter 5, arguing that it is here where we can start to see that the management of disasters, including disease outbreaks, was predicated on different methods and based on different understandings of the relationship between contagion and the environment. Although the Lisbon earthquake of 1755 is often credited with instigating new intellectual inquiry into the nature of environmental disasters, Ermus shows that we should look instead to the Plague of Provence for the origins of this change in mentality. What sets the response to this large outbreak apart from those of previous eras is less the street-level actions taken to manage the disease than its highly centralized nature – with the regent in Paris deploying military commanders with unlimited authority to manage the crisis under martial law, thereby bypassing and overruling municipal efforts – and underlying thought processes about the nature of contagion. This was an era of vociferous debate between those who continued to believe that diseases arose in polluted environments that gave rise to corrupted air, called miasma, and those who believed more stridently in contagion and the possibility that disease was transmitted from person to person. The contagionists ultimately won the day, and their push for centralized trade embargoes, sanitary lines, and quarantines marked a distinctive shift in how disease outbreaks were managed in the decades and centuries to come.

In Chapter 6, Guillaume Linte further explores the theme of foreign disease environments by examining the early modern development of medical literature on exotic diseases, a key concern of which was the health of Europeans living in hot countries or climates. From the sixteenth century, overseas voyages to the south and east required travelling through the so-called Torrid Zone, located between the Tropics of Cancer and Capricorn. Not only did explorers pass through the region, but colonies and trading posts, meant for the spice and slave trades, were also established within it. A variety of environments – the West African coasts, the Caribbean islands, and the Indian peninsula – then witnessed a growing European presence over the following centuries. Yet this tropical region embodied difficult living conditions, and it logically ensued that the health of those who travelled or settled there would be negatively affected. At the crossroads of medicine and geography, literature on exotic diseases, produced primarily by physicians and surgeons who served aboard ships or in the colonies, provided key inputs for contemporary understanding of intertropical environments – and particular the rain that was deemed to be especially disease-inducing.

Recurrent plague was one of the many reasons traditional environmental notions frayed across the centuries, and it affected how contemporary European writers perceived diseased spaces elsewhere. Modern study of those recurrent outbreaks, in turn, gave rise to another dramatic intellectual reversal in the twentieth century: prominent medievalists and early modernists up to the end of the 1990s who had argued that *Yersinia pestis* (the pathogen that causes plague) could not have caused the massive and recurrent epidemics in Europe were proven incorrect. Their arguments were based largely on the apparently different manifestations (seasonality, mortality, speed of transmission) of the disease in the European past and the more recent (i.e., late nineteenth century) Asian outbreaks, as well as the fact that no sizeable epidemics had occurred in Europe since the 1700s (for a summary, see Green 2014 and Little 2011). The ideas invented in the early modern era (Chapters 4 and 5) that plague was repeatedly imported from the East and that new ideas of public health control (Chapter 5) – in contrast to longstanding medieval healthscaping efforts (Chapters 1–3) – finally freed Europeans of this menace, remained popular among historians until very recently. So too were ideas that foreign environments were especially unhealthy (Chapters 4 and 6). Many of these ideas are now being discarded, with modern science in many respects furnishing new information that enables us to revisit historical "facts." Jones ended Chapter 4, for example, with the recognition, emerging from recent studies, that local environments most likely did figure prominently in the generation of recurrent plague outbreaks across medieval and early modern Eurasia. Wild animal reservoirs of *Y. pestis* plausibly became established in a variety of regions, each comprising a different animal species suited to a locally specific environment. Furthermore, diverse local ecologies and climates both generated new strains of plague and caused it to behave differently from one place to another (Green 2020).

This turn to modern science leads us into Section 3, "Science Meets Historical Disease Environments." The three chapters in this final section address the "now what?" predicament – how do we need to think about the past and its dramatic pestilences now that we know with certainty that *Y. pestis* was involved in large-scale outbreaks? How do we need to think about the relationship between other diseases and the environment in the past? We return to the urgency, not just because the technologies and possibilities for scientific analysis are amazing, but because we now are ourselves held down by a tenacious pandemic.

Gérard Chouin's work in Chapter 7 acts as a bridge between all three sections of this volume. It first considers the origins and persistence of a longstanding narrative that entwines Africa, diseased environments, and death. He begins by revisiting European travelogues about the early modern Atlantic world, probing them as historical sources and reflecting critically on their contribution to the deeply rooted perception that tropical Africa represented the world's most dangerous environment. Early modern travellers' accounts are full of horrendous stories about the deadly or debilitating illnesses that awaited Europeans in Atlantic Africa. By unpacking the travellers' accounts, however, Chouin dismantles what he calls the narrative "smokescreen" and points towards a much more complex picture than that offered by a superficial reading of the socially and culturally constructed seventeenth-century travel stories. He then flips the narrative on its head and takes an anthropological perspective to explore how Africans themselves conceptualized and managed their own environment and its diseases before the nineteenth century.

As we saw with the medieval European cases, African understanding of the "environment" – and of disease causation – was far more extensive than how we think of it today: it embodied not only the physical landscape but also the spiritual and social realms. Managing the multiple spheres that comprised the environment meant that pre-modern Africans had developed a complex variety of disease mitigation techniques, each targeting the suspected origin of disease.

Chouin ends his chapter with an exploration of his working hypothesis about the making, demise, or subsistence of diseases in selected regions of the African continent's environment. Focussing on malaria and plague in particular, the former first arising in Africa and the latter being an imported disease, Chouin demonstrates how working cross-disciplinarily and bringing together evidence from the humanities and the sciences – including research on ancient DNA – allows us to slowly build a clearer picture of the intricate relationship between diseases and the environment in the past.

In Chapter 8, Nükhet Varlık explores these issues further as they apply to Anatolia, in modern-day Turkey. As elsewhere across Eurasia, plague arrived in Anatolia and its surroundings in the mid-fourteenth century on the heels of political, social, and environmental crises. As the region that hosted the disease for the longest time during the Second Plague Pandemic – a full 600 years – understanding what kept its plague reservoirs continuously active when they appear to have died out in Europe may help us to better comprehend the disease's long-term rhythms, expansion, and contraction. In short, Varlık asks, what social, economic, and, especially, environmental conditions were conducive to the persistence and later disappearance of plague from this region? As she demonstrates in this chapter that engages with historical and scientific literature, we need to be looking at how reservoirs, and the wild rodent populations that comprised them, expanded and contracted over time in reaction to climatic, environmental, and human-induced change.

In Chapter 9, Sharon DeWitte returns us to where we began: medieval Europe. Instead of looking at how communities addressed concerns with diseased environments, DeWitte demonstrates what bioarchaeological research can teach us about the impact of inter-related crises – including dramatic climate and environmental change, plague epidemics, and massive animal die-offs – on individual and community survivorship and health. That people's standards of living improved following the Black Death is already well known; however, as DeWitte's research shows, apparent gains in general health and survival might have been lost as the population and available resources achieved a new environmental equilibrium in the face of increasing urbanization and shifting climatic conditions. These findings demonstrate the dramatic effects that the interaction of natural forces (e.g., climatic conditions and disease epidemics) and anthropogenic factors (e.g., urban environments and socioeconomic disparities) had on human health in past populations.

The longstanding trend towards increasing urbanization and ongoing destruction of the natural habitat across the world means that the unhealthy conditions faced by our ancestors continue to affect us even today, evidenced by the threat posed by diseases breaking out of historically limited geographic regions and by emerging infectious diseases (Bouchard et al. 2019; Duik-Wasser et al. 2021; Hassell et al. 2017; Kilpatrick et al. 2017; Mackenstedt et al. 2015; Vanwambeke et al. 2019). These threats are now appearing at a more rapid pace, evidenced by our numerous twenty-first century epidemic disease experiences: SARS (global, 2002–04), H1N1 influenza (global, 2009–10), Ebola (West Africa, 2014–16), plague (Democratic Republic of the Congo, 2020; Madagascar, 2014–15, 2017–18), Zika (Americas, 2015–16), yellow fever (Africa, 2016), and now COVID-19 (global, 2019–ongoing).

As we attempt to understand how "our" disease outbreaks happened, exploring the intersection between human culture and practices and naturally occurring phenomena is critical; applying our lens of enquiry to the past is equally critical if we want to understand both how the "environment" was conceived historically and how and why it (and its management) changed over time (Hoffmann 2014). This includes how and why diseases erupted where they did and from whence they spread (Green 2017).

As the nine chapters in this volume demonstrate, the literal meaning of research – to re-search – allows us to look where we have looked repeatedly, not quite seeing what we once saw. This dialogue with the recent past is especially relevant in our modern pandemic moment, but even more so with the certainty of changing environmental conditions at a planetary scale. We particularly need to understand ourselves as actors and to comprehend the ideas that inform our assumptions and our actions. Our place in the environment is as old as we are as a species, and it is by looking to the past and understanding how our thinking about disease and the environment has changed over time, and with what successes and with what failures, that we might find our way forward into the future.

References

Akyeampong, Emmanuel. 2006. "Disease in West African History." In *Themes in West Africa's History*, edited by Akyeampong, Emmanuel, 33–51. Oxford, Athens and Accra: James Currey, Ohio University Press, and Woeli Publishing Services.

Arnold, David. 1991. "The Indian Ocean as a Disease Zone, 1500–1950." *South Asia: Journal of South Asian Studies* 14, no. 2: 1–21.

Barrett, Ron and George Armelagos. 2013. *An Unnatural History of Emerging Infections*. Oxford: Oxford University Press.

Ben Ari, Tamara, Simon Neerinckx, Kenneth L. Gage, Katharina Kreppel, Anne Laudisoit, Herwig Leirs, and Nils Chr. Stenseth. 2011. "Plague and Climate: Scales Matter," *PLoS Pathogens* 7, no. 9: e1002160.

Betsinger, Tracy K. and Sharon N. DeWitte, eds. 2020. *The Bioarchaeology of Urbanization: The Biological, Demographic, and Social Consequences of Living in Cities*. Cham: Springer.

Borsch, Stuart. 2005. *The Black Death in Egypt and England: A Comparative Study.* Austin: University of Texas Press.

Bos, Kirsten I., Alexander Herbig, Jason Sahl, Nicholas Waglechner, Mathieu Fourment, Stephen A. Forrest, Jennifer Klunk, Verena J. Schuenemann, Debi Poinar, Melanie Kuch, G. Brian Golding, Olivier Dutour, Paul Keim, Wagner, David M., Holmes Edward C., Johannes Krause, and Poinar Hendrik N. 2016. "Eighteenth-Century *Yersinia pestis* Genomes Reveal the Long-Term Persistence of an Historical Plague Focus." *eLife* 5: e12994. https://doi.org/10.7554/eLife.12994.

Bouchard, C., A. Dibernardo, J. Koffi, H. Wood, P. A. Leighton, and L. R. Lindsay. 2019. "N Increased Risk of Tick-borne Diseases with Climate and Environmental Changes." *Canada Communicable Disease Report* 45, no. 4: 83–89.

Braudel, Fernand. 1949. *La Méditerranée et le Monde Méditerranéen à l'Epoque de Philippe II.* 3 vols. Paris: Armand Colin.

Braudel, Fernand. 1972–73. *The Mediterranean and the Mediterranean World in the Age of Philip II.* 2 vols, 2nd rev. ed., translated by Siân Reynolds. New York: Harper & Row.

Bretelle-Establet, Florence, Marie Gaille, and Mehrnaz Katouzian-Safadi, eds. 2019. *Making Sense of Health, Disease, and the Environment in Cross-cultural History: The Arabic-Islamic World, China, Europe and North America.* Cham: Springer.

Brooke, John L. 2014. *Climate Change and the Course of Global History: A Rough Journey.* New York: Cambridge University Press.

Cagle, Hugh. 2015. "Beyond the Senegal: Inventing the Tropics in the Late Middle Ages." *Journal of Medieval Iberian Studies* 7, no. 2: 197–217.

Campbell, Bruce M. S. 2016. *The Great Transition: Climate, Disease and Society in the Late-Medieval World.* Cambridge: Cambridge University Press.

Campbell, Bruce M.S. and Francis Ludlow. 2020. "Climate, Disease and Society in Late-Medieval Ireland." *Proceedings of the Royal Irish Academy: Archaeology, Culture, History, Literature* 120: 159–252.

Carmichael, Ann G. 2014. "Plague Persistence in Western Europe: A Hypothesis." *The Medieval Globe* 1: 157–91.

Ciecieznski, N. J. 2013. "The Stench of Disease: Public Health and the Environment in Late-Medieval English Towns and Cities." *Health, Culture and Society* 4, no. 1: 92–104.

Coomans, Janna. 2021. *Community, Urban Health and Environment in the Late Medieval Low Countries.* Cambridge: Cambridge University Press.

Crosby, Alfred W. 1972. *The Columbian Exchange: Biological and Cultural Consequences of 1492.* Westport, CT: Greenwood.

Crosby, Alfred W. 1986. *Ecological Imperialism: The Biological Expansion of Europe, 900–1900.* Cambridge: Cambridge University Press.

Curtin, Philip. 1998. *Disease and Empire: The Health of European Troops in the Conquest of Africa.* Cambridge: Cambridge University Press.

Davis, Diana K. 2007. *Resurrecting the Granary of Rome: Environmental History and French Colonial Expansion in North Africa.* Athens, OH: Athens University Press.

Derr, Jennifer. 2019. *The Lived Nile: Environment, Disease, and Material Colonial Economy in Egypt.* Palo Alto, CA: Stanford University Press.

Dey, Arnab. 2018. *Tea Environments and Plantation Culture: Imperial Disarray in Eastern India.* Cambridge: Cambridge University Press.

Diuk-Wasser, Maria A., Meredith C. VanAcker, and Maria P. Fernandez. 2021. "Impact of Land Use Changes and Habitat Fragmentation on the Eco-epidemiology of Tick-borne Diseases." *Journal of Medical Entomology* 58, no. 4: 1546–64.

Dobson, Mary J. 1997. *Contours of Death and Disease in Early Modern England*. Cambridge: Cambridge University Press.

Elvin, Mark and Liu Ts'ui-jung, eds. 1998. *Sediments of Time: Environment and Society in Chinese History*. Cambridge: Cambridge University Press.

Eroshenko, Galina A., Nikita Yu Nosov, Yaroslav M. Krasnov, Yevgeny G. Oglodin, Lyubov M. Kukleva, Natalia P. Guseva, Alexander A. Kuznetsov, Sabyrzhan T. Abdikarimov, Aigul K. Dzhaparova, and Vladimir V. Kutyrev. 2017. "*Yersinia pestis* Strains of Ancient Phylogenetic Branch 0.ANT Are Widely Spread in the High-Mountain Plague Foci of Kyrgyzstan." *PLoS ONE* 12, no. 10: e0187230.

Fay, Isla. 2015. *Health and the City: Disease, Environment and Government in Norwich, 1200–1575*. Woodbridge: Boydell Press.

Gelter, Guy. 2013. "Healthscaping a Medieval City: Lucca's *Curia viarum* and the Future of Public Health History." *Urban History* 40, no. 3: 395–415.

Geltner, Guy. 2019. *Roads to Health: Infrastructure and Urban Wellbeing in Later Medieval Italy*. Philadelphia: University of Pennsylvania Press.

Geltner, Guy. 2020. "The Path to Pistoia: Urban Hygiene Before the Black Death." *Past & Present* 246, no. 1: 3–33.

Glacken, Clarence J. 1967. *Traces on the Rhodian shore: Nature and Culture in Western Thought from Ancient Times to the End of the Eighteenth Century*. Berkeley: University of California Press.

Gratien, Chris. 2017. "The Ottoman Quagmire: Malaria, Swamps, and Settlement in the Late Ottoman Mediterranean." *International Journal of Middle East Studies* 49, no. 4: 583–604.

Green, Monica H. 2014. "Taking 'Pandemic' Seriously: Making the Black Death Global." *The Medieval Globe* 1: 27–62.

Green, Monica H. 2017. "The Globalisations of Disease." In *Human Dispersal and Species Movement: From Prehistory to Present*, edited by Nicole Boivin, Rémy Crassard, and Michael D. Petraglia, 494–520. Cambridge: Cambridge University Press.

Green, Monica H. 2018. "Climate and Disease in Medieval Eurasia." In *Oxford Research Encyclopedia of Asian History*. Oxford: Oxford University Press.

Green, Monica H. 2020. "The Four Black Deaths." *The American Historical Review* 125, no. 5: 1601–31.

Green, Monica H. and Lori Jones. 2020. "The Evolution and Spread of Major Human Diseases in the Indian Ocean World." In *Disease Dispersion and Impact in the Indian Ocean World*, edited by Gwyn Campbell and Eva-Maria Knoll, 25–57. Cham: Palgrave MacMillan.

Harper, Kyle. 2016. "Invisible Environmental History: Infectious Disease in Late Antiquity." *Late Antique Archaeology* 12, no. 1: 116–31.

Harper, Kyle. 2017. *The Fate of Rome: Climate, Disease and the End of an Empire*. Princeton, NJ: Princeton University Press.

Hassell, James M., Michael Begon, Melissa J. Ward, and Eric M. Fèvre. 2017. "Urbanization and Disease Emergence: Dynamics at the Wildlife–Livestock–Human Interface." *Trends in Ecology & Evolution* 32, no. 1: 55–67.

Hoffmann, Richard C. 2014. *An Environmental History of Medieval Europe*. Cambridge: Cambridge University Press.

Jørgensen, Dolly. 2013. "The Medieval Sense of Smell, Stench, and Sanitation." In *Les cinq sens de la ville du Moyen Âge à nos jours*, edited by Ulrike Krampl, Robert Beck, and Emmanuelle Retaillaud-Bajac, 301–13. Tours: Presses Universitaires Francois-Rabelais.

Kausrud, Kyrre Linné, Mike Begon, Tamara Ben Ari, Hildegunn Viljugrein, Jan Esper, Ulf Büntgen, Herwig Leirs, Claudia Junge, Bao Yang, Meixue Yang, Lei Xu, and Nils Chr Stenseth. 2010. "Modeling the Epidemiological History of Plague in Central Asia: Palaeoclimatic Forcing on a Disease System over the Past Millennium." *BMC Biology* 8, no. 1: 1–14.

Kenny, Charles. 2021. *The Plague Cycle: The Unending War Between Humanity and Infectious Disease.* New York: Scribner.

Kilpatrick, A. Marm, Andrew D. M. Dobson, Taal Levi, Daniel J. Salkeld, Andrea Swei, Howard S. Ginsberg, Anne Kjemtrup, Kerry A. Padgett, Per M. Jensen, Durland Fish, Nick H. Ogden, and Maria A. Diuk-Wasser. 2017. "Lyme Disease Ecology in a Changing World: Consensus, Uncertainty and Critical Gaps for Improving Control." *Philosophical Transactions of the Royal Society B: Biological Sciences* 372, no. 1722: 20160117.

King, Charlotte L., Siân E. Halcrow, Nancy Tayles, and Stephanie Shkrum. 2017. "Considering the Palaeoepidemiological Implications of Socioeconomic and Environmental Change in Southeast Asia." *Archaeological Research in Asia* 11: 27–37.

Lamb, Hubert Horace. 1966. *The Changing Climate: Selected Papers.* London: Methuen.

Lamb, Hubert Horace. 1977. *Climate: Past, Present and Future.* Vol. 2. London: Methuen.

Lambin, Eric F., Annelise Tran, Sophie O. Vanwambeke, Catherine Linard, and Valérie Soti. 2010. "Pathogenic Landscapes: Interactions Between Land, People, Disease Vectors, and Their Animal Hosts." *International Journal of Health Geographics* 9, no. 1: 1–13.

Le Roy Ladurie, Emmanuel. 1967. *Histoire du climat depuis l'an mil.* Paris: Flammarion.

Le Roy Ladurie, Emmanuel. 1981. "A Concept: The Unification of the Globe by Disease (Fourteenth to Seventeenth Centuries)." In *The Mind and Method of the Historian.* Translated by Siân Reynolds and Ben Reynolds, 28–83. Chicago, IL: Chicago University Press.

Le Roy Ladurie, Emmanuel. 2004–2009. *Histoire humaine et comparée du climat.* 3 volumes. Paris: Fayard.

Little, Lester K., ed. 2007. *Plague and the End of Antiquity: The Pandemic of 541–750.* Cambridge: Cambridge University Press.

Little, Lester K. 2011. "Plague Historians in Lab Coats." *Past & Present* 213, no. 1: 267–90.

Luterbacher, J., T. P. Newfield, E. Xoplaki, E. Nowatzki, N. Luther, M. Zhang, and N. Khelifi. 2020. "Past Pandemics and Climate Variability across the Mediterranean." *Euro-Mediterranean Journal for Environmental Integration* 5, no. 46. https://doi.org/10.1007/s41207-020-00197-5

Mackenstedt, Ute, David Jenkins, and Thomas Romig. 2015. "The Role of Wildlife in the Transmission of Parasitic Zoonoses in Peri-Urban and Urban Areas." *International Journal for Parasitology: Parasites and Wildlife* 4, no. 1: 71–9.

Marks, Robert. 1998. *Tigers, Rice, Silk, and Silt: Environment and Economy in Late Imperial South China.* Cambridge: Cambridge University Press.

Marks, Robert B. 2017. *China: An Environmental History.* Lanham, MD: Rowman & Littlefield.

McCandless, Peter. 2011. *Slavery, Disease, and Suffering in the Southern Lowcountry.* Cambridge: Cambridge University Press.

McMichael, Anthony. 2017. *Climate Change and the Health of Nations: Famines, Fevers, and the Fate of Populations.* Oxford: Oxford University Press.

McNeill, John Robert. 2003. "Observations on the Nature and Culture of Environmental History." *History and Theory* 42, no. 4: 5–43.

McNeill, John Robert. 2010a. "The State of the Field of Environmental History." *Annual Review of Environment and Resources* 35, no. 1: 345–74.

McNeill, John Robert. 2010b. *Mosquito Empires: Ecology and War in the Greater Caribbean, 1620–1914.* Cambridge: Cambridge University Press.

Mikhail, Alan. 2012. *Nature and Empire in Ottoman Egypt: An Environmental History.* Cambridge: Cambridge University Press.

Morozova, Irina, Artem Kasianov, Sergey Bruskin, Judith Neukamm, Martyna Molak, Elena Batieva, Aleksandra Pudło, Frank J. Rühli, and Verena J. Schuenemann. 2020. "New Ancient Eastern European *Yersinia pestis* Genomes Illuminate the Dispersal of Plague in Europe." *Philosophical Transactions of the Royal Society B* 375, no. 1812: 20190569.

Newfield, Timothy P. 2016. "Mysterious and Mortiferous Clouds: The Climate Cooling and Disease Burden of Late Antiquity." *Late Antique Archaeology* 12, no. 1: 89–115.

Public Health England. 2019. "Emerging Infections: How and Why They Arise." https://www.gov.uk/government/publications/emerging-infections-characteristics-epidemiology-and-global-distribution/emerging-infections-how-and-why-they-arise

Rascovan, Nicolás, Karl-Göran Sjögren, Kristian Kristiansen, Rasmus Nielsen, Eske Willerslev, Christelle Desnues, and Simon Rasmussen. 2019. "Emergence and Spread of Basal Lineages of *Yersinia pestis* during the Neolithic Decline." *Cell* 176, no. 1–2: 295–305.

Rawcliffe, Carole. 2013. *Urban Bodies: Communal Health in Late Medieval English Towns and Cities.* Woodbridge: Boydell Press.

Rawcliffe, Carole and Claire Weeda, eds. 2019. *Policing the Urban Environment in Premodern Europe.* Amsterdam: Amsterdam University Press.

Reisen, William K. 2010. "Landscape Epidemiology of Vector-Borne Diseases." *Annual Review of Entomology* 55, no. 1: 461–83.

Robbins Schug, Gwen, ed. 2020. *The Routledge Handbook of the Bioarchaeology of Climate and Environmental Change.* London: Routledge.

Sallares, Robert. 2002. *Malaria and Rome: A History of Malaria in Ancient Italy.* Oxford: Oxford University Press.

Sallares, Robert. 2006. "Role of Environmental Changes in the Spread of Malaria in Europe during the Holocene." *Quaternary International* 150, no. 1: 21–27.

Selassie, Yohannes Gebre. 2011. "Plague as a Possible Factor for the Decline and Collapse of the Aksumite Empire: A New Interpretation." *ITYOPIS—Northeast African Journal of Social Sciences and Humanities* 1: 36–61.

Seifert, Lisa, Ingrid Wiechmann, Michaela Harbeck, Astrid Thomas, Gisela Grupe, Michaela Projahn, Holger C. Scholz, and Julia M. Riehm. 2016. "Genotyping *Yersinia pestis* in Historical Plague: Evidence for Long-Term Persistence of *Y. Pestis* in Europe from the 14th to the 17th Century." *PLoS ONE* 11, no. 1: e0145194.

Sivaramakrishnan, Kavita. 2011. "Recasting Disease and Its Environment: Indigenous Medical Practitioners, the Plague, and Politics in Colonial India, 1898–1910." In *Cultivating the Colonies: Colonial States and their Environmental Legacies,* edited by Christina Folke Ax, Niels Brimnes, Niklas Thode Jensen, Karen Oslund, 191–213. Athens: Ohio University Press.

Spyrou, Maria A., Marcel Keller, Rezeda I. Tukhbatova, Christiana L. Scheib, Elizabeth A. Nelson, Aida Andrades Valtueña, Gunnar U. Neumann et al. 2019. "Phylogeography of the Second Plague Pandemic Revealed through Analysis of Historical *Yersinia pestis* Genomes." *Nature Communications*10, no. 1: 1–13.

Tabak, Faruk. 2008. *The Waning of the Mediterranean, 1550–1870: A Geohistorical Approach.* Baltimore, MD: Johns Hopkins University Press.

Vanwambeke, Sophie O., Catherine Linard, and Marius Gilbert. 2019. "Emerging Challenges of Infectious Diseases as a Feature of Land Systems." *Current Opinion in Environmental Sustainability* 38: 31–6.

Varlık, Nükhet. 2015. *Plague and Empire in the Early Modern Mediterranean World: The Ottoman Experience, 1347–1600.* Cambridge: Cambridge University Press.

Walter, Brittany S. and Sharon N. DeWitte. 2017. "Urban and Rural Mortality and Survival in Medieval England." *Annals of Human Biology* 44, no. 4: 338–48.

Warren, James Francis. 2020. "Climate, Weather and Pestilence in the Philippines Since the Sixteenth Century." In *Disease Dispersion and Impact in the Indian Ocean World*, edited by Gwyn Campbell and Eva-Maria Knoll, 105–127. Cham: Palgrave MacMillan.

Wear, Andrew. 2008. "Place, Health, and Disease: The *Airs, Waters, Places* Tradition in Early Modern England and North America." *Journal of Medieval and Early Modern Studies* 38, no. 3: 443–65.

Wear, Andrew. 2011. "The Prospective Colonist and Strange Environments: Advice on Health and Prosperity." In *Cultivating the Colonies: Colonial States and their Environmental Legacies*, edited by Christina Folke Ax, Niels Brimnes, Niklas Thode Jensen, and Karen Oslund, 19–46. Athens: Ohio University Press.

Webb, James L. A. 2018. "Climate, Ecology, and Infectious Human Disease." In *The Palgrave Handbook of Climate History*, edited by Sam White, Christian Pfister, and Franz Mauelshagen, 355–65. London: Palgrave Macmillan.

Webster, Emily. 2021. "Microbial Empires: Changing Ecologies and Multispecies Epidemics In British Imperial Cities, 1837–1910." PhD diss., University of Chicago.

White, Sam. 2010. "Rethinking Disease in Ottoman History." *International Journal of Middle East Studies* 42, no. 4: 549–67.

Zaneri, Taylor and Guy Geltner. 2020. "The Dynamics of Healthscaping: Mapping Communal Hygiene in Bologna, 1287–1383." *Urban History*, 1–26.

Ziegler, Michelle. 2016a. "Landscapes of Disease." *Landscapes* 17, no. 2: 99–107.

Ziegler, Michelle. 2016b. "Malarial Landscapes in Late Antique Rome and the Tiber Valley." *Landscapes* 17, no. 2: 139–155.

Section I

Cleansing and Managing Local *Airs, Waters, and Places*

1 "For the Good and Pacific State of the People and the Commune"

Healthscaping in Bologna and Siena before the Black Death (c. 1100–1348)

Anna M. Peterson and Courtney Krolikowski

Introduction

Popular culture has conditioned us to imagine the medieval city as a place of crowded, filthy streets and dank alleys where disease ran rampant and death was everywhere.[1] While this may make for gritty storytelling, it does not accurately reflect a world that sought to improve and understand its environmental surroundings. This fictionalized landscape is largely a product of the Victorian era, which, amid unrestrained industrialization, was battling its own public health crisis (Rawcliffe 2013, 17–25). In reality, medieval cities, along with their assistive institutions, sought to maintain a healthy urban environment, both physically and spiritually, through a combination of legislation, urban planning, and charity. This is especially evident in Italy where, between 1000 and 1300 CE, the peninsula's population increased from approximately 5.2 million to 12.5 million people. It also became one of the most urbanized and commercially successful regions in Europe (Campbell 2016, 61). At a local level, municipalities began to issue and enforce law codes, established bureaucracies, and expanded their authority over urban and the surrounding areas alike. However, these changes also brought new challenges as populations continued to swell and cities expanded rapidly (Wickham 2016, 121–69). Comprehensive and effective healthscaping measures were made possible, and necessary, by the changes experienced in cities during the thirteenth century.

Medieval medical literature, religious practices, and civic legislation all show deep concern for cleanliness and contamination (Rawcliffe 2013, 20). Officials in cities such as Bologna and Siena looked to science and medicine to improve the lives of their people and their urban environments; so too did they desire to prevent corruption, support charitable activities, and promote civic religious life – all of which were closely tied to their local identity.

DOI: 10.4324/9780429055478-3

Taken together, these actions were part of a system of practices that can be categorized as healthscaping, a term that has only recently been applied to the medieval period. Guy Geltner, who spearheaded the use of healthscaping in his study of medieval public health, defines it as "a physical, social, legal administrative and political process of providing [urban] environments with the means to safeguard and improve residents' wellbeing" (Geltner 2013, 396). The flexibility of this term is emblematic of local authorities' non-linear approach to the care and protection of their populaces; it also makes clear that contemporary medical theories and practices impacted how urban centres approached healthscaping. The extant evidence, however, often makes it difficult to determine how effective these policies actually were. This challenge does not make the exploration of healthscaping any less valuable for historians seeking to understand how city officials cared for their populations.

This chapter discusses how various healthscaping policies and practices were conceived and enacted in two northern Italian cities between the twelfth and mid-fourteenth centuries: Bologna and Siena. These two cities make for fertile comparison since each was both a powerful commercial hub in its respective region and an important religious centre. The political trajectory of the two cities was also similar as each developed strong municipal legislative bodies in the thirteenth century, including comprehensive law codes. The healthscaping policies that emerged in Bologna and Siena were largely shaped by contemporary understandings of health and disease and demonstrate how various aspects of civic life were impacted by the desire to keep urban spaces clean and respectable, and to ensure the health of all, no matter their social class or status. The chapter begins with a brief introduction to medieval medical theories and the governing bodies charged with public health in each city. Next, it explores the built environments, using food and water to illustrate how healthscaping worked in practice. Finally, it analyses how the charitable practices undertaken by each commune and assistive institution embraced the spiritual aspect of healthscaping. A good city was a healthy city – morally, spiritually, and physically – and both Bologna and Siena aimed to be just that.

Medieval Medicine and Healthscaping

While the concept of healthscaping is a modern historiographical construct, the model helps historians to contextualize how contemporary medical theories, even superficially, influenced the ways in which officials in Bologna and Siena approached the care of their respective populations. During the Twelfth-Century Renaissance, the works of Hippocrates (d. c.370 BCE), Galen (d. 216 CE), and other renowned Greek and Arab physicians were, in a sense, "rediscovered," translated from Arabic to Latin, and circulated throughout Europe. These texts helped to revolutionize the study and practice of medicine; through them, physicians and scholars came to understand that the maintenance of health depended upon a system of "comprehensive, but essentially simple, holistic principles" (Rawcliffe 2013, 55). The universe was understood to be comprised of four elements (earth, air, fire, and water) and the human body, as its microcosm, included four humours (black bile, blood, yellow bile, and phlegm) that each manifested two basic qualities (hot or cold and wet or dry). In this system, blood was warm and moist, like air; yellow bile was hot and dry, like fire; black bile was cold and dry, like earth; and phlegm was cool and wet, like water. Furthermore, each person had an individual complexion, meaning a unique configuration of the humours that was specific to them (Demaitre 2013, 16). In a healthy body, the humours were in balance; an excess of any humour was expelled through urine, faeces, hair, or mucus before they could cause harm. Illness or disease meant that the body was suffering from the overproduction, corruption, or retention of one or more humours. This system became known as humouralism, and it remained the dominant theoretical model of health and disease into the nineteenth century.

Unfortunately, the human body rarely remained healthy. According to Galenic theory, the six *res non naturales* (non-naturals) affected the humoural balance and, thus, a person's health (Berryman 2012, 210; García Ballester 1993, 105–15). Non-naturals were the external forces and behavioural factors that influenced the body: air, food and drink, exercise and rest, sleep and wakefulness, secretion and excretion, and mental affections or emotions. Medieval medical science also taught that the absorption of images and scents through the sensory organs significantly impacted the body. Pleasing sights and clean air were beneficial to health, while bad smells from rotting corpses, old foodstuffs, excrement, and stagnant water would infect the air and cause anyone who was exposed to it to suffer from its corruption (Ciecieznski 2013, 92). It was believed, therefore, that through the careful manipulation of the non-naturals and the environment it was possible to mitigate disease (Gil Sotres 1998, 298–314).

The influence of Galenic theory can be observed in the healthscaping policies issued by the municipalities in Bologna and Siena, as well as elsewhere in Europe. Legislation addressing hygiene and sanitation put medieval medicine into practice (Ciecieznski 2013, 92). Significant effort was put into cleaning streets, waterways, and markets in hopes of preserving the city's health and beauty (Bocchi 1990, 72–76; Geltner 2014, 307–11). For example, human and animal waste, refuse from tanneries or butchers, and household trash were all issues that European cities sought to regulate and control (Coomans 2019, 88–93; Geltner 2013, 399–402; 2014, 311–16; Rawcliffe 2012, 177–95). Anything that hindered the supply or quality of public necessities was of particular interest to both Bologna's and Siena's governments. Since it was impossible to eliminate many sources of pollution, as they often went hand in hand with the industries vital to the city's economy, governments sought to contain their effects as much as possible, often through legislation and penalties if such laws were broken.

Governing Bologna and Siena

The conjuncture of the institutionalization of medieval society, the growth of administrative and governmental bodies, and the rise of healthscaping policies in the thirteenth century was not a coincidence. As towns and cities experienced an influx of people, wealth, and trade and as the role and authority of local officials began to grow, healthscaping became essential (Wickham 2016, 164). By exerting more control over the regulation and development of the urban environment, municipal bodies were able to directly respond to the needs of their cities, specifically through healthscaping policies. During the thirteenth and fourteenth centuries, Bologna and Siena each introduced a significant amount of health-related legislation that impacted the use of public spaces and regulated private behaviour. These sanitary laws were not "hollow threats or hopeless ambitions" because violators were actively punished (Coomans 2019, 86). Before discussing these measures, though, it is important to understand what institutions and administrative frameworks were tasked with creating and enforcing them.

In Bologna, the end of the twelfth century witnessed conflict within the city's oligarchy. This culminated in 1195 when the structure of the commune's government was changed. Now led by the *podestà*, a foreign-born man[2] with legal training (Vigueur 2000), and a council of judges, collaborators, *milites* (knights), and notaries, the government aimed to reform the city's financial offices. The council adopted the name *Consiglio di credenza*, ultimately growing to include one hundred representatives from the wealthier segments of society. The *Consiglio* was responsible for electing all communal officials who, in turn, comprised a *curia* that worked alongside the *podestà*. In 1217, the *Consiglio Generale* was formed, which allowed representatives of the popular class to be directly involved in the local government. However, by the middle of the thirteenth century, the government structure changed once again. This shift resulted in Bologna being run predominantly by corporate associations and popular societies, namely, guilds and arms societies. Together, they formed the *popolo*, a political group that aimed to protect the interests of commoners – who, in many cases, were wealthy businessmen and merchants – against the city's nobility. In 1255, the position of the *Capitano del Popolo* (captain of the *popolo*) was officially recognized as the head of the *popolo*'s political structure. Together, these groups and individuals became tremendously powerful and influential in the city's operation.

This chapter focuses primarily on the Bolognese *Statuti* (city statutes) enacted between 1248 and 1335. Statutes regulating the Bolognese Commune were written and collected as early as the twelfth century, addressing the norms issued by the *podestà*, *Capitano del Popolo*, and other communal bodies. The *Statuti* were cohesive, organized, and structured volumes, with the first extant volume dating to 1248. When viewed as part of the *ius commune* – a constantly changing, growing, and evolving body of Roman civil, canon, and feudal laws that had a "transterritorial applicability" – the *Statuti* fit into a larger, universal understanding of medieval law and legal tradition (Kirshner 2015, 3–4). By examining Bologna's *Statuti,* it is possible to follow the development of the city's approach to healthscaping through its management of infrastructure and civilian life. Analysing the statutes that pertain to the commune's health between 1248 and 1335, thus, allows us to discover and decipher not only the mechanisms of civic practice but also the prevailing social ideology concerning health, disease, and their place in the commune.

Similar governmental structures existed in Siena, although there are some notable differences. From the mid-thirteenth century onwards, Siena's chief magistrate was, as in Bologna, a foreign-born *podestà*. Alongside him was the Captain of the *Popolo* who represented the *populares* – the artisans and working population (Ascheri and Franco 2020, 33). By the late thirteenth century, power to govern lay with the *Consistroro*, the city's signory, which consisted of the *Nove*, the four *Provveditori* of the *Biccherna* (the central financial institution), the four Consuls of the *Mercanzia* (merchant guild), and the three Consuls of the *Milites* (Bowsky 1981, 23–24, 28). The *Nove* (Nine), which was in power from 1290 until 1355, and other iterations of this council were dedicated to upholding the "good and pacific state of the people and the Commune" (*pro bono et pacifico statu populi et comunis*) (Zdekauer 1897, 72, n. 1a, hereafter COST 1262).[3] While it could not unilaterally issue ordinances or direct the city's finances, the *Nove* called council meetings, ruled on conflicting statutes, and, on Thursdays, heard petitions from the people (COST 1262, 72; see also Bowsky 1981; Waley 1991, 46–48). Further, the *Consiglio Generale* was the city's main legislative body that advised the *Nove* on foreign and local issues and took care of statutory requirements that arose every January and July (Ascheri and Franco 2020, 47; Bowsky 1981, 85, 88–89).

Siena's governance was informed by the *Constituto*, the earliest extant version of which is dated to 1262. The *Constituto* is divided into five thematic *distinctiones* (sections): (i) Church and charity (*De fide catholica*), (ii) civil procedure (*De iudiciis*), (iii) communal jurisprudence (*De rebus et negotiis comunitatis*), (iv) behaviour of the people (*De rebus et negotiis privatorum*), and (v) the penal code (*De penis*). Healthscaping policies fell mainly in the first, third – which accounts for much of the regulations regarding waste, water, and food – and fifth sections. The pointed and precise language found in the *Constituto* likely resulted from rulings issued by the *Consiglio Generale* addressing specific issues from petitioners (Dani 2015, 161–66). When required, the statutes were enforced by committees comprising three or more men from each *terzo* (Kucher 2005b, 512). Additionally, new editions of the *Constituto* were circulated to ensure that the Sienese were kept abreast of updates and, in May 1309, a vernacular version was made available to the public to increase the document's accessibility (Elsheikh 2002, vol. 1, 120–22, hereafter COST 1309; see also Bowsky 1981, 95). The commune thus was committed not only to preserving the health of the population and the city but also to ensuring that everyone had the opportunity understand how they were being governed.

It is evident from the *Statuti* in Bologna and the *Constituto* in Siena that officials in both cities, despite internal and external conflict, understood that a healthy city was one that attempted to balance the physical and spiritual. However, they also knew that their healthscaping measures would not be carried out thanks to goodwill; rather, they would require enforcement and penalties.

Healthscaping and Managing the Urban Environment

The Built Environment

Two structures dominate Siena's skyline: the cathedral's dome and the tower of the Palazzo Pubblico. The commune purposefully crafted how people viewed and experienced the city, presenting it as a uniform and efficiently built environment that protected and cared for its people. Its commitment to a strict built environment has been described as a "fanatical desire for orderliness" (Braunfels 1988, 67); whether or not that was true, there is a sense of purpose to everything. The fact that the tower and the dome are the two most visible structures was by design, as they highlight the two main powers in the city: the commune and the bishop (Braunfels 1988, 63–66). This "fanatical desire" to monitor and control the built environment also existed when it came to regulating environmental and social pollution (Rees Jones 2010, 284–85). Nowhere is this more evident than in the extant editions of the *Constituto* that clearly demonstrate a push to deal with those kinds of pollution that are reminiscent of the non-naturals, not only in public spaces like roads, squares, and fountains but also in private ones, such as people's homes and even their bodies.

In Bologna, the guiding hand of government is also evident in the city's construction and maintenance. While the leaning Due Torri (two towers) are both the symbol of and a main tourist attraction in the city, the iconic porticos and arcades of Bologna have an equally interesting history. Clearly, the commune saw the benefits of arcades, as their cover and paved walkways permitted easy travel throughout the city. Furthermore, merchants could conduct business no matter the weather and craftsmen could use the space as an extension of their workshops to promote their wares. In 1288, a statute ordained that the owners of all houses or buildings were required to construct porticos if there were no pre-existing ones; they were also responsible for the porticos' maintenance "in perpetuity" (Bocchi 1990, 63–78; Fasoli and Sella 1937, 163, hereafter Statuti 1288). Although owned and maintained by individuals, the porticos and arcades were meant for public use and, as such, were highly regulated spaces. For example, streets had to be uniformly paved to prevent accidents and "everyone must remove, from the street in front of his house mud, earth, grape-skins [...] and all other dirt" (Dean 2002,

53). These measures from 1288 are still enforced to this day, although only through custom.

It was paramount that the city remained clean and free of both visual and odorous contamination. By the thirteenth century, medical theories about the nature and impact of odours, based on Galenic medicine, were widespread and insisted that clean air and the avoidance of foul sights would encourage health (Robinson 2019, 113). In 1288, city officials mandated that no one should throw "into the piazza of the commune of Bologna or in the crossroads at the Porta Ravennate, any stinking or dead animals or rotten fish or shellfish or any filthy or stinking thing or food scraps, sweepings, dung or prison filth." Similarly, another stated that it was prohibited to toss "grape-skins or dung or horses, asses, dead meat or other filth along the walls or into the city ditches." Offenders were fined 20 *solidi* (Dean 2002, 50–52). As rotting meats or fish produce pungent scents, it is clear that the statutes were concerned with the impact of foul odours on health. The hefty fine served as a deterrent to repeat offenders.

In 1256, the office of the *fango*, the Bolognese notary responsible for streets, waterway, and dirt, was established. The officeholder was paid to preserve and enforce sanitary measures, suggesting that the population might have been prone to "attend[ing] to their own needs first [...] and those of the city haphazardly at best" (Geltner 2014, 309, 311). In July 1320, for example, Guido de Calcaria of San Tommasso was reported to the *fango* for throwing "dung and other trash and filth [...] harmfully and maliciously" into a local well (Geltner 2014, 311). Guido's actions clearly violated the statutes, and it was the *fango*'s job to investigate and deal with him. Bologna's healthscaping practices, including creating a salaried position, targeted environmental pollution in an effort to prevent foul odours or other avenues of contamination from taking root in the city.

Similar provisions appear in Siena, especially for markets. Although markets were a key part of commerce and ensured that foodstuffs were accessible to the population, they were also a significant source of pollution. At the end of the day, leftover food and refuse was not only unsightly but also attracted unwanted vermin. In a contract dated 9 October 1267, Campi Fiori was to be cleaned by a man with one pig and four piglets that would eat the refuse (Balestracci 1998, 348–49; Zdekauer 1967, 44, 117). Pigs, too, were heavily regulated, largely because they produced large quantities of faeces or "dirt," to the point that the commune employed a man just to drive them from the city. Furthermore, in the fourteenth century, the *Consiglio Generale* ruled that fish that were not sold during the market day were to be thrown on the ground so that anyone could take them for free; ironically, this was meant to ensure freshness (Balestracci 1998, 347, 349).

Butchering animals posed a significant risk to the environment not only because it required livestock to be kept within the city but also because the slaughter, leftover blood, and viscera created smells and sounds that contaminated the streets and water. The commune struggled to regulate the butchers' guild, largely because its members were wealthy, powerful, and supplied the city with a critical resource. Their actions purportedly also resulted in social pollution, wherein, by restricting the number of places where they could work, butchers were able to inflate the costs and engage in price-fixing (Zupko and Laures 1996, 75–76). Good intentions were not enough to ensure enforcement: it was clear that economics could be at odds with the city's healthscaping policies.

Death also fell within the remit of healthscaping. Deathcare would usually have been the responsibility of the deceased person's family. However, as more people flocked to cities from the twelfth century onwards, they often no longer had a traditional familial network on which to fall back. In such instances, the dead were buried in parish churches or monasteries, in accordance with their final testament or wishes (Cohn 1988, 60–61). In the absence of kin or a will to provide direction, other options were needed. This was especially true for the poor whose burial often fell to hospitals or other assistive institutions. Having a stranger prepare the corpse was, from the twelfth century onwards, one of the regulated acts of mercy (Tobit 12:12). Perhaps this was a necessary response to changing demographics, but it could also have been a means to destigmatize those who handled remains. Whatever the case, deathcare became a charitable act. As both Bologna and Siena grew, appropriately disposing of human remains became a crucial aspect of maintaining a healthy city.

What happened to the deceased who had no family? In Bologna, the *confoteria* of Santa Maria della Morte, formally founded in 1336, visited criminals in the city's prison and buried their bodies after execution (Terpstra 1995, 10). Interestingly, this was the first Italian example of a *confoteria* – a lay confraternity dedicated to caring for the imprisoned and condemned. In Siena, if someone died in one of the hospitals, the body was washed and prepared for burial by a staff member of the same gender (Alexandre-Bidon 2010, 109–33). The 1262 *Constituto* dictated that a committee of three men, one from each *terzo*, was to be convened in March to build a tomb, paid for by the city, to house the dead respectfully (COST 1262, 34). A marginal annotation, added sometime between 1264 and 1269, states that the rector of the city's largest hospital, the Ospedale di Santa Maria della Scala, should purchase a house or land nearby to build tombs or a pit. Naturally, class still applied in death: higher status corpses were interred in the piazza, while the rest were buried in a communal site (COST 1262, 32; Peterson 2021a, 183). The rector must have complied since archaeological digs have confirmed the presence of a large pit filled with skeletal remains under the Piazza del Duomo (Bianchini et al. 1991, 210). Having a burial site so close to the Ospedale, especially during times of plague, helped mitigate anxiety regarding pollution: burying the dead so close by meant that any remaining corruption lingering on the body would not be carried through the city.

Whether it was dirt or death, Bologna and Siena, along with local institutions, worked to mitigate the issues associated with environmental pollution.

As evidenced by the office of the *fango* and the role of the Ospedale, as well as the efforts of the citizens, healthscaping required significant municipal and public engagement.

Food and Water

Among the non-naturals, food and drink influenced health directly and, unsurprisingly, received a significant amount of attention from both medieval physicians and city governments. The quality of food and/or drink was of utmost importance because contamination was thought to bring about disease. As a result, city officials were keen to enact legislation and police markets to curb the sale of anything that could disrupt the well-being of either their people or their environments.

Officials in Siena, located in one of the driest parts of Tuscany, were very conscious of residents' ability to reliably access clean water. Seventeen fountains, many of which are still active today, were spread strategically throughout the city to supply people and industries with water. They were primarily fed by underground aqueducts, which carried water from the limestone, or tufa, beneath the hills (Kucher 2005b, 505–507). Water was used for drinking, to provide power, aid in industrial tasks, and remove waste. Waste was deposited in subterranean pits that were cleaned periodically. Perhaps, surprisingly, the *Constituto* contained virtually no regulation regarding drinking water, except that wells and fountains should be built in places easily accessible to pilgrims (Kucher 2005b, 524–25). However, the 1262 *Constituto* did mandate that private individuals were required to cover their drains to prevent the spread of disease through corrupted air (COST 1262, 277–87, 307–308; see also Bocchi 1990, 73). The city used the aforementioned committees to make reports about damages or to evaluate, as they did in 1309, the construction of a new laundry basin at the city's expense (Kucher 2005b, 512–13). Additionally, butchers were not permitted to work near fountains. If caught, they were fined 20 *solidi* (COST 1262, 322). Tanners likewise were prohibited from working outside their shops to prevent foul-smelling runoff (Balestracci 1998, 351–52).

Water was allocated according to need. For example, one statute gave those engaged in the wool industry access to overflow from the aqueduct that fed Fonte Branda, in the *terzo* of Camollia. They were not, however, permitted to use any of the water basins, such as the ones found near Fonte Branda. This was meant to prevent cross contamination (Kucher 2005a, 42). What of wastewater? Tanning and slaughtering animals were messy work and the resulting waste posed a health risk. These activities were undertaken downstream of all other industries so that wastewater would accumulate in purposefully dug ditches located far from potable water. The effluence would then flow outside the city's walls, where it could be absorbed into the ground or nearby streams (Kucher 2005b, 521–23). Despite the care with which the city officials treated water, it is impossible to know how effective their measures were in practice (Kucher 2005a, 96). Again, their agenda was often challenged by the guilds that leveraged serious political and economic power in the city.

Bologna prohibited the dumping of waste in public areas. Waterways and sites that drained into them were similarly regulated and policed. The same statute that prohibited the dumping of refuse along the city walls or in ditches, noted that a penalty of 20 *solidi* applied to those who skinned animals on the bridge or by the Aposa waterway (Dean 2002, 52). Another statute ordered that "all water of dye-works, or anything else pertaining to dying that contains filth [...] or tanners' waste [...] is not to be disposed of in the city or the suburbs except into the Aposa or Savena, when it flows, and then only at night" (Dean 2002, 51). Offenders of this statute were met with a particularly steep fine of 100 *solidi*, half of which went to the commune and half to the person who reported the infraction. Clearly, it could be profitable to report infractions. The statute further noted that all citizens were required to report any such offences that, if they failed to do so, they would be fined 20 *solidi* (Statuti 1288, 138). While these two statutes seem contradictory, they drew on the same desire to protect citizens from contaminated water. In the statute regarding skinning animals, it is likely that the carcass would have remained in or near the river. This would mean that corruption from the animal's body – through the draining of its blood and eventual decay – would remain a source of pollution in the river for a long time. In the second statute, dumping industrial by-products was permitted, but only at night. This ensured that the waterways were clear of potential sources of contamination during the daytime when citizens might need access to water. Finally, that a fine was incurred both for the action of polluting the waterway and failing to report it is telling of just how important this statute was.

In Siena, food was not just about nourishment: it was also charity. The city's hospitals and leprosaria were by far some of the most important assistive institutions. Hospitals acted as a food bank, especially in the case of the Ospedale di Santa Maria della Scala and the Casa della Misericordia. The Ospedale had significant agrarian landholdings, including orchards, vineyards, and fields in the surrounding area collectively known as the *grancie* (Epstein 1986). Leftover food and broken bread from staff meals were distributed weekly (Pellegrini 2005, 115–16). The Ospedale's wealth and commitment to community service is probably best exemplified by the events of 12 May 1329 when a violent riot erupted during market day in the Piazza del Campo due to a combination of grain shortages and the skyrocketing price of foodstuffs. The *Nove*, unable to supply the grain itself, reached out to the Ospedale and the Casa for assistance. Both opened their stores to supplement the market and end the unrest (Dean 2002, 173–74). The commune knew that it could turn to its hospitals in times of need and not be rebuffed, because their purpose was to feed not only the poor but all of Siena.

Additionally, the Casa della Misericordia facilitated a city-wide outreach program. While the brothers did care for the sick at the Casa, they also went around Siena performing acts of charity that are clearly laid out in the Casa's earliest extant rule from 1331. For example, on Mondays and Wednesdays, the brothers distributed an unspecified amount of *limosina* (alms) to the poor, and on Fridays, they gave bread to prisoners (Banchi 1886, 39). Only men performed this kind of external outreach. Women, like those who had taken vows to care for the pregnant women and sick at Ospedale dei Monna Agnese, would likely not have been permitted to do in-house care. Men, however, could move freely around the city distributing alms and food. They brought not only medicines and syrups from their apothecary but also meat, grains, sugar, and almonds to the sick poor. In reality, anyone could ask the Casa for assistance (Banchi 1886, 41–42; Peterson 2021a, 186–87, 189), and their freedom allowed the brothers to attend not only to the poor but also to pregnant and postpartum women in their homes. The 1331 statutes allowed the brothers to provide foodstuffs for these women (Brunetti 2005, 60–61) who, especially while breastfeeding, needed an iron-rich diet (Bullough and Campbell 1980, 322–24). Therefore, fifteen days after childbirth, the brothers brought them bread, wine, chicken, eggs, oil, and cooking lard. The foodstuffs provided appear to be in line with prevailing medical discourse regarding diet and pregnancy. By reaching out to the poor and postpartum women of the city, the brothers were providing a much-needed lifeline. A proper diet was critical for the nourishment of both body and soul. On a larger scale, healthscaping policies in both Bologna and Siena sought to maintain the cities' humoural balance, a task that required constant attention and innovation.

Charity as Healthscaping

In the eyes of the communes of Bologna and Siena, charity was a natural extension of healthscaping because there was little distinction between spiritual and physical health. Serving those in need was a celebrated virtue in the Middle Ages. As a tangible expression of religious devotion, charity manifested in many ways, most notably the corporeal acts of mercy: nourishing the hungry and thirsty, clothing the naked, providing shelter, visiting the sick and imprisoned, and deathcare (D'Andrea 2019, 177; Matthew 25:31–46; Tobit 12:12). Encouraged by religious decrees, sermons, and concerns that their growing wealth may put their soul at risk, laity across the medieval West sought to donate their time and money to the sick poor, orphaned, and destitute, collectively known as the *miserabiles personae* (miserable persons) (Brodman 2009, 10, 15), in an effort to gain social and spiritual capital. The communes were well equipped to care for the soul and body of their citizenry, although residency was a critical factor in gaining access to these services. Not only did the municipality use legal avenues but also tapped into the extensive networks or care and assistive institutions that existed in Bologna and Siena.

The municipality was not the only establishment that existed to promote the health and well-being of the commune. The purpose of medieval assistive institutions, specifically hospitals and leprosaria, was to provide care and protection to the city's most vulnerable members. Medieval hospitals were public-facing institutions that provided predominantly short-term care for the poor, sick, and pilgrims, whereas leprosaria provided long-term care for the incurable. Both institutions were staffed most often by laymen and women who took oaths of poverty and obedience. Historiographically, the period between 1130 and 1260 is known as the Charitable Revolution (Vauchez 1978, 152–53), which coincides with part of the boom in the establishment of assistive institutions. There were three main waves of foundations between the eleventh century and the Black Death.[4] It is not a coincidence that during this same period healthscaping became a priority since local governments not only had enough power to write and enforce legislation but also had the assistance of institutions like hospitals and leprosaria to realize these policies.

How did municipalities blend charity and healthscaping? One way that the Bolognese supported the sick poor was by giving foodstuffs and/or money to select institutions throughout the city. One such recipient of the commune's support was the city's leprosarium, San Lazzaro, which is first mentioned in a property sale from 1214 but was clearly well established by that point. According to the statutes of 1248, 1250, 1252, 1259, 1264, and 1288, the leprosarium was granted twenty-five baskets (*corbe*) of grain (*hospitali misellorum XXV corb. frumenti*) (Frati 1869, 42 hereafter Statuti 1245–67). While the leprosarium was not the recipient of the largest donations made by the city – the Cistercian convent of Santa Maria della Misericordia, for example, received between twenty-five and sixty baskets of corn or grain and between fifty and 150 lire annually during this period – twenty-five baskets seem to have been a common bequest to institutions that received support from the *anziani* (the executive body of the *popolo*) (Statuti 1245–67, 46). Whereas the donations granted to convents, like Santa Maria della Misericordia, and other monastic houses differed from year to year, the leprosarium received a consistent stream of aid from the commune. No matter the motivations for providing this kind of charity, it is clear that the commune felt a desire to help citizens who had become *miserabiles personae*.

It was not just the Bolognese government that wanted to encourage the city's spiritual health. Citizens formed private associations and confraternities that allowed men and women from both the urban elite and humbler backgrounds to participate in the public practice of patronage, hospitality, charity, and mutual assistance (D'Andrea 2019, 177). For example, in 1289, a confraternity, later known as Santa Maria della Vita, built a hospital in the city centre to house and care for pilgrims, derelicts, and the sick (Terpstra 1995, 6). Beginning in the twelfth century, many of Bologna's confraternities were consolidated and, by the turn of the fifteenth century, essentially managed the hospitals (Tura 2017, 38). Between 1317 and 1327, five confraternities established six hospitals, and almost all of their foundations stipulated that they would be financed by donations. Most served specialized purposes; for example, the confraternity of San Francesco founded a hospital for female pilgrims in 1324. This boom in hospitals over such a short period clearly reflects the city's growing prosperity and the importance of its location for pilgrims (Terpstra 1995, 10).

In Siena, the Ospedale di Santa Maria della Scala was one of medieval Western Europe's most famous hospitals. Founded by the cathedral chapter, it was first mentioned on 29 March 1090 and remained operational late into the twentieth century. Aside from the city's two leprosaria, there were two other significant hospitals. The first was the Casa della Misericordia, founded before 1251 by the civic saint Andrea Gallerani (Catoni 1989, 3; Nardi 2004, 65). Despite coming from one of Siena's most powerful magnate families, confession and charitable works were at the heart of Gallerani's story. He had committed murder, been exiled, and then returned to Siena to devote his life to caring for the sick poor (Carli 1964, 246). The other was the Ospedale dei Monna Agnese, founded by a woman of the same name sometime before 1275. Monna Agnese's hospital catered to pregnant woman, a group that was often excluded from hospitals due to the stigma surrounding unwed mothers. Monna Agnese was a very active founder. In December 1278, she asked the *Consiglio Generale* for fifty *libri* to provide care and beds for forty of the sick poor. She remained the *hospitalitrix and gubernatrix* (rectress) until 1314. There was clearly a need for the hospital's services. In 1299, Rinaldo, bishop of Siena, granted forty days of indulgences to anyone who donated to the house. While he did not refer to fact that the women in question were pregnant, he pointed out, with a clear air of judgement, that the hospital was very crowded (Brunetti 2005, 39, 60). Hospitals and leprosaria, and their staff, were often given tax breaks, leading to concerns that they were abusing their position (Osheim 1983, 386–87). In 1292, the commune exempted the Casa, Monna Agnese, and the Ospedale from paying the *gabella* (an indirect tax) on corn, wine, and other sundries for the service of the poor (Bowsky 1970, 119; Brunetti 2005, 4). The Sienese government also donated money, linens, straw mattresses, and even building materials (COST 1262, 35; COST 1309, 60–70; see also Brunetti 2005, 39– 40) to the hospitals and leprosaria to support them while also reaping spiritual and social capital.

Charity did come with some strings attached, as evidenced by the communes' approach to lepers. Being a Bolognese or Sienese citizen ensured that people diagnosed with leprosy were eligible to enter their respective city's leprosarium; foreigners, however, could not. Membership, whether of a city or a leper house, mattered. According to both civic and ecclesiastic authorities across Europe, lepers essentially fell into two categories: "wild" and "tame." This dichotomy conveniently allowed civic and ecclesiastic powers to reconcile the "otherwise contradictory ideas about the disease," as "wild" lepers were thought to be sexually voracious and sinful. "Tame" lepers, or those who entered a leprosarium, were understood to have satisfied their religious role as an intercessor (Peterson 2021b, 327–36; Rawcliffe 2006, 284). These ideas are incorporated into the regulation of leprosy sufferers in both cities. In Bologna's 1252 *Statuti*, a statute states that poor, leprous persons "if s/he is of the city" (*si est de civitate*) would be provided with the eight *lire* entrance fee to facilitate their admission to the city's leprosarium. However, if they were foreign, it was up to their native city to support them financially (Statuti 1245–67, 256). Perhaps foreign lepers were also seen to be more contaminating than local ones.

Siena took a similar approach. There were two leprosaria located on opposite sides of the city: San Lazaro, which first appears in a land sale in August 1229, and Corpo Santo, which is first mentioned in the 1262 *Constituto* (Peterson 2020, 28–29). Lepers were not permitted to live within the city walls, and the municipality hired three men, one from each *terzo*, tasked with finding lepers. If successful, these men could fine the property owner and remove the sick individual. From there, the leper, if he or she had the money or with financial assistance from the city, could enter a leprosarium. The fine was likely put in place to deter family members from sheltering their sick relatives and thereby prevent the disease from spreading in such close quarters (Zdekauer 1894, 137–38). The Sienese did allow foreign lepers into the city, but only during Holy Week, which was one of Siena's most important religious celebrations.

Additionally, lepers from San Lazaro were exclusively permitted to ring bells within the walls to attract alms (COST 1262, 51; COST 1309, 44–45; see also Demaitre 2021, 208–66; Peterson 2020, 40–42; Rawcliffe 2006, 14, 99). Despite what superficially reads as a contradictory approach to the welfare of lepers, the commune knew that abandoning them was not an option. Providing for lepers not only gave the ill a space where they could be cared for and protected but also helped to ensure the continued health of the city's populace and its urban environment. Regulating movement was crucial to maintaining a healthy and clean city. The communes were clear in their intentions: their efforts were for the care of *their* population, regardless of their status or health.

Hospitals and leprosaria thus were one of the many actors that helped to make healthscaping policies a success, especially when it came to protecting and caring for marginalized groups such as women, foundlings, and leprosy sufferers. Charitable efforts, not only of these institutions but also of the communes were crucial to the continued welfare of the cities' respective populations. It was not only a matter of clean streets and water but also a matter of addressing issues that impacted the soul.

Conclusion

Healthscaping is a relatively new field of research, one that will continue to enrich medieval studies as a whole by providing insight into the multifaceted ways in which communities and governments sought to protect and promote public and environmental health. Ultimately, neither Bologna nor Siena was unique in wanting to protect and promote communal health through healthscaping measures; this sentiment can be found throughout medieval

Europe (Geltner 2012, 231–45). One thing that is crucial to understand is that officials in both Bologna and Siena were interested in maintaining and promoting the health of their cities long before the arrival of the Black Death in 1348. Plague is often pointed to as the watershed moment of public health when municipalities and individuals alike first started to care about issues of hygiene and sanitation. As this chapter has shown, however, these fourteenth-century efforts were built on a strong foundation of pre-existing healthscaping policies. The approach was twofold: legislation and the support of assistive institutions. While the extant documentation makes it difficult to examine how healthscaping policies played out in practice, even if these statutes were the ideal, it shows that residents of communes knew that they were responsible for the health and well-being of their city and the broader population. Urban environments could, in other words, be properly managed to prevent disease and ill health. The medieval world was far from reactionary, and municipalities often aimed to maintain health instead of restoring it after the fact.

Notes

1 We would like to thank Dr. Lori Jones for her comments and encouragement. We greatly appreciate the advice and counsel of Prof. Faith Wallis, Dr. Sasha Pfau, Dr. John Haywood, and Dr. Fernando Arias Guillén. All translations are ours unless otherwise indicated.
2 The office of the *podestà* was filled by a foreigner in order to protect the office from local factionalism.
3 The number of members was always divisible by three so that each *terzo* (administrative district) – San Martino, Camollia, and Città – was represented equally.
4 The first wave coincides with a period of growing urbanization within Europe, while the second occurred as the laity became more active in religious life and had more disposable wealth. The third wave took place as medieval society began to institutionalise, witnessing an increase in municipal involvement in the oversight of hospitals and leprosaria (Brodman 1998, 47–49; Caille 1978, 31–32, 37, 42; Keyvanian, 2016, 6–7).

References

Alexandre-Bidon, Danièle. 2010. *La mort au Moyen Âge XIIIe-XVIe siècle*. Paris: Pluriel.

Ascheri, Mario, and Bradley Franco. 2020. *A History of Siena: From Its Origins to the Present Day*. London: Routledge.

Balestracci, Duccio. 1998. "The Regulation of Public Health in Italian Medieval Towns." In *Die Vielfalt der Dinge: Neue Wege zur Analyse mittelalterlicher Sachkultur*, edited by Helmut Hundsbichler, Gerhard Jaritz, and Thomas Kühtreiber, 345–57. Vienna: Verlag Der Österreichischen Akademie der Wissenschaften.

Banchi, Luciano, ed. 1886. *Statuti de la Casa di Santa Maria de la Misericordia di Siena, volgarizzati circa il MCCCXXXI*. Siena: Bernardino.

Berryman, Jack W. 2012. "Motion and Rest: Galen on Exercise and Health." *The Lancet* 380, no. 9838: 210–11. https://doi.org/10.1016/S0140-6736(12)61205-7.

Bianchini, G., Enrica Boldrini, R. Corsi, D. de Luca, F. Gabbrielli, and A. Mennucci. 1991. "La lettura stratigrafica." In *Santa Maria della Scala: Archeologia ed edilizia sulla piazza dello Spedale*, edited by Enrica Bolbrini and Roberto Parenti, 179–247. Florence: Edizioni All'Insegna del Giglio.

Bocchi, Francesca. 1990. "Regulation of the Urban Environment by the Italian Communes from the Twelfth to the Fourteenth Century." *Bulletin of the John Rylands Library* 72, no. 3: 63–78.

Bowsky, William M. 1970. *The Finances of the Commune of Siena 1287–1355*. Oxford: Oxford University Press.

Bowsky, William M. 1981. *A Medieval Italian Commune: Siena under the Nine, 1287–1355*. Berkley: University of California Press.

Braunfels, Wolfgrang. 1988. *Urban Design in Western Europe: Regime and Architecture, 900–1900*. Translated by Kenneth J. Northcott. Chicago, IL: Chicago University Press.

Brodman, James. 1998. *Charity and Welfare: Hospitals and the Poor in Medieval Catalonia*. Philadelphia: University of Pennsylvania Press.

Brodman, James. 2009. *Charity and Religion in Medieval Europe*. Washington, DC: The Catholic University of America Press.

Brunetti, Lucia. 2005. *Agnese e il suo Ospedale, Siena, XIII–XV Secolo*. Pisa: Pacini Editore.

Bullough, Vern and Cameron Campbell. 1980. "Female Longevity and Diet in the Middle Ages." *Speculum* 55, no. 2: 317–25.

Caille, Jacqueline. 1978. *Hôpitaux et charité publique à Narbonne au Moyen Âge de la fin du XIe à la fin du XVe siècle*. Toulouse: Privat.

Campbell, Bruce M. S. 2016. *The Great Transition: Climate, Disease and Society in the Late-Medieval World*. Cambridge: Cambridge University Press.

Carli, Enzo. 1964. "Considerazioni e notizie sul B. Andrea Gallerani e sulla sua famiglia." *Economia e storia* 2: 253–62.

Catoni, Giuliano. 1989. "Gli oblati della Misericordia a Siena: Poveri e benefattori a Siena nella prima metà del Trecento." In *La società del bisogno: Povertà e assistenza nella Toscana medievale*, edited by Giuliano Pinto, 1–17. Florence: Salimbeni.

Ciecieznski, N. J. 2013. "The Stench of Disease: Public Health and the Environment in Late-Medieval English Towns and Cities." *Health, Culture and Society* 4, no. 1: 92–104. https://doi.org/10.5195/hcs.2013.114.

Cohn, Samuel K. 1988. *Death and Property in Siena, 1205–1800: Strategies for the Afterlife*. Baltimore, MD: Johns Hopkins University Press.

Coomans, Janna. 2019. "The King of Dirt: Public Health and Sanitation in Late Medieval Ghent." *Urban History* 46, no. 1: 82–105. https://doi.org/10.1017/S096 392681800024X.

D'Andrea, David. 2019. "Cities of God or Structures of Superstition: Medieval Confraternities and Charitable Hospitals in the Early Modern World." In *A Companion to Medieval and Early Modern Confraternities*, edited by Konrad Eisenbichler, 176–93. Leiden: Brill.

Dani, Alessandro. 2015. *Gli Statuti dei Comuni della Repubblica di Siena (secoli XIII-XV): Profilo di una cultura comunitaria*. Siena: Edizioni Il Leccio.

Dean, Trevor, ed. and trans. 2002. *The Towns of Medieval Italy in the Later Middle Ages*. Manchester: Manchester University Press.

Demaitre, Luke. 2013. *Medieval Medicine: The Art of Healing, From Head to Toe*. Santa Barbara, CA: Praeger.

Demaitre, Luke. 2021. "The Clapper as '*vox miselli*': New Perspectives on Iconography." In *Leprosy and Identity in the Middle Ages: From England to the Mediterranean*, edited by Elma Brenner and François-Oliver Touati, 208–66. Manchester: Manchester University Press.

Elsheikh, Mahmoud S., ed. 2002. *Il Costituto del Comune di Siena, volgarizzato nel MCCCIX-MCCCX.* 3 vols. Siena: Fondazione Monte dei paschi di Siena.

Epstein, Stephan. 1986. *Alle origini della fattoria Toscana: l'Ospedale della Scala di Siena e le sue terre (metà '200- metà '400).* Florence: Salimbeni.

Fasoli, Gina and Pietro Sella, eds. 1937. *Statuti di Bologna dell'anno 1288.* Vatican City: Biblioteca Apostolica Vaticana.

Frati, Luigi, ed. 1869. *Statuti di Bologna dall'anno 1245 all'anno 1267.* 3 vols. Bologna: Regia Tipografia.

García Ballester, Luis. 1993. "On the Origin of the 'Six Non-Natural Things' in Galen." In *Galen und das hellenistische Erbe*, edited by Jutta Kollesch and Diethard Nickel, 105–15. Stuttgart: Franz Steiner Verlag.

Geltner, Guy. 2012. "Public Health and the Pre-Modern City: A Research Agenda." *History Compass* 10, no. 3: 231–45. https://doi.org/10.1111/j.1478-0542.2011.00826.x.

Geltner, Guy. 2013. "Healthscaping a Medieval City: Lucca's *Curia viarum* and the Future of Public Health History." *Urban History* 40, no. 3: 395–415.

Geltner, Guy. 2014. "Finding Matter Out of Place: Bologna's 'Dirt' (*Fango*) Officials in the History of Premodern Public Health." In *The Far-Sighted Gaze of Capital Cities: Essays in Honor of Francesca Bocchi*, edited by Rosa Smurra, Hubert Houben, and Manuela Ghizzoni, 307–21. Rome: Viella. https://doi.org/10.1017/S0963926813000321.

Geltner, Guy. 2017. "Public Health." In *A Companion to Medieval and Renaissance Bologna*, edited by Sarah R. Blanshei, 103–28. Leiden: Brill.

Gil Sotres, Pedro. 1998. "The Regimens of Health." In *Western Medical Thought from Antiquity to the Middle Ages*, edited by Mirko D. Grmek, 291–318. Cambridge, MA: Harvard University Press.

Giusberti, Fabio, and Francesca R. Monaco. 2018. "Economy and Demography." In *A Companion to Medieval and Renaissance Bologna*, edited by Sarah R. Blanshei, 145–84. Leiden: Brill.

Green, Monica. 2001. *The Trotula: A Medieval Compendium of Women's Medicine.* Philadelphia: University of Pennsylvania Press.

Hessel, Alfred. 1975. *Storia della città di Bologna dal 1116 al 1280.* Translated by Gina Fasoli. Bologna: Alfa.

Hyde, John K. 1972. "Commune, University and Society in Early Medieval Bologna." In *Universities in Politics: Case Studies from the Late Middle Ages and Early Modern Period*, edited by John W. Baldwin and Richard A. Goldthwaite, 17–46. Baltimore, MD: Johns Hopkins University Press.

Jones, Sarah Rees. 2010. "The Regulation of 'Nuisance': Civic Government and the Built Environment in the Medieval City." In *Evolucao de Paisagem Urbana Sociedade e Economia*, edited by Maria do Carmo Ribeiro and Arnaldo Sousa Melo, 283–94. Braga: Centro de Investigação Transdiciplinar "Cultura, Espaço e Memória."

Keyvanian, Carla. 2016. *Hospitals and Urbanism in Rome, 1200–1500.* Leiden: Brill.

Kirshner, Julius. 2015. *Marriage, Dowry, and Citizenship in Late Medieval and Renaissance Italy.* Toronto: University of Toronto Press.

Kucher, Michael P. 2005a. *The Water Supply System of Siena, Italy: The Medieval Roots of the Modern Networked City.* New York: Routledge.

Kucher, Michael P. 2005b. "The Use of Water and its Regulation in Medieval Siena." *Journal of Urban History* 31, no. 4: 504–36. https://doi.org/10.1177/00961442 04274398.

McVaugh, Michael. 2002. *Medicine Before the Plague: Practitioners and Their Patients in the Crown of Aragon, 1285–1345.* Cambridge: Cambridge University Press.

Mundy, John Hine. 1955. "Hospitals and Leprosaries in Twelfth and Early Thirteenth-Century Toulouse." In *Essays in Medieval Life and Thought: Presented in Honor of Austin Patterson Evans*, edited by John H. Mundy, Richard W. Emery, and Benjamin N. Nelson, 181–205. New York: Columbia University Press.

Nardi, Paolo. 2004. "Origini e sviluppo della Casa della Misericordia dei secoli XIII e XIV." In *La Misericordia di Siena attraverso i secoli della Domus Misericordie all'Arciconfraternita di Misericordia*, edited by Mario Ascheri and Patrizia Turrini, 176–93. Siena: Protagon editori toscani.

Osheim, Duane J. 1983. "Conversion, *Conversi*, and the Christian Life in Late Medieval Tuscany." *Speculum* 58, no. 12: 368–90.

Pellegrini, Michele, ed. 2005. *La Comunità Ospedaliera del Santa Maria della Scala e il suo più antico statuto (Siena, 1305).* Pisa: Pacini Editore.

Peterson, Anna M. 2020. "Beyond the City's Walls: The Lepers of Narbonne and Siena before the Black Death." In *Tracing Hospital Boundaries: Integration and Segregation in Southeastern Europe and Beyond, 1050–1970*, edited by Jane Stevens Crawshaw, Irena Benyovsky, and Kathleen Vongsathorn, 25–45. Leiden: Brill.

Peterson, Anna M. 2021a. "Public Health and Hospitals in Medieval Siena before the Black Death." In *A Companion to Late Medieval and Early Modern Siena*, edited by Santa Casciani and Heather Richardson Hayton, 175–94. Leiden: Brill.

Peterson, Anna M. 2021b. "Connotation and Denotation: The Construction of the Leper in Narbonne and Siena Before the Plague." In *Leprosy and Identity in the Middle Ages: From England to the Mediterranean*, edited by Elma Brenner and François-Oliver Touati, 323–43. Manchester: Manchester University Press.

Rawcliffe, Carole. 2006. *Leprosy in Medieval England.* Woodbridge: Boydell Press.

Rawcliffe, Carole. 2012. "Sources for the Study of Public Health in the Medieval City." In *Understanding Medieval Primary Sources: Using Historical Sources to Discover Medieval Europe*, edited by Joel T. Rosenthal, 177–95. New York: Routledge.

Rawcliffe, Carole. 2013. *Urban Bodies: Communal Health in Late Medieval English Towns and Cities.* Woodbridge: Boydell Press.

Robinson, Katelynn. 2019. *The Sense of Smell in the Middle Ages: A Source of Certainty.* New York: Routledge.

Siraisi, Nancy G. 1981. *Taddeo Alderotti and His Pupils: Two Generations of Italian Medical Learning.* Princeton, NJ: Princeton University Press.

Terpstra, Nicholas. 1995. *Lay Confraternities and Civic Religion in Renaissance Bologna.* Cambridge: Cambridge University Press.

Tura, Diana. 2017. "Archival Sources: Governmental, Judicial, Religious, Familial." In *A Companion to Medieval and Renaissance Bologna*, edited by Sarah R. Blanshei, 26–41. Leiden: Brill.

Vauchez, André. 1978. "Assistance et charité en occident, XIIIe-XVe siècle." In *Domanda e consumi. Livelli e strutture (nei secoli XII-XVII)*, edited by Vera Barbagli Bagnoli, 151–62. Florence: Olschki.

Vigueur, Jean-Claude Maire, ed. 2000. *I podestà dell'Italia Comunale: Reclutamento e circolazione degli ufficiali forestieri (fine XII sec. -metà XIV sec.).* 2 vols. Rome: École française de Rome.

Waley, Daniel. 1991. *Siena and the Sienese in the Thirteenth Century.* Cambridge: Cambridge University Press.

Wallis, Faith. 2010. *Medieval Medicine: A Reader.* Toronto: University of Toronto Press.

Wickham, Chis. 2016. *Medieval Europe.* New Haven, CT: Yale University Press.

Zaneri, Taylor, and Guy Geltner. 2020. "The Dynamics of Healthscaping: Mapping Communal Hygiene in Bologna, 1287–1383." *Urban History,* 1–26. https://doi.org/10.1017/S0963926820000541.

Zdekauer, Ludovico. 1894. "Il frammento degli ultimi due libri del più antico Constituto senese, 1262–1270," *Bullettino Senese di Storia Patria* 1: 131–35, 271–84.

Zdekauer, Ludovico. 1895. "Il frammento degli ultimi due libri del più antico Constituto senese, 1262–1270." *Bullettino Senese di Storia Patria* 2: 137–44, 315–22.

Zdekauer, Ludovico. 1896. "Il frammento degli ultimi due libri del più antico Constituto senese, 1262–1270." *Bullettino Senese di Storia Patria* 3: 79–92.

Zdekauer, Ludovico, ed. 1897. *Il Constituto del Comune di Siena dell'anno 1262.* Milan: Ulrico Hoepli.

Zdekauer, Ludovico. 1967. *La Vita Pubblica dei Senesi nel Dugento: Conferenza tenuta il 10 Aprile 1897.* Bologna: Arnaldo Forni Editore.

Zupko, Ronald E., and Robert A. Laures. 1996. *Straws in the Wind: Medieval Urban Environmental Law, the Case of Northern Italy.* Boulder, CO: Westview Press.

2 "*The Nourishment of Infections*"

Disease and Waterscape in Late Medieval Valencia

Abigail Agresta

Introduction

Water was one of the greatest advantages with which a medieval city could be blessed.[1] In a prologue to his 1384 tract on the public good, *Regiment de la Cosa Publica*, the Valencian theological writer Francesc Eiximenis praised his native city, which "abound[ed with] springs, rivers, and very good waters with which the whole land is irrigated, and is therefore very fertile and beautiful" (Eiximenis (1383) 2009, 62).[2] But all water was not created equal. Some years earlier, the municipal council of the same city had complained about nearby "stagnant water" flooding rice fields. Such water, it declared, caused infections, illness, and death throughout the city and the surrounding countryside (Archivo Municipal de Valencia (hereafter AMV) A–3, fol. 101v).

Medical writers also described the two faces of water on the landscape. Physician Jacme d'Agramont, whose 1348 *Regiment de preservació de pestilència* was the earliest treatise written in response to the Black Death, devoted particular attention to environmental features that might cause plague to arise in a city. Chief among them was if a city "[had] around it many swamps and channels or canals full of unmoving water" (Agramont (1348) 2015, 57).[3] Such water would corrupt the air around it, forming a noxious miasma that led to disease. Medical professionals across medieval Europe took a similarly dim view of stagnant water, and city governments sought accordingly to purge it from urban and suburban landscapes (Rawcliffe 2013, 188–97). These measures were part of broader efforts on the part of municipal governments to create healthful environments within and around their cities, efforts that historians of medieval public health have begun to term "healthscaping." Coined in a modern public health context, healthscaping refers to practices that create environments conducive to health: designing, cleaning, and maintaining public and semi-public spaces and infrastructure to serve public health goals. In the Middle Ages, public health was intimately tied to morality and public order and so was very dear to the hearts of most city rulers. Medieval municipal healthscapers operated within a Galenic framework, focusing on the external factors (the "six non-naturals") that influenced health, particularly on the

DOI: 10.4324/9780429055478-4

quality of air and food (Geltner 2020, 2019). Stagnant water (just like garbage and waste matter) fell into the former category: it was a problem mainly because it could corrupt the air around it, and this, in turn, could cause disease in those who lived or worked nearby.

The city government of Valencia, like other cities, sought to promote health through a variety of means, but the scale of its engagement with water is particularly striking. Valencia stood amidst a landscape of watercourses. A network of canals that irrigated the land around the city made it one of the richest agricultural areas around the generally arid Mediterranean. Branches of these same canals flowed through the city and around its walls. Managing health and disease on the Valencian landscape was largely a matter of encouraging and maintaining water flow. Running water was vital to the city's population – turning the mill wheels that ground the city's flour and irrigating the crops that brought the city wealth – but water that stood still threatened the city's well-being.

Valencia is, therefore, an excellent case study with which to investigate public health efforts against stagnant water in the late medieval period. This chapter will show not only municipal attempts to eliminate stagnant water but also the limits of those efforts and the conflicts that they engendered. Medieval cities have long had a reputation for filth and indifference to hygiene. Recent scholarship has made it abundantly clear that this reputation is undeserved. In fact, urban governments valued cleanliness for both medical and political reasons. Mayors and city councils across Europe passed legislation to prohibit filth, waste, and stagnation in their jurisdictions; they also hired officials to clean their streets and police the habits of their residents (Fay 2015; Geltner 2019; Geltner and Coomans 2013; Jørgensen 2010; Rawcliffe 2013). Yet despite the fervent efforts of city government officials, medieval observers often found that urban hygiene and public health left much to be desired. As early as 1335, the Valencian council forbade the placement of trash heaps around the city's main gates. By 1397, after several generations of such bans, the dumps around the city's river-facing gates had become so large that they impeded passage, "from which ensues great inconvenience and ugliness and furthermore stench and corruption, for the broken pottery, trash and filth are in such quantity that they remain here in mountains and heaps that grow from day to day" (AMV A–21, fol. 121v).[4]

The shortcomings of medieval municipal public health efforts were not the result of ignorance, indifference, or incompetence. Rather, these struggles were due to meagre enforcement capabilities, competing economic interests, and jurisdictional limits. None of these issues was unique to the Middle Ages. Medieval city governments did not struggle with filth and stagnation because they were medieval, but rather because they were municipal. The challenges that they faced in eliminating health hazards also confront local governments today. In other words, although belief in stagnant water as a primary health risk was particular to premodern Europe, this story fits into a larger, continuous history of municipal efforts to maintain and improve environments for the sake of public health.

Managing Water for Health in Valencia

The kingdom of Valencia, which became part of the Christian kingdom of the Crown of Aragon with Jaume I's conquest in 1238, was famous in the medieval period for its fertile agricultural land. That fertility was due less to the gifts of nature than to what the Valencian council called "the works and arts of men" (AMV g3–16, fols. 98r–100v).[5] In the years after the eighth-century Islamic conquest, communities of Andalusi farmers had created networks of irrigation canals (called *hortas*) across the Valencian plain. Surrounding the city of Valencia was one such system: the *horta* of Valencia. Major or "mother" canals diverted water from the River Guadalaviar (today known as the Túria) into smaller canals and irrigation ditches north and south of the riverbed (Glick 1970, 175–77). In the years after Jaume's conquest, Catalan settlers modified and intensified this network so that it watered nearly every field within the *horta* boundaries (Torró 2009, 83–101). Thus, although the Valencian plain receives barely 400 mm of annual rainfall, the river (which has its headwaters in the rainier mountains of the kingdom's interior) supplied enough water for extensive crop irrigation. The canal system also extended into the city itself. One of the major canal branches, Na Rovella, flowed in and out of the walls, merging with the city's moats and sewers, powering its mills, and carrying away its waste. Just outside the city, towards the sea, coastal wetlands absorbed this runoff (Map 2.1).

Carol Rawcliffe (2013, 216–22) has observed that water channels served as the venous system of medieval cities. This was particularly true of Valencia and its canals. The city council's authority to manage water extended across the city's urban and suburban environments. In times of drought, the council sought mainly to ensure that enough water reached the city. This precious resource, however, could also be a hazard. Excess water, or water that ceased to flow, was considered a source of stagnation and thus of disease.

In the later medieval period, the city council of Valencia made it its business to protect the water flowing around the city from blockage and neglect. The actual cleanliness of the urban water was much less of a concern than its movement. This, again, was not because medieval people had no notion of water purity. Rather, their standards prioritized different attributes than do modern ones. While modern water quality is judged largely on the basis of microbial or chemical content – phenomena invisible to the naked eye – medieval notions of water quality were based on visible factors: clarity, odour, and to some extent temperature. Clean water was clear, cold, and did not smell bad (Squatriti 1998, 36–41). For drinking and cooking, water had to be clean. In Valencia, these needs were for the most part served by private wells. The city also maintained and built a few fountains and drinking troughs, which tended to draw from springs rather than from the irrigation

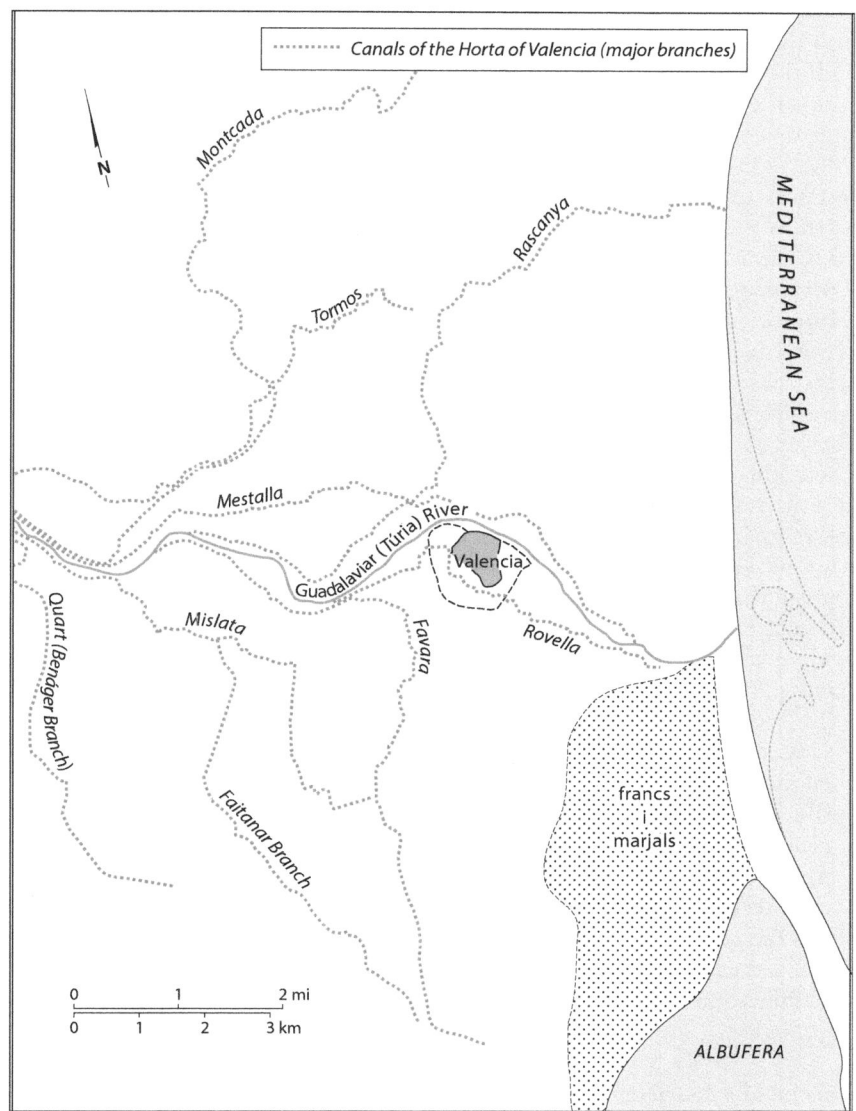

Map 2.1 The city of Valencia and its environs. Map by Bill Nelson.

system. Clean water was also required for some industrial uses. In 1453, the first paper mill in the city of Valencia was under construction, and its owner found that the river water was too "reddish and murky" for papermaking. Mindful of the "great benefit and honour" that a paper mill would bring to the city, the municipal government decided to fund the necessary equipment (water wheel, pond, and sink) that would give the water the necessary clarity (AMV A–35, fols. 312v–13r). For most industrial uses, the cleanliness of the water was irrelevant. The Na Rovella canal that ran through the city was known as the "depths of blood and fire" (*molla de sang i foc*), because it was used to clean the butcheries and to fight fires (Sanchis Ibor 2002, 93–5).

Dirty water did not corrupt the air as long as it was moving. According to custom, every week from vespers on Saturday to vespers on Sunday, all of the water in the Na Rovella was allowed to run through the sewer network to clean it (AMV A–4, fol. 412r). This moving water was thought to carry "corruptions and infections" away from the city. Once again, the analogy here was to the body's venous system, which in medieval medical theory carried non-circulating blood from the centre to the extremities of the body, where it was absorbed. Just as blockages in the body would cause blood to pool, stagnate, and corrupt, blockages in the canals would turn water into a disease hazard (Rawcliffe 2013, 221). It was vital to the health of the whole organism that the system was kept flowing.

To that end, the city council of Valencia declared the necessity to periodically clean the moats around the city wall, into which the urban sewers flowed:

> It was proposed that […] the moats [should be cleaned] to remove corruptions and infections by which the air becomes corrupted and many illnesses have occurred and are in the city. And if the moats are not cleaned, the main channels of the sewers of the city will not be able to drain, nor will the filth be able to get out, because of the obstruction of the great filth and obstructions that are in the said moats. For which reason the council ordains and establishes that all of the moats of the city be cleaned and rebuilt to remove the said filth and bad vapours and to dispel sickness and corruption.
>
> (AMV A–6, fol. 37v)[6]

From the late fourteenth century on, this work was organized through the Board of Walls and Sewers, an independently funded municipal body devoted to infrastructure in and around the city. As with water purity, corruption was a noticeable phenomenon: stagnant water was detectable by smell. Indeed, no firm distinction existed between odours and corruption: the bad smell was a signal that corruption was entering the body (Rawcliffe 2013, 120).

Blockage alone could cause corruption, but it was an even greater hazard when the water was noxious in the first place. In 1418, the council complained that the moats were so badly blocked that "they could give irreparable damage and ruin to the houses of the city, besides the bad influences which they produce." The matter was particularly urgent "in the tanners' quarter, as already the filth running through the canals is rising and overflowing such that the tanners cannot work in their workshops" (AMV A–27, fol. 65r).[7] Tanners were usually the agents rather than the victims of filthy water. Tanning hides was one of the foulest industries in medieval towns, and city governments tended to locate tanneries well downstream of the city (Guillerme 1988, 78–9). In Valencia, however, the tanners' quarter was located in the upstream suburbs, which allowed the prevailing winds to blow its stench out of the city rather than into it. Although the quarter was upriver of the city, the tanners dumped their effluent below the diversion point for the Na Rovella canal that supplied water to the rest of the city's industries, thereby protecting the general water supply.

Throughout the later medieval period, the council also banned the dumping of waste into the urban canals. In 1322, the council forbade throwing sheep and goat stomachs into the Na Rovella canal, along with various other types of household and industrial waste (AMV A–1, fol. 189r). In 1327, no one was to throw "stones or trash or dead animals or any other type of filth into the canals" (AMV A–2, fol. 12r).[8] Later, bans included salt fish, broken pottery, and blood (AMV A–6, fols. 56v–7v; A–3, fol. 133r). The council was concerned not only about waste that would putrefy in the water but also about objects that would choke the canals and prevent the water from flowing. Washing clothes in the canals was banned in 1327, on the grounds that it would clog the canals; the ban was subsequently reversed in 1373 (AMV A–2, fols. 27r–v; A–16, fol. 170v). The official charged with enforcing these bans was known as the *mostaçaf*. This office, inherited from the previous Islamic municipal administration, was in charge of market regulations (weights and measures, prices, and quality), matters of public morality (blasphemy, working on holy days), and the built environment (street cleaning, building maintenance, and construction permits). With so many responsibilities and the entire city to police, the *mostaçaf* must have relied on complaints from neighbours as well as his own observations, as similar officials did in other cities. Unfortunately for historians, the *mostaçaf*'s judgements were summary and given orally, leaving no record of usual practices, offences, or punishments (Glick 1971).

Ordinary Valencians were also concerned with water flow and described its hazards in much the same way that municipal officials did. In 1401, the confraternity of Sant Jaume and the inhabitants of the nearby neighbourhood (*pobla*) of En Vicent Desgraus (within the walls near the present-day Pilar Square) petitioned the council to construct a sewer "to receive the filth of that area, from which the residents [...] receive great infections and stenches." These occurred "on account of a pool where water collects in times of rain, and which, not having an outlet, putrefies and produces a great and grave stench" (AMV A–22, fols. 121v–22r).[9] The council did approve this project, although it ultimately decided to reimburse the residents for constructing the sewer themselves rather than undertake the work directly, in order to avoid "the fraud of excessive cost or paying more than the cost is" (AMV A–22, fols. 127r–v).[10] Likewise, in 1415, residents on the Street of the Freneria complained that the cover of the sewer that ran under their street was broken, leaving the channel open to the sky. Blocked by trash, this channel overflowed and pooled around the foundations of nearby houses, causing them to rot. The foul vapours that emerged, moreover, made passersby sick (AMV Protocolos Francesc Scola 3/1, fols. 101r–4r). The council again agreed to assist although, in this case, the Board of Walls and Sewers undertook the repair work (AMV d3-24, fols. 141r–53r).

Despite the clarity with which council and residents perceived the danger of stagnant water, the elimination of these hazards could be complicated. In 1380, residents of the parish of Santa Creu, just south of the tanners' quarter, complained about a row of workshops in a neighbourhood that belonged to the Shoemakers' Guild. The shoemakers were,

> on account of their leather-working, almost continually throwing a great quantity of waste into the moat [which ran in front of their shops], in such a manner that it is often ruined and it is necessary to clean it many times, not without corruption of the area and discord among the neighbours and damage to the public good.
>
> (AMV Notals II.6, fol. 87r)[11]

Municipal officials had for several years been warning these shoemakers to "avoid this ruin and public and private damage [...] and throw this waste elsewhere" (AMV Notals II.6, fol. 87r).[12] The shoemakers challenged this characterization of public good and public damage. "Their trade," they argued, "was useful and necessary to the public good of this city, and consequently the aforesaid use of their workshops and of the moat was necessary to the public good, because the curing of hides in this trade cannot be done in another manner, nor is there another place where one can throw the filth" (AMV Notals II.6, fol. 87r).[13]

Although blockage and stagnant filthy water were widely recognized as health hazards, residents and craftsmen in Santa Creu had different ideas about how these circumstances affected the public good. The shoemakers did not contest the nuisance they were causing; rather, they asserted that the value of the output was more important than the damage caused by the process.

After much debate back and forth, members of the council joined the present and past *mostaçafs* to inspect the site. A solution was then proposed: in the space between the wall of the workshops and the moat, which was about twenty-two *palms* (4.6 m) wide, the shoemakers were to construct two pools "of good cement, fully watertight." Each pool would have a drain leading into the moat, fitted with an iron grille or net to strain the trash out of the water. Beside the pools, the shoemakers were to build a small cement channel with a similar grille to flush the moat with clear water from their workshops "if and when it is necessary or convenient" (AMV Notals II.6, fol. 87r).[14] The rest of the space between the wall and the moat was to become a corral or trash heap opening onto the workshops. In this way, when the pools themselves needed to be cleaned, the waste could go first into the heap and then be hauled away and disposed of elsewhere.

As a solution, this seems to have satisfied all parties: the shoemakers were able to dispose of their waste, the neighbours were spared infection from a clogged moat, and the city was relieved from the effort and expense of repairs. The shoemakers were essentially asked to construct a private segment of the sewer system, one that allowed water to flow freely while keeping waste from blocking the public channel. Because the water from the pools continued to flow into the moat and could be easily flushed with clean water from the workshops, it no longer presented a health hazard to others nearby. The elaborate nature of this fix was a consequence of the difficulty of enforcement. Successive *mostaçafs* had been trying for years to require the shoemakers simply to dispose of their waste elsewhere. Even with the cooperation of the neighbours, the city government appears not to have had the capacity to police these health hazards. Hence, the pools: more expensive for the shoemakers, but much easier for the council to enforce. Once municipal officials ensured their construction, the collective pools would have offered a more convenient dumping site than the moat. The shoemakers could be relied on to use them, and the *mostaçaf* relieved of the burden of policing this area. Less than three weeks after the initial agreement, the shoemakers informed the council that the construction was complete. City official Francesc Urgells inspected the site and informed the council that all was in order (AMV Notals II.6, fol. 87r). The council, facing conflicting claims about the impact of the shoemakers' waste on the public good, brokered a compromise that allowed it to sidestep a regulatory headache.

Environmental Water Hazards Beyond the City

Stagnant water was of greatest concern in the crowded urban core, where infections might easily spread to passersby. Yet the council also sought to eliminate such hazards in the countryside. Starting in the late fourteenth century, the council sponsored efforts to drain and settle the marshes that were located to the southeast of the city, in part, "because of the infection which [ensued]" from the water that stood there (Archivo Catedral de Valencia, Libro 3518, fols. 167(bis)r–170r, with reference to Glick 1970, 99–100).[15] These efforts were only moderately effective in the long term, mostly because the marshes could not attract a dense enough settler population to maintain the drainage canals that the city so optimistically constructed (Agresta 2022). Nonetheless, the council insisted for decades that the project was "a thing most necessary to the health of the people of the city" (AMV A–32, fols. 17bisv–18bisr).[16]

The council reserved its fiercest ire for stagnant water hazards created by human beings. As noted at the start of this chapter, rice cultivation was one such hazard. Rice had been a popular crop in Iberia since its introduction (along with sugar cane, artichokes, and other crops of Indian origin) in the wake of the eighth-century Islamic conquest (Watson 1983, 1974). Although rice was less central to Christian gastronomy than wheat, it continued to be widely cultivated under Christian rule, particularly in well-watered areas like Valencia and the Ebro delta (Franklin-Lyons 2022).

In medieval Valencia, rice seedlings were sown in the spring and harvested in the fall. In late spring, farmers flooded the rice fields and left that water standing throughout the summer months to irrigate the plants and discourage the growth of weeds. The municipal government repeatedly banned rice irrigation throughout the late medieval period, partly because of the excessive water usage, but primarily because "the water [that stands in the rice fields] is infected and corrupt, and from it ensues infection and corruption in the boundaries of the city" (AMV A–3, fol. 101v.)[17] In 1402, the council contributed funds to the nearby village of Albuixec so that its residents could drain their marshes, "which are the nourishment of infections." The sum of fifty gold florins was paid on condition that rice not be grown in the former marshlands (AMV A–22, fols. 218r–v).[18]

Concerns about infection could even trump other environmental hazards. In 1392, in order to avert flooding, the council sponsored the diversion of the city's river, the Guadalaviar, away from the port at the river's mouth. But by August 1394, residents of the port area complained to the council that outflow from the canals was pooling in the now-empty riverbed. These stagnant pools were a source of infection, as "experience [had] shown through the excessive illnesses among the inhabitants of the said port" (AMV A–20, fols. 191r–v).[19] On these grounds, the council of 1394 permitted the residents to undo the river diversion of 2 years earlier although it declined to pay for the reversal out of the city coffers.

It is tempting to attribute these stories of unhealthy marshes and local outbreaks of disease near stagnant pools to malaria or other water- or mosquito-borne illness. Modern medicine too associates stagnant water with certain kinds of disease risk. The evidence, however, is far from sufficient for such an exercise. Pools of stagnant water would have smelled and looked foul regardless of the vectors or pathogens they fostered. It would have been easy for both residents and the local government to blame a wetland, a flooded field, or a muddy riverbed for any illnesses or deaths perceived to exceed the norm. The surviving documents, meanwhile, tell us nothing about the circumstances of these illnesses and deaths. While the city council of Valencia may have had good reason (in modern epidemiological terms) to be suspicious of stagnant water, we cannot assume that modern disease risks lay behind medieval mentions of "infection."

Like rice, flax was a profitable commodity whose production threatened local public health. To be processed into linen, the stalks of the flax plant had to be "retted": soaked in water until the rest of the plant rotted away. This was exactly as unpleasant as it sounds, and the resulting liquid was so noxious as to be lethal to aquatic organisms. Most medieval European cities restricted flax-retting on nuisance or public-health grounds (Hoffman 2014, 226, 264–65).[20] Valencia was no different.

In August 1376, the council complained that the flax- and hemp-retting pools located below the royal palace (across the river from the city) had proliferated in recent years and were now emitting "stench and infection or corruption in damage to the public good." The council mandated that the new pools be dismantled, and only the "earlier or original" ones be allowed to remain (AMV A–17, fol. 65v).[21] At the start of the next summer retting season, however, the royal bailiff, Francesc Marrades, appeared before the council to protest these restrictions. The king collected a tithe on the revenue from the pools, as on other enterprises within the *horta*. Therefore, Marrades argued, restricting them was prejudicial to the royal patrimony. But Marrades went even further: he claimed that the council had exaggerated the danger of disease. "Some small stench" did issue from the pools, he acknowledged, "but it was only smelled [when one was] very close to [them]." As for disease, he continued, "no infection had [in fact] occurred in the city" (AMV A–17, fol. 103v.)[22]

City officials retorted that while the stench had indeed been tolerable when there were only a few pools, "little by little these pools had increased in number and in size, such that they retted much of the flax and hemp produced in the area." And now, "during the retting-season – that is the summer months – one smells such odour coming from these pools first in the palace and then in the city that it appears a great corruption, particularly when the wind blows from the east" (AMV A–17, fol. 104r).[23] While it was never their intention to deprive the king of revenue, the officials added, surely "this ordinance would at least bring profit to the Lord [King] through the health and well-being of his palace." The pools could be rebuilt elsewhere, where they would be less of a nuisance (AMV A–17, fol. 104r).[24] The council then proposed to the bailiff that "worthy men, particularly doctors" go to inspect the site and make a final determination (AMV A–17, fol. 104v).[25]

While, as a general matter, the association between stench and infection was accepted, it was still possible to debate the specifics of a particular case. The incentives on either side are clear: the bailiff's business was to protect royal revenue, while the council, with little financial stake in the pools, could prioritize the "health and well-being" of the local population. Both parties here seem to have agreed that the degree of stench emitted by the flax pools was commensurate with the degree of "corruption" or danger to health, and that the area put at risk was the area where the smell reached. Marrades, therefore, sought to establish that the stench existed only in the immediate vicinity of the pools, while the municipal officials argued that it spread across the river to the city. Each side also marshalled different evidence. Marrades argued that an absence of illness could be taken as an absence of hazard: if no one had actually gotten sick from these pools, how could they be a cause of disease? The council, by contrast, called in doctors to assess the danger. Unlike town governments in Italy at this time, the Valencian city council did not employ municipal doctors, nor did it routinely rely on their advice.[26] When council documents mention professional medical expertise, it is generally to lend rhetorical weight to what was assumed to be common knowledge.[27] The council's call for a medical assessment of the flax pools was an effort to back up its claims. Municipal officials believed that they knew a health hazard when they saw (or smelled) one.

Conclusion

The city council of Valencia, like city councils elsewhere in Europe, focused considerable energy on efforts to ban or eliminate stagnant water in the city and its environs. Stagnant water was widely understood as a disease hazard: by medical experts, governmental authorities, and the general public. Despite this consensus, various sources of stagnant water remained an ongoing problem, in Valencia as elsewhere. The ultimate outcome of many of the fights discussed above was unknown, and many involved both conflict and compromise. As these examples have shown, the municipal government's fight against stagnant water was often limited in its reach and funding. This is, of course, more or less the historical norm for municipal governments, which continue to be limited in their enforcement capabilities. Modern cities likewise struggle to control pollution in their rivers and to provide clean water to their inhabitants. Municipal officials in Valencia also faced opposition in their efforts to eliminate certain types of stagnant water from the city. Its opponents spanned the social scale, from residents to royal representatives. This, too, is unsurprising. Those who are profiting from a nuisance tend to see its downsides differently than those who are not. Enforcement difficulties do not mean that medieval people did not care about urban hygiene. Rather, these cases remind us that, then as now, public health concerns were inevitably enmeshed in a range of other issues. Concerns about the hazards of stagnant water coexisted with economic interests and political and fiscal realities. The public health problems that cities faced in the medieval period are not so different from those that cities face today.

Notes

1 The author sincerely thanks Ellen Arnold and Lori Jones for their comments on this article. This research was funded by the Fulbright Commission.
2 "...ací abunden les fonts, els rius i molt bones aigües amb què es rega tota la terra, i així és més fèrtil i més bella..."
3 "...ha entorn de si e de prop molts estaynns e molts braçals ho céquies plenes d'aygua no movible..."

4 "de que segueix gran embargament & legea & encara pudor & corruptio major-
    ment com lo testam terra broça & sutzures son en tant quantitat que reten aqui
    munts & montons & crexen de dia en dia."
5 "...los treballs e arts de les homens..."
6 "...Encara fon proposat en lo dit consell que molts vegades sens parlat & rahonat
    enaquell que bo seria que los valls en torn lo mur de la Ciutat fossen escurats per
    tolre corrupcions & infeccions per les quals laer seu corromp & moltes malalties
    ha hauds & ha en la Ciutat. E si los dits valls nos escuraven les mars dels dits
    albellons de la dita Ciutat no porien exaguar no les mundicies daqui exir per
    lenbargament dels grans inmundicies & enbargaments que son en los dits valls.
    Per tal lo dit consell ordena & establi que tots los valls de la Ciutat sien scurats &
    adobats per tolre les dits inmundicies & mals vapors & per lunyar malalties &
    corrupcions."
7 "...porien dar reeperable dan e roina als alberchs de la dita Ciutat ultra les males
    influencies que donen e com los dits valls en alguna part specialment davant los
    blanquers, haien mester prest e in açps soccors e adob car ja munten mes e sobre
    pujen les immundicies que les mares alli discorrents en tant quels dits blanquers
    no poden fer exerci en lurs adoberies..."
8 "...pedres o basures o besties mortes ne negunes altres altres [sic] immundicies en
    lo dits valls."
9 "...una mare per rebre les inmundicies de aquella part en la qual los vehins d'aqui
    reeben grans infeccions & pudors per rao duna passa on a temps pluvials se fa
    congregacio daygues & com no haien un decorrer podrexen se & donen gran &
    greu fetor."
10 "...per esquivar frau de excessiu cost o de pagar mes que no seria lo cost."
11 "... per adop de lur cuyram quasi continuament gitassen grans e moltes in-
    mundicies en lo dit vall de manera que aquell senrunava soven. E covenia aquell
    escurar moltes vegades no sens corrupcio daquella partida e envig de les dites sin-
    gulares persones vehines de la dita partida e dan de la cosa publica de la Ciutat."
12 "a esquivar lo dit enrunament de dan publich e privat [...] a giter les imundicies
    dessus dites en altra part."
13 "lur offici era a utilitat e neccessitat de la cosa publica de la dita Ciutat e per con-
    seguent lo dit aemprament dadoberies e de vayll era necessari a la cosa publica,
    com en altre manera ladop del cuyram per obs del dit offici no pogues haver
    perfeccio ne haguessen altra part on gitar poguessen les dites inmundicies."
14 "si e quant obs o expedient sera."
15 "... la infeccio que sen segueix ..."
16 "cosa molt necessaria ala salut del poble de la dita Ciutat."
17 "les aygues que exien daquelles correnties eren infectes & corruptes per la qual
    infeccio & corrupcio se son enseguides en lo terma de la Ciutat."
18 "nodriment de infeccions."
19 "E allo havia demostra experencia per massa malalties dels habitadors del dit
    Grau."
20 Guillerme (1988, 100–1) suggests that flax-retting was not environmentally
    important. Hoffman (1996) contradicts this. On surviving flax-retting pools in
    Aragon, see Gerrard (2011, 18).
21 "pudor e infeccio o corrupcio en dan de la cosa publica."
22 "daquelles o dels lins o canems qui daquelles se trahien isques alcuna poca pudor,
    empero solament era sentida allen prop les dits basses e no en la Ciutat ne sen
    seguia alcuna infectio."
23 "en apres poch a poch les dites basses eren estades crescudes en nombre e en gra-
    nea en tent que grans res dels lins e canems de la orta si ameraven, e seguias en
    lo temps del amerament daquells (ço es, en lestiu) que tanta pudor se sentia de les

dites basses e lins e canems, principalment e primera en lo Real del Senyor Re, e apres en la dita Ciutat, e specialment a temps que fos o corregues vent de levant, que paria una gran corrupcio."

24 "la dita ordenacio ans sen seguia profit al dit Senyor almenys per sanitat e bon estatge del Seu Real."

25 "alcuns promens, specialment metges."

26 Milan, by contrast, did have doctors on the municipal payroll (Carmichael 1998).

27 See, for example, an outbreak of plague in 1383, when the council cited "the report and assertion of doctors" (*relacio & assercio de les metges*) to confirm that plague was already spreading in the city. AMV A–18, fols. 16v–17r.

References

Archival Sources

Archivo Catedral de Valencia
Archivo Municipal de Valencia

Printed Sources

Agramont, Jacme d'. 2015. *Regiment de preservació de pestilència (1348)*, edited by Joan Veny, Introduction by Francesc Cremades. Barcelona: Colleció Scripta.

Agresta, Abigail. 2022. *The Keys to Bread and Wine: Faith, Nature, and Infrastructure in Late Medieval Valencia*. Ithaca, NY: Cornell University Press.

Carmichael, Ann G. 1998. "Epidemics and State Medicine in Fifteenth-Century Milan." In *Medicine from the Black Death to the French Disease*, edited by Roger French, Jon Arrizabalaga, Andrew Cunningham, and Luis García-Ballester, 221–47. Aldershot: Ashgate.

Coomans, Janna and Guy Geltner. 2013. "On the Street and in the Bathhouse: Medieval Galenism in Action?" *Anuario de Estudios Medievales* 43, no. 1: 53–82.

Eiximenis, Francesc. 2009. *Regiment de la cosa pública* (1383). Edited by Lluís Brines and Josep Palomero. Alzira: Bromera.

Fay, Isla. 2015. *Health and the City: Disease, Environment and Government in Norwich, 1200–1575*. York: York Medieval Press.

Franklin-Lyons, Adam. 2022. *Shortage and Famine in the Late Medieval Crown of Aragon*. State College, PA: Penn State University Press.

Geltner, Guy. 2019. *Roads to Health: Infrastructure and Urban Wellbeing in Later Medieval Italy*. Philadelphia: University of Pennsylvania Press.

Geltner, Guy. 2020. "The Path to Pistoia: Urban Hygiene Before the Black Death." *Past & Present* 246, no. 1: 3–33.

Gerrard, Chris. 2011. "Contest and Co-operation: Strategies for Medieval and Later Irrigation Along the Upper Huecha Valley, Aragón, North-east Spain." *Water History* 3, no. 1: 3–28.

Glick, Thomas F. 1970. *Irrigation and Society in Medieval Valencia*. Cambridge, MA: The Belknap Press of Harvard University Press.

Glick, Thomas F. 1971. "'Muhtasib' and 'Mustasaf': A Case Study of Institutional Diffusion." *Viator* 2: 59–82.

Guillerme, André. 1988. *The Age of Water: The Urban Environment in the North of France, AD 300–1800*. College Station: Texas A&M University Press.

Hoffman, Richard. 1996. "Economic Development and Aquatic Ecosystems in Medieval Europe." *The American Historical Review* 3: 631–69.

Hoffman, Richard. 2014. *An Environmental History of the Middle Ages.* Cambridge: Cambridge University Press.

Jørgensen, Dolly. 2010. "All Good Rule of the Citee: Sanitation and Civic Government in England, 1400–1600." *Journal of Urban History* 36, no. 3: 300–15.

Rawcliffe, Carole. 2013. *Urban Bodies: Communal Health in Late Medieval English Towns and Cities.* Woodbridge: Boydell Press.

Sanchis Ibor, Carles. 2002. "Acequia, Saneamiento y Trazados Urbanos in Valencia." In *Historia de la ciudad II. Territorio, sociedad y patrimonio,* edited by Sonia Dauksis Ortolá and Francesco Taberner Pastor, 92–105. Valencia: Publicacions de la Universitat de Valencia.

Squatriti, Paolo. 1998. *Water and Society in Early Medieval Italy, AD 400–1000.* Cambridge: Cambridge University Press.

Torró, Josep. 2009. "Field and Canal Building after the Conquest: Modifications to the Cultivated Ecosystem in the Kingdom of Valencia, ca. 1250–ca.1350." In *Worlds of History and Economics: Essays in Honour of Andrew M. Watson,* edited by Brian Catlos, 77–108. Valencia: Publicacions de la Universitat de Valencia.

Watson, Andrew. 1974. "The Arab Agricultural Revolution and Its Diffusion, 700–1100." *The Journal of Economic History* 34, no. 1: 8–35.

Watson, Andrew. 1983. *Agricultural Innovation in the Early Islamic World: The Diffusion of Crops and Farming Techniques, 700–1100.* Cambridge: Cambridge University Press.

3 From Helpful Gardens to Hateful Words

Moral and Physical Healthscaping in the Late Medieval Rhineland

Lucy C. Barnhouse

Introduction

Medieval public health may sound to some like a contradiction in terms.[1] Monty Python's vision of the medieval city – in which a cart stacked with plague victims trundles down a dung-filled street, while muddy brawlers roll into a pile of straw – spoofs an enduring stereotype. In a world in which a king can be recognized because "he hasn't got shit all over him," the approach of the city-dweller trying to hide from it all in a basket may seem eminently reasonable (White et al. 2001). In reality, however, communal and individual health was carefully managed in medieval cities. Waste was managed using culverts and canals, and neighbourhoods were organized to minimize air and water pollution (Brimblecombe 1976; Jørgensen 2013). Moreover, urban environments were thought of as places where moral as well as physical health needed to be cultivated; in other words, bashing a not-yet-dead sick person over the head, as in Monty Python's plague-ridden environment, would be a threat to the morality as well as the peace of the community (Rexroth 2007; White et al. 2001).

In this chapter, I use the cities of the central Rhineland, located in a prosperous trading zone in what is now Germany, to examine how medieval public health was conceptualized and managed, even in communities without central public health policy. Mainz, Worms, and Speyer were linked to each other by both civic and ecclesiastical law (Stadtarchiv Mainz 32/10). None of these cities had the centralized governmental structure found in late medieval England or the Italian republics of the same period. But business agreements, civic laws, and records of disputes all show that their officials were intentional and diligent in creating and maintaining healthy urban environments. I use the term "healthscaping," coined by Guy Geltner, throughout this chapter to describe such holistic efforts (Geltner 2013). Healthscaping encompasses regulations and practices that may not align with modern, policy-based definitions of public health, but which were seen by medieval people as necessary for managing the health of communities and the spaces they used. Following Geltner's example, I look at a wide range of practices and laws – from neighbourhood design and industrial management to

DOI: 10.4324/9780429055478-5

laws about cursing – pertaining to the definition and maintenance of healthy environments in Mainz, Worms, and Speyer in the thirteenth and fourteenth centuries. Healthscaping offers insight into how medieval theories of holistic health were applied to collective regimens and how growing cities negotiated tensions between individual and collective rights. The cities of the central Rhineland undertook complex and multifaceted efforts at urban healthscaping and the management of natural resources. For the most part, however, these did not originate with the civic government or other central authorities. Instead, maintaining public health was viewed as a collective responsibility.

This chapter considers three main areas of healthscaping in the cities of the late medieval Rhineland: the legal condition of sickness and the unhealthful effects of moral pollution; the upkeep of gutters and canals, and access to water; and the regulation of baths and bathhouses. The rights of individuals and groups, and how private rights and the public good were negotiated, were intimately bound up with these spheres of health regulation. First, this chapter examines the city as a conceptual zone of health, exploring how urban spaces were organized and regulated for the sake of individual and communal health. According to medieval medical theory, the atmosphere had a direct effect on an individual's humoural balance (Carmichael 2010; Karras 2005). Creating and maintaining a healthy environment, therefore, was key for all the city's residents. In examining individual and institutional approaches to health, I then discuss the role of bathing and bathhouses. Contrary to the durable cliché about medieval people wallowing in (and sometimes harvesting) filth, bathhouses were common institutions in late medieval cities, sites of sometimes contentious social interaction, but also serving as places of relaxation and physical cleansing (Clay 1909; Weigl 2013). Lastly, continuing to explore the uses of water in city healthscapes, I examine how Speyer, Worms, and Mainz dealt with regulating access to wells in increasingly crowded urban environments, and with managing space and resources.

Peregrine Horden, Carole Rawcliffe, and François-Olivier Touati are but a few of the historians who have explained holistic medieval theories of health in recent years (Horden 2019; Rawcliffe 2013; Touati 2004). Insofar as such concepts have been associated with public health, however, it has usually been in relation to coherent centralized policies, whether in England, Italy, or prosperous imperial cities such as Nürnberg (Rawcliffe 2013b). The records of Mainz, Worms, and Speyer, however, reveal that conceptual links between moral and physical well-being did not necessarily result in centralized infrastructure, even when urban communities were prosperous and stable. In the later Middle Ages, urban growth brought new uses of social spaces, as well as new needs for such space. Amid rapid change to existing neighbourhoods and expansion into new ones, lack of cohesive regulation should not be viewed as synonymous with indifference on the part of municipal authorities. In response to the changing needs of their populations, each of these cities of the Upper Rhineland developed different customs and laws concerning public health and environmental management.

My data are drawn from the charters of Mainz, Worms, and Speyer. Charters functioned as business agreements, laying out the rights and responsibilities of individuals and institutions. Most, but not all, of these legal documents were issued by civic authorities, sometimes in response to petitions. I have also drawn on the records of hospitals, which were often more scrupulous than other institutions in recording details about water access. The civic law codes of Mainz and Speyer offer additional insight into how health and sickness were viewed and managed. Since the quantity and proportion of surviving sources vary from city to city, I have used the records of the papal penitentiary dealing with the region for comparative evidence. A lack of centralized regulation, I contend, does not indicate that municipal authorities were indifferent to concerns with healthful resource management, or powerless to enact relevant legislation. Rather, public health regulation and environmental management were incorporated into city customs that were adapted to accommodate the rights of individual citizens.

Sickness and Health

In early July 1404, a dispute between Eberhard Riese and his neighbour Morhenne, proprietor of a bathhouse, was finally closed. The 2 men had been at odds over both the channel [Rinnel] carrying wastewater from the baths and the channel through Eberhard's house (or possibly tavern) known as the Unicorn. The *Baumeister* [building inspectors] of Mainz, Henne Bumbrecht and Clesichen Scharte, had been to view the centrally located property in their official capacity. They had then testified to their findings in court, together with two municipal carpenters. The *Baumeister* concluded that the channel leading from Morhenne's bathhouse could remain as it was since it had lain there "von alders wegen" – for a long time (Hessisches Staatsarchiv Darmstadt C1 A Nr. 89). Eberhard, for his part, should construct at his own cost a gutter into which the water falling from his roof could be led. Although tradition, rather than utility, is referred to explicitly in the resolution of the dispute, there is an emphasis on due professional process having been observed. The authoritative letter testifying to the result is itself referred to as a kind of channel: "We have each affixed our seals hereto," write Henne and Clesichen, "in testimony of the fact that all insidiousness [gevêrde] and malice [Arglist] should flow out into this letter" (Hessisches Staatsarchiv Darmstadt C1 A Nr. 89).

This record shows not only the tension between Morhenne and Eberhard, but several tensions characteristic of public health initiatives in Mainz and other cities of the Rhineland and beyond in the later Middle Ages. Tradition is seen as authoritative, but officials are charged with giving their expert opinion based on up-to-date observation. The construction and upkeep of water channels, while acknowledged as affecting the public good, is entrusted to private initiative. The image of the charter itself as conveying order and peace the way a good channel carries water is an unusual but illuminating one. For people in the growing cities of late medieval Europe, both public order and public health were important concerns. The collective well-being of the community was thought of as dependent on good relationships as well as good policies (Geltner 2012; Hyams 2003; Rawcliffe 2013b).

The connection between moral and physical health may not seem an obvious one to us. But as the letter designed to drain Eberhard and Morhenne's anger (as well as to regulate their drainage systems) shows, medieval records often show the two as linked. From the classical period of Greek medicine onwards, individual characteristics were discussed as both affecting regimens – customized programs of diet and activity – and being affected by them. Medieval medical theory held that good health was both highly personalized and dependent on the environment (Horden 2007). The quality of the atmosphere was a matter of moral as well as physical well-being. According to medieval medical theory, the health of the soul and the health of the body were always interconnected. Demons could infect the air like miasma from rotting food. And anger and foul words were bad not only for an individual's health but also for the well-being of the city as a whole, introducing unhealthful emotions into shared public spaces (Bernau 2010). So the quality of air, water, and social interactions were each crucial to the state of public health in late medieval cities (Rexroth 2007).

The cities of the late medieval Rhineland were organized in ways to facilitate communal health. Hospitals that had been around for a few centuries were usually located near the centre, while institutions founded to accommodate the growing populations of the later Middle Ages might find themselves in peripheral locations. Mainz's Heilig Geist Spital, dating from the mid-twelfth century, was first located next to the cathedral, before being moved to the new city walls in 1236 (Gudenus 1743). When the hospital brothers went to inspect the hospital property and collect rents in the fourteenth century, they stepped out into a bustling commercial district, with the city hall and a shopping centre (Kaufhaus) as their near neighbours (Dobras 2015). Their route through the city took them along the Rhine, which gave the hospital running water. They passed the hospital chapel, a bake house, and several other houses before entering the butchers' district. Turning west, away from the river, they walked through the semi-agricultural belt along the Ambach, another stream. This provided water for the dyers' trade, the lepers' chapel, the brothers of St. Anthony and their pigs, and the new hospital, which was managed by the sisters of St. Agnes (Hessisches Staatsarchiv Darmstadt C1 A Nr. 89). In this neighbourhood, religious houses could grow food for themselves, and potential health hazards like the pigs, the butchers, and the pungent dyers were kept in their own district, with plenty of fresh air. The same principle applied to the lepers' chapel, a 15 minutes walk from the leper hospital outside the walls (Demaitre 2007; Laqua 2011; Digitales Häuserbuch Mainz). Here, the potentially contagious sick could receive care without posing a health hazard to the other residents of Mainz (Rawcliffe 2006). Turning back into the city, the hospital staff responsible for the rents would continue

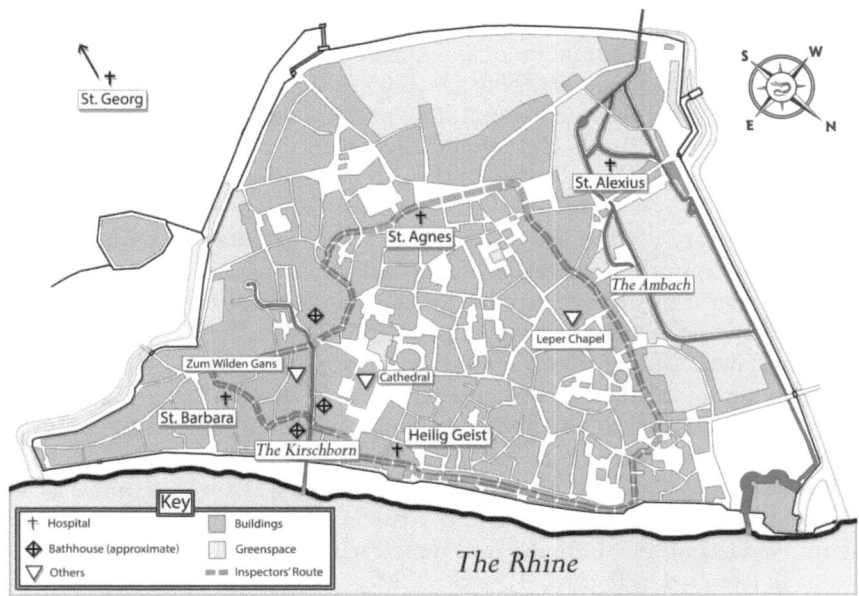

Map 3.1 Late medieval Mainz. Map by John Wyatt Greenlee, SEH Mapping.

through the prosperous patricians' houses into the markets and bathhouses of the new city (Stadtarchiv Mainz 33/1; Lester 2010). Among the bathhouses, all of the city's hospitals held rents in the house "of the wild goose," which may have served as a guesthouse for travellers (Hessisches Staatsarchiv Darmstadt C1 A Nr. 89).

In Speyer, the city's oldest hospital was situated in the shadow of the cathedral itself, as was common for twelfth-century foundations. The leper hospital, too, had been around for so long that the city had grown up around it. It was located in the city's commercial district, in the street of the salt merchants, a few streets away from the cathedral. In Worms, meanwhile, all three identified hospitals were located at or outside the walls, by the gate of St. Martin, the gate of St. Andreas, and in the fields. Regardless of location, the hospitals served as orientation points in their neighbourhoods, landmarks in the healthscapes of their cities.

Providing for the physical health of the individual was considered to be crucial to the moral health of the community as a whole. Not only through the support of hospitals but also through the provision of food, drink, and clothing for the poor, medieval city councils and private individuals demonstrated a commitment to public health that saw individual and communal well-being as intimately connected. This negotiation of individual and civic obligations is also demonstrated in the law codes of Mainz and Speyer. Even the severe legal punishment of banishment could be mitigated by the condition of sickness, which conferred a special legal status. An illness severe enough to confine a person to bed resulted in special exemptions. Those banished from Mainz who became ill ("bettesiech") were permitted to re-enter the city until they were convalescent (or for a term not exceeding 14 days). Re-entry on the same terms was also permitted if their close family members became "bettesiech." If such illness was caused by a wound, special punishments were enjoined on the striker (Stadtarchiv Mainz 32/10).

The legal codes of both Mainz and Speyer are concerned with communal as well as individual health. Both are thematically organized, with verbal and physical violence viewed as threats against the health of the body politic as well as individuals. In Speyer, insults and slanders are grouped with assault and wounding as offences against well-being. Some medieval manuscripts have clear rubrics, red text marking out distinct sections. Speyer's civic code lacks such organizational signposts but offences against health are clearly grouped together, having been codified at the same time in 1328 (Stadtarchiv Speyer 001 A/006). Individual punishments for wounding and swearing are mixed in together, suggesting that they were viewed as comparable. Moreover, drawing a weapon to make a threat was viewed as a punishable offence in itself: even if no individual was thereby wounded, the good health of the community still could be (Stadtarchiv Speyer 001 A/006). Mainz's Friedebuch – a collection of statues known as a Peace Book – describes the offences of swearing and insults as "filling the air with bad words," suggesting a moral miasma polluting the air (Stadtarchiv Mainz 32/10). The fact that both cities grouped their statutes in this way suggests that criminal offences were seen as a danger to the ideal health of the city and to the order and peace which officials stepped in to restore. It is tempting to see legal codes as performing a parallel function for the city to that which medicinal regimens did for the individual, with preventative and corrective measures for maintaining ideal balance (García Ballester 2002).

The decentralized approach to regulating public health in Mainz, Worms, and Speyer was no mere default for lack of resources. Goodwill and good knowledge of the law are both presented as desirable for individuals. Mediating a conflict over a gutter in 1414, the *Baumeister* of Mainz advised that both parties should have been better informed. Civic authorities, whether appointed professionals like the *Baumeister* or council members, responded to the concerns of citizens and intervened in unusually complex or acrimonious cases, or in those likely to affect large numbers of people. They did so as part of a system governed by custom as well as law, where personal relationships not only shaped legal proceedings but also were recognized in legal theory. The ways in which concepts of health guided urban legislation and influenced legal decisions provide material for reassessing how public health was conceptualized and valued by medieval communities.

Bathhouses

Bathhouses were common not only in Mainz, Worms, and Speyer, but in smaller towns in their respective dioceses. Bathing was used as a preventative as well as curative measure, and the bathhouses dedicated to fulfilling these needs for the urban population also functioned as multipurpose social spaces (Tuchen 2003; Weingärtner 1981). Municipal charters reveal that bathhouse revenues were held not only by laypersons but also by religious individuals and institutions. Rents in three separate bathhouses in Worms were given by a married couple to the church of St. Andreas in 1299; one of the houses was identified by location (near the gate of the Jews), one as "of Saint Paul," and one as belonging to Magister Wido (Boos 1890). Wido is elsewhere given rents on the other two houses, suggesting that he had duties of supervision over all of them (Boos 1890). Clearly, Magister Wido was viewed as competent and trustworthy. This evidence for baths providing ecclesiastical income also indicates that, contrary to clichés, bathhouses were not, at least in the late thirteenth century, viewed as morally suspect (Coomans 2018; Miller 1997; Weingärtner 1981).

Further evidence for the integration of bathhouses in late medieval cities is found in the fact that hospitals appear as especially attentive administrators of bathhouses. Hospital administrators were clearly aware of how – and by whom – the baths were being run (Stadtarchiv Mainz 33/1 and 33/2). They may have had an unusually direct interest in the competent management of such institutions, as baths often formed part of regimens of hospital care. At the outset of the fourteenth century, the master of Mainz's Heilig Geist Spital even ran his own bathhouse (Hessisches Staatsarchiv Darmstadt C1 A Nr. 78). Worms had at least six bathhouses over the course of the period under study. Mainz had as many as ten by the latter fourteenth century, and by the reckoning of Richard Dertsch, medieval Mainz had eighteen separate bathhouses, though not all simultaneously (Dertsch 1962). A paucity of topographical or onomastic identifiers for the baths of Speyer makes it difficult to estimate their number, although they appear in civic charters throughout the first half of the fourteenth century (Hilgard 1885). Baths were important enough in Speyer that those responsible for them ("Beder") are found in a list of water-using professions in the civic statutes of 1343 (Stadtarchiv Speyer 001 A/006). In all three cities, those responsible for bathhouses, like Magister Wido, are often referred to as "magistri," indicating that bathhouse management was viewed as a profession requiring specialized training (Baas 1931).

One testament from Worms records the installation of a bath in a private courtyard, but most bathhouses provided places for social interaction as well as the support of individual health regimens (Boos 1890). The papal penitentiary records indicate that Johannes Pinteme, an acolyte of Mainz, went to the bathhouse in Arnezloben with a friend of his, a scholar named Wigand. A servant was stationed at the door of the baths with a dog, suggesting managerial concern to prevent undesirable clientele or conduct. The dog attacked

Wigand, who responded by throwing stones at it. The servant, in turn, struck Wigand over the head with a rod; the argument escalated, with blows and strong words on both sides. Eventually, Pinteme struck the bathhouse servant on the head with a sword. The commission exonerating him concluded that the servant had "to some degree recovered" and his death six weeks later might have occurred "because of a bad regimen, or other infirmity, or indeed from that same wound," indicating medically knowledgeable inquiry (RPG V 02043). Another supplicant who wrote to the papal penitentiary for absolution was Johannes Aufdemwerde, described as a "poor priest" of the diocese of Mainz. He turned to baths while attempting an exorcism for a certain Katherina of Baldersheim, who was possessed by multiple demons. Katherina, however, died, "having been tied up in a bath for a long time" (RG IV 06355). Clearly, Aufdemwerde saw this as a reasonable treatment for the symptoms that he had diagnosed as those of demon possession. The limited evidence of the procedure, which went so disastrously wrong, certainly begs the question why Aufdemwerde left his patient *bound* in a bath. His instruction and experience in therapeutic practice appear to have been limited. Nevertheless, he did receive his absolution (RG IV 06355). The penitentiary's record demonstrates, not incidentally, that the priest – and perhaps Katherina as well – perceived a connection between spiritual and bodily cleanliness.

Private Wells, Public Good: Accessing Water

Access to clean water was highly valued in Mainz, Worms, and Speyer, which strikes another blow against the resilient myth that clean water was virtually unknown to medieval town-dwellers, let alone valued by them (Rawcliffe 2013b). Charters affirming rights or resolving disputes reveal that such access was often determined by private property rights. Klaus Grewe has identified private wells as "the standard way of supplying water in many [late medieval] cities"; while new cities often included networks of pipes and wells, such infrastructure was only gradually introduced in established cities such as Mainz, Worms, and Speyer (Grewe 2000). Bishops and councils often took responsibility for public networks, while many used private wells (Zupko and Laures 1996). Latrines appear more seldom than wells; while over twenty mentions of latrines can be found, most of these are preserved in hospital records (Stadtarchiv Mainz 33/4 and 33/3; Hessisches Staatarchiv Darmstadt C1 A Nr. 89 and A2 168/310; Bayrisches Staatsarchiv Würzburg MBVI 17).

Charter evidence of wells, often mentioned in connection with the rights over their access, peaks in different decades for each of the 3 cities: from the 1280s–1310s in Speyer; from the 1290s–1320s in Worms; and from the 1320s–1350s in Mainz (Stadtarchiv Mainz Q 62 20, U/1293, U/1345 April 6 / II, U/1352 June 27, U/1356 May 11, and 33/2; Hessisches Staatsarchiv Darmstadt A2 168/321, A2 168/627, and C1 A Nr. 89; Stadtarchiv Worms U/1309 April 23 and 0431/1; Stiftsbibliothek Aschaffenburg MS Perg 26). This may be attributable to separate periods of urban growth when new buildings led to competition for space and new ownership led to ambiguity over rights. In each of the cities, property descriptions are often oriented according to water sources. As Anne E. Lester has shown, such relational descriptions reveal what spaces were viewed as the focal points of neighbourhoods (Lester 2010). From the examples of arrangements among neighbours brought before municipal authorities, a culture of active negotiation may be inferred.

Facilitating the growth and the protection of water supplies was a priority for institutional and individual property holders. The importance of water access is demonstrated by numerous leases made on condition that wells be built within a certain period from when the tenant took possession. Conflict over access, or the desire to prevent it, could be caused by transfer of ownership, as in a 1345 contract from Mainz. A priest won rights over ten houses, with the specification that all inhabitants had, from time immemorial, access to a well on the property via a path "wide enough for one person with two urns" (Stadtarchiv Mainz U/1345 April 6 / II). In other instances, the catalyst for dispute remains unknown, and we see only the results: in Mainz, a woman named Else won rights including "a path [to a well] that may not be closed"; or a contract between the Clarissans and a married couple decreeing that water could not be drawn from the nuns' well without permission; otherwise, the well before the gate should be used (Stadtarchiv Mainz U/1352 June 27 and U/1352 August 28). An unusually acrimonious example of struggles over water accessibility comes from 1396. Johann Kannengiesser, a tinker, obtained from the judges of Mainz a charter certifying that he and his wife had won conditional access to a well adjacent to his cellar but separated from his house by a wall belonging to the dean and chapter of the prosperous foundation of Maria ad Gradus. The wall was a fairly recent creation, and Johannes and his wife are permitted to make a door through it, "for their needs (zu ihrem Notdurft)" on the understanding that the dean and chapter may, at their will, wall up the well again (Stadtarchiv Mainz U/1396 May 13).

In Speyer, issues of accessing wells and canals are conspicuous by their absence. In none of the fourteenth-century civic statutes compiled in the Friedebuch does water regulation appear except in relation to the tradespersons required to use it responsibly, "for the cultivation of peace" (Stadtarchiv Speyer 001 A/006). The council's 1343 city ordinances group together all water-using professions, including bathhouse managers (Stadtarchiv Speyer 001 A/006). The council of Speyer did issue case-specific ordinances in response to pressing concerns, including a decree of 1355 "on the public pipes" (Stadtarchiv Speyer 001 A/006). Private citizens were reprimanded for diverting the water from this system for private use, and a graduated series of penalties was devised. The council's assertion that such abuses were widespread and scandalous is clearly hyperbolic, but the fact that using diverted water for multiple fields was seen as a possibility speaks both to the scale of infractions and to the dimensions of the project itself.

Examining the records of Worms gives us some clues as to how such a system was maintained. A main canal flowing through its centre served the city; the rights of the burghers over it are confirmed in multiple royal privileges over the course of the fourteenth century (Boos 1890). Disagreements between different groups, however, frequently arose over the canal's use and maintenance. By the time the city judges mediated an agreement between the cloister of St. Paul and the millers' guild in 1400, a stalemate had prevailed for some time. St. Paul wanted the millers to take on regular cleaning of the canal, and the guild insisted that it was owed payment for doing so. In the end, the cloister was ordered to make a one-time payment to the millers, while the latter agreed that they had to keep the canal clear (Boos 1890). A 1303 agreement on the construction of a bridge near the leper hospital chapel, also from Worms, includes conditions on how water supply and access would be maintained over generations (Boos 1890). Central authorities created effective legislation for water access, especially in periods of urban growth; but they did so in response to concerns raised by individuals or groups, rather than on independent initiative. We need not conclude, however, that dissatisfaction and conflict were the norm in managing urban water supply. Rather, the pretext of conflict was often used to settle long-standing problems or reach compromises, especially when ecclesiastical and secular groups both held interests, as in the case of St. Paul and the millers' guild (Schofield and Vince 2003).

Private property rights – and the custom assuring them – were cherished as a component of civic identity. In Mainz, city custom itself enshrined the endurance of a decentralized system; charters delineating the responsibility of tenants for the upkeep and repair of urban property do so in accordance with" city's law and custom" [recht und gewohnheit] (Hessisches Staatsarchiv Darmstadt C1 A Nr. 89 and A2 168/527; Stadtarchiv Mainz U/1401 June 29 II and U/1468 March 28). Extant records suggest a very decentralized approach to obtaining fresh water and handling the disposal of waste. Although the law codes of Speyer and Mainz contain no prescriptions for explicitly hygienic measures, they show sensitivity to questions of health. Such questions, as we have seen, were resolved in a variety of ways not only through law and custom but also through individual negotiations.

Conclusion

For the officials, institutions, and individuals of late medieval cities, complex questions of public health were of great importance. This did not mean, however, that they attempted to solve these questions with centralized policy. It was not just civic officials who were concerned with regulating water access, taking care of the sick, and making sure the air was healthy. Religious communities, artisans' guilds, and ordinary residents of the city all appear in late medieval court records, actively involved in maintaining their rights to manage and use clean water, clean streets, and clean air. Hospital officials, in navigating the urban environment, took special note of water sources, public latrines, and bathhouses. That the residents of Mainz, Worms, and Speyer not only used but valued clean water is shown by the numerous business agreements in which water access is carefully regulated. The thirteenth and fourteenth centuries were times of change. In the central Rhineland, no single set of ordinances or governing body controlled public health policy. But through the carefully negotiated maintenance and use of bathhouses and gutters, wells and canals, the residents of Mainz, Worms, and Speyer all participated in healthscaping.

Note

1 I am indebted to the Fulbright Commission for funding the research on which this chapter is based, to Dr. Guy Geltner for his feedback and encouragement on an early version of this work presented at the meeting of the European Association for Urban History in Lisbon, 2014, and to Dr. Wendy Turner for her thoughtful comments on an earlier draft.

References

Archival Sources

Bayrisches Staatsarchiv Würzburg, Mainzer Bücher Verschiedenen Inhalts 17
Hessisches Staatsarchiv Darmstadt
Stadtarchiv Mainz
Stadtarchiv Speyer
Stadtarchiv Worms
Stiftsbibliothek Aschaffenburg MS Perg 26

Printed Sources

Baas, Karl. 1931. *Mittelalterliche Gesundheitsfürsorge im Gebiet des heutigen Rheinhessens*. Sonderdrück. Veröffentlichungen aus dem Gebiete der Medizinalverwaltung. Berlin: Richard Schoetz.
Bernau, Anke. 2010. "Bodies and the Supernatural: Humans, Demons, and Angels." In *A Cultural History of the Human Body in the Medieval Age*, edited by Linda Kalof, 99–120. London: Bloomsbury.
Brimblecombe, Peter. 1976. "Attitudes and Responses Towards Air Pollution in Medieval England." *Journal of the Air Pollution Control Association* 26: 941–45.
Boos, Heinrich, ed. 1890. *Urkundenbuch der Stadt Worms*. 2 vols. Berlin: Dunker & Humblot.
Carmichael, Ann. 2010. "Health, Disease, and the Medieval Body." In *A Cultural History of the Human Body in the Medieval Age*, edited by Linda Kalof, 39–58. London: Bloomsbury.
Clay, Rotha Mary. 1909. *The Medieval Hospitals of England*. London: Methuen.
Coomans, Janna. 2018. "The King of Dirt: Public Health and Sanitation in Late Medieval Ghent." *Urban History* 46, no. 1: 82–105.

Demaitre, Luke. 2007. *Leprosy in Pre-Modern Medicine: A Malady of the Whole Body.* Baltimore, MD: Johns Hopkins University Press.

Dertsch, Richard, ed. 1962–3. *Die Urkunden des Stadtarchivs Mainz: Regesten.* Beiträge zur Geschichte der Stadt Mainz 20. 3 vols. Mainz: Stadtarchiv.

Digitales Häuserbuch Mainz. http://www.mainz.de/microsite/digitales-haeuserbuch/kartenteil/digitales-haeuserbuch-kartenteil.php.

Dobras, Wolfgang. 2015. "Verfassung, Gesellschaft und Wirtschaft in Mainz im 14. Jahrhundert." In *Mittelalterliche Kaufhäuser im europäischen Vergleich* (Mainzer Vorträge Bd. 16), edited by Franz Josef Felten, 31–54. Stuttgart: Steiner Verlag.

García Ballester, Luis. 2002. "The Origin of the Six Non-Natural Things in Galen." In: *Galen and Galenism: Theory and Medical Practice from Antiquity to the European Renaissance*, edited by Jon Arrizabalaga et al., 35–42. Farnham: Ashgate.

Geltner, Guy. 2012. "Public Health and the Pre-Modern City: A Research Agenda." *History Compass* 10: 231–45.

Geltner, Guy. 2013. "Healthscaping a Medieval City: Lucca's *Curia viarum* and the Future of Public Health History." *Urban History* 40: 395–415.

Grewe, Klaus. 2000. "Water Technology in Medieval Germany." In *Working with Water in Medieval Europe: Technology and Resource-Use*, edited by Paolo Squatriti, 129–60. Leiden: Brill.

Gudenus, Valentin Ferdinand. 1743. *Codex diplomaticus: exhibens anecdota ab anno DCCCLXXXI ad MCCC Moguntiaca, ius Germanicum, et S.R.I. historiam illustrantia I.* Göttingen: Sumptu Regiae Officinae Librar. Academ.

Hilgard, Alfred, ed. 1885. *Urkunden zur Geschichte der Stadt Speyer.* Strassburg: Trübner.

Horden, Peregrine. 2007. "A Non-Natural Environment: Medicine without Doctors and the Medieval European Hospital." In *The Medieval Hospital and Medical Practice*, edited by Barbara S. Bowers, 133–47. Farnham: Ashgate.

Horden, Peregrine. 2019. *Cultures of Healing: Medieval and After.* London: Routledge.

Hyams, Paul. 2003. *Rancor and Reconciliation in Medieval England.* Ithaca, NY: Cornell University Press.

Jørgensen, Dolly. 2013. "The Medieval Sense of Smell, Stench, and Sanitation." In *Les cinq sens de la ville du Moyen Âge à nos jours*, edited by Ulrike Krampl, Robert Beck and Emmanuelle Retaillaud-Bajac, 301–13. Tours: Presses Universitaires Francois-Rabelais.

Karras, Ruth Mazo. 2005. *Sexuality in Medieval Europe: Doing Unto Others.* New York: Routledge.

Laqua, Benjamin. 2011. *Bruderschaften und Hospitäler während des hohen Mittelalters: Kölner Befunde im westeuropäisch-vergleichende Perspektive.* Stuttgart: Hiersemann.

Lester, Anne E. 2010. "Crafting a Charitable Landscape: Urban Topographies in Charters and Testaments from Medieval Champagne." In *Cities, Texts, and Social Networks, 400–1500: Experiences and Perceptions of Medieval Urban Space*, edited by Caroline Goodson, Anne E. Lester, and Carol Symes, 125–48. Farnham: Ashgate.

Miller, Timothy S. 1985. *The Birth of the Hospital in the Byzantine Empire.* Baltimore, MD: Johns Hopkins University Press.

Rawcliffe, Carole. 2006. *Leprosy in Medieval England.* Woodbridge: Boydell & Brewer.

Rawcliffe, Carole. 2013a. "'Less Mudslinging and More Facts': A New Look at an Old Debate about Public Health in Late Medieval English Towns." *Bulletin of the John Rylands University of Manchester Library* 89: 203–21.

Rawcliffe, Carole. 2013b. *Urban Bodies: Communal Health in Late Medieval English Towns and Cities*. Rochester, NY: Boydell and Brewer.

Repertorium Germanicum Online, RG IV 06355, URL: http://rg-online.dhi-roma.it/RG/4/6355

Repertorium Germanicum Online, RPG V 02043, URL: http://rg-online.dhi-roma.it/RPG/5/2043

Rexroth, Frank. 2007. "Zweierlei Bedürftigkeit. Armenhäuser und selektive caritas im England des 14. bis 16. Jahrhundert." In *Sozialgeschichte Mittelalterlicher Hospitäler*, edited by Neithard Bulst and Karl-Heinz Spiess, 11–37. Ostfildern: Jan Thorbecke Verlag.

Schofield, John, and Alan Vince. 2003. "The Environment of Medieval Towns." In *Medieval Towns: The Archaeology of British Towns in their European Setting*, 2nd ed., 212–42. Leicester: Leicester University Press.

Touati, François-Olivier. 2004. "La géographie hospitalière médiévale." In *Hôpitaux et maladreries au moyen âge: espace et environnement: actes du colloque international d'Amiens-Beauvais, 22, 23 et 24 novembre 2002*, edited by Pascal Montaubin, 7–20. Rouen: CAHMER.

Tuchen, Birgit. 2003. *Öffentliche Badhäuser in Deutschland und der Schweiz im Mittelalter und der frühen Neuzeit*. Petersberg: Imhof Verlag.

Weigl, Herwig. 2013. "Städte und Spital, Arme und Almosen: Beobachtungen aus dem späten Mittelalter: Ein Vorspann." In *Orte der Stadt im Wandel vom Mittelalter zur Gegenwart*, edited by Lukas Morscher, Martin Scheutz, and Walter Schuster, 407–46. Innsbruck: Studien Verlag.

Weingärtner, Elke. 1981. *Das Medizinal- und Fürsorgewesen der Stadt Trier im Mittelalter und der frühen Neuzeit*. Trier: Porta Alba Verlag.

White, Michael, Graham Chapman, John Cleese, Eric Idle, Terry Gilliam, Terry Jones, Michael Palin, John Goldstone, Mark Forstater. 2001. *Monty Python and the Holy Grail*, directed by Terry Gilliam and Terry Jones. Special ed., Widescreen ed. Burbank, CA: Columbia TriStar Home Entertainment.

Zupko, Ronald E. and Robert A. Laures. 1996. "Protecting the Water." In: *Straws In The Wind: Medieval Urban Environmental Law--the Case Of Northern Italy*, 59–72. London: Routledge.

Recalibrating *Airs, Waters, and Places*

New Environments, New Mentalities

4 "*Turkey is Almost a Perpetual Seminary of the Plague*"
Relocating Pathogenic Plague Environments

Lori Jones

Introduction

As a deadly plague outbreak engulfed the Mediterranean port city of Marseille and beyond in 1720, English physician Richard Mead sought to explain both what conditions generated this still feared disease and whence it came.[1] Mead believed that plague had been absent from London, if not from England as a whole, for several generations. It no longer appeared as a cause of death in the publicly available Bills of Mortality; official records likewise had not recorded a single plague death since 1679. Although that official record conflicts with recent epidemiological work, which reveals that the autumnal mortality spike associated with plague actually continued around London after 1665 until the late 1720s (Cummins, Kelly, and Ó Gráda 2016, 5), in Mead's professional opinion, the disease's long absence meant that it was not a local – in modern terms endemic – disease. Instead, he wrote, it was "a satisfaction to know that the *Plague* is not a Native of our country" (Mead 1720, 20).

Plague had been a hot topic in London throughout the latter half of the seventeenth century and into the eighteenth, as newspaper stories about foreign outbreaks appeared regularly. The threat that even far away epidemics posed to English interests overseas – or to the public at large should an infected ship arrive in a domestic port – ensured that journalists and newspaper sellers had a ready readership for such stories (Siena 2019, 49–51; Slack 1985, 245). Despite knowing that repeated outbreaks had devastated London and other English towns for centuries, to Mead and other early modern newspaper readers, the threat posed by plague largely came from insalubrious environments outside the kingdom.

As an esteemed, if somewhat controversial, Fellow of the Royal College of Physicians and the Royal Society, Mead's opinions held sway among medical writers and readers. To him, it was obvious that plague was contagious, transmitted via corrupted air, by contact with infected persons through their touch and breath, and in commercial goods transported from contaminated ports.[2] Moreover, based on what he called the evidence of "the Natural History of several Countries" and the observations of "the ancientist and best Authors of

DOI: 10.4324/9780429055478-7

Physick," he claimed that underlying outbreaks were the specific environmental and climatic features of foreign regions of the world (Mead 1720, 2–3). Then, once the disease invaded an English port, it inevitably became a domestic disease "of the *Poorer* sort, among whom this Evil generally begins" (Mead 1720, 38).

Two opposing environments are implicated in Mead's understanding of, and advice for controlling, plague: foreign disease-generating ones and domestic disease-receiving ones (see Figures 4.1 and 4.2). In his telling, it was the particular combination of stagnant bodies of water, deep crevices, poorly managed burial practices, and very hot, humid, and rainy climate found in the eastern and southern parts of the world that gave rise to plague outbreaks that were then spread through commerce. The most obvious place for plague's origin, Mead asserted, was Turkey, which he deemed to be almost "a perpetual *Seminary*" of the disease (Mead 1720, 18). Worse, the contagious poison of plague "maintains it self there [in Turkey] by circulating from *Infected* Persons to Goods; which is chiefly owing to the Negligence of the People... who are stupidly Careless in this Affair" (Mead 1720, 18). In the Ottoman Empire, it seemed, one could find the perfect combination of precipitating factors: a consistently hot and sultry climate, a stagnant landscape, and a population that apparently had little sense of how to maintain a healthy environment or contain disease outbreaks. The best – most "highly reasonable" in Mead's words – preventative action, in this case, was "that whatever

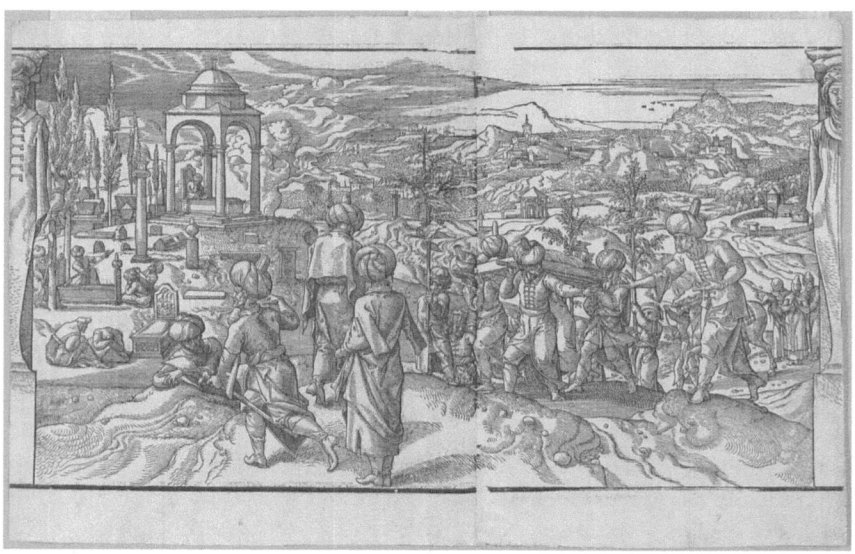

Figure 4.1 A Turkish funeral from the frieze *Ces Moeurs et fachons de faire de Turcz*. Woodcut after Pieter Coecke van Aelst, 1553. The landscape, customs, and habits of Turks were blamed for plague by the seventeenth century. The Met, Public Domain.

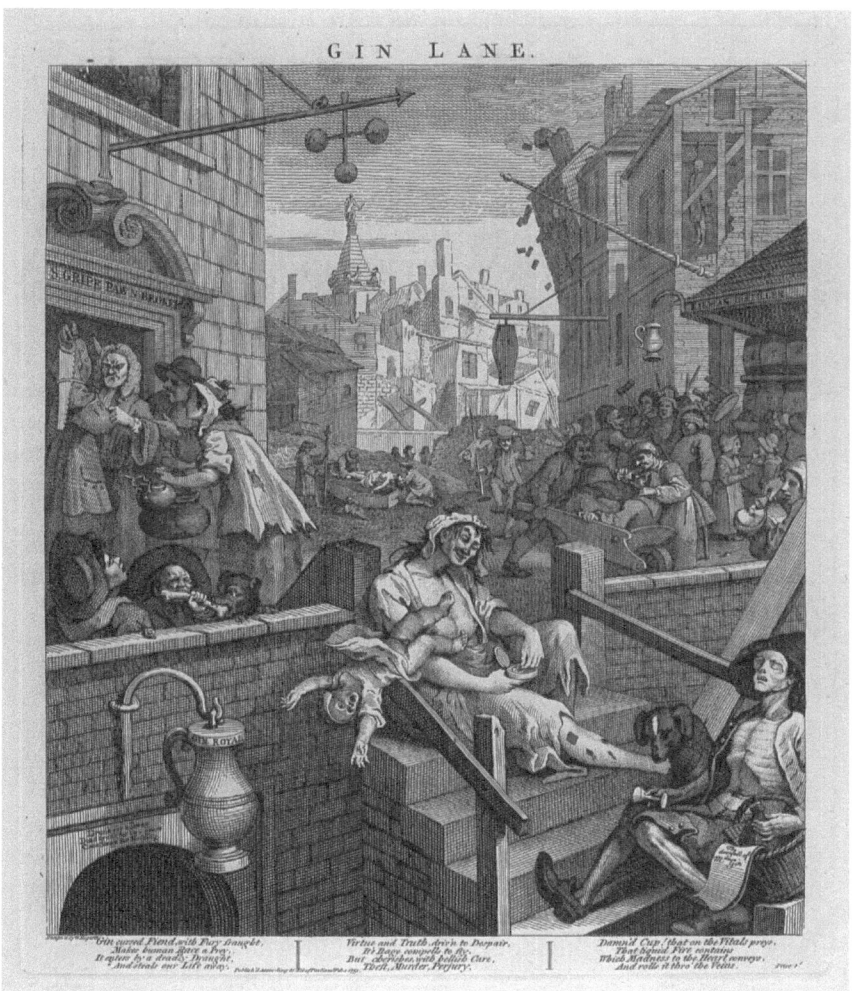

Figure 4.2 A poor London street strewn with hopeless drunkards and lined with gin shops and a flourishing pawnbroker. Engraving after W. Hogarth, c. 1751. Although later than the period addressed here, the image captures the widespread belief that the poor were predisposed to plague because of their living conditions. Wellcome Collection, Public Domain Mark.

Cotton is imported from that Part of the World, should at all Times be kept in *Quarantine*" (Mead 1720, 27–8).

In Britain, by contrast, Mead believed that "there is [not] any one Instance of a *Pestilential* Disease among us of great Consequence, which we did not receive from other *Infected* Places" (Mead 1720, 5). In a later edition of the same work, he claimed that the cool climate and changing seasons in his homeland actually mitigated the negative effects of any potentially unhealthy local environments, making the "Air of our climate … so far from being ever the Original of the true plague" (Mead 1744, 71). The threat of disease, therefore, came from beyond the borders. Yet, it was obvious that plague sometimes did appear in this much more salubrious island, imported through commerce before taking hold amongst the poorer residents of port cities whose own hygienic and living habits left much to be desired. In these poor neighbourhoods, Mead called for mandatory sanitary and medical inspection, evacuation, and cleansing whenever an epidemic seemed likely. He also advised, to widespread consternation, that *cordons sanitaires* be placed around infected towns and neighbourhoods, that suspected cases be isolated and removed to plague hospitals, and even that the death penalty be considered for resisters (Slack 1985, 326–37).

Richard Mead's ideas reflected the still-influential Hippocratic *On Airs, Waters, and Places* tradition. This treatise suggested that a clear relationship existed between particular geographies, climates, and their diseases. Yet, unlike earlier medical writers who had interpreted this tradition to identify local plague-generating environments, Mead used the Hippocratic arguments to support his belief that plague could not possibly be endemic in England but instead arose elsewhere, notably in Turkey. Other early-eighteenth-century medical writers also pointed with suspicion to the Ottoman Empire. The docking of the *Grand-Saint-Antoine* in Marseille with a purportedly plague-infected cargo picked up in an Eastern Mediterranean port seemed to replicate the arrival of plague-infested ships into Mediterranean cities from the Levant centuries earlier. By the nineteenth century, the notion that the entire Eastern Mediterranean was a particularly dangerous pathogenic environment was well entrenched in European medical, travel, and literary writing.

Mead's deterministic epidemiological thinking marked the near endpoint of long-term speculation about where – in which environments and among which peoples – plague epidemics arose. It had been evident to centuries of medical writers, for example, that plague resided or erupted in particular geographic spaces. Appraisals of which plague environments were naturally pathogenic and which were accidental aftermaths of spreading epidemics, however, evolved over time as longstanding Hippocratic ideas about the respective unhealthiness of particular environments and people were reworked in response to changing medical norms and contemporary socio-cultural and political considerations. Such issues included, among other things, increasing (and increasingly concentrated) urban poverty, religious conflict, and global trading and diplomatic relationships. Underlying these largely domestic factors was a significant increase in European travel and in the resultant production of popular travelogues and narratives. Witnessing – or at least reading about – regular outbreaks of disease in the faraway Levant must have given Europeans with decreasing plague experience at home (and often little tangible knowledge of the region itself) the sense that the entire

Eastern Mediterranean under Ottoman rule was, and perhaps always had been, disease-ridden.

This chapter explores how contemporary medical writers, particularly but not exclusively those in England and France, explained recurrent plague outbreaks by adapting theories that linked natural environments and disease. In particular, it demonstrates that while belief in the overall environment–disease relationship remained largely intact, portrayals of where those diseased places were located changed over time, with local "plaguescapes" ultimately being replaced by definitively foreign ones (Jones 2022a, 2016).

Diseased *Airs, Waters, and Places*

Few medical authors who wrote about plague after the Black Death would have rejected the idea that outbreaks of the disease emerged from unhealthy environments.[3] In this line of thinking, they drew upon a 2,000-year-old medical tradition that overtly linked local environments, diseases, and people's state of health.

As early as the fifth century BCE, Greek natural philosopher Alcmaeon of Croton argued that disease is "sometimes affected by … certain waters or a particular site" (quoted in Freeman 1948, 40–1). The Hippocratic treatise *On Airs, Waters, and Places* elaborated considerably on the idea that environment and climate both affect the presence or prevalence of certain diseases and define people's health status in any given location. For example, the treatise recommends that upon entering a city for the first time, one should pay particular attention to its orientation, the nature of its waters and landscape, and its seasons and climate in order to know "the diseases peculiar to the place, or the particular nature of common diseases" as well as "what epidemic diseases will attack the city, either in summer or in winter" (Hippocrates 1886, 157). Furthermore, winds could spread diseases generated in one landscape to another: the Greeks believed that the hot and humid winds blowing across the Mediterranean Sea from the North African coast, for example, carried moist chronic diseases, such as fluxes, diarrhoeas, dysenteries, and epilepsy (Hippocrates 1886, 158–61). Other sections in the *On Airs, Waters, and Places* treatise explain not only the different environments found in "Europe" and "Asia" – by which is imputed the eastern Mediterranean region and beyond – but also perceived differences in the physical and mental health of the people who lived there. In short, "the forms and dispositions of mankind … correspond with the nature of the country" in which a populace lives (Hippocrates 1886, 182).

Subsequent medical authorities incorporated aspects of *On Airs, Waters, and Places* into their own theories. Central to Galen of Pergamon's writings in the third century CE, for example, was the idea that an invisible poisonous vapour called miasma could generate disease when it entered people's bodies and disturbed their humoural balances. Miasma, or corrupted air, was believed to arise from particular features of the environment, such as stagnant water, marshes and swamps, ditches, deep valleys, and the cracked surfaces of the earth. Rotting corpses, enclosed, stale spaces, and extreme heat could also generate corrupted air. Galen noted that whereas some diseases were transmitted directly, from one individual to another, others affected people who lived far apart because once corrupted, poisoned air spreads through the wind from one place and people to another (Jouanna 2001; 2012, 130). In all cases, the bodies of those most susceptible to the ill effects of polluted air were naturally inclined to attract its corruption or were unable to counteract it.

These ideas were put into practice to explain more than theoretical epidemics. The First Plague Pandemic (c.541 CE to mid-eighth century), also known as the Justinianic Plague, was first recorded at the port city of Pelusium, on the eastern Nile Delta, in July 541. (This does not mean, of course, that the pandemic actually began there: since plague is not normally a human disease, its "first appearance in Pelusium thus may be an artefact of human perception [and written records], rather than historical and scientific fact" (Green and Jones 2020, 44)). Near-contemporary medical writers, such as Stephanus of Athens, relied on Galenic principles and assumed that the inhalation of pestilential or putrefied air arising from an insalubrious environment was behind the pandemic (Mulhall 2021). In the seventh century, Isidore of Seville similarly explained that the quickly spreading *pestilentia* arose from air that had been corrupted; according to Isidore, people exposed to corrupted air blown by the wind were just as likely to be infected by disease as those who lived directly beside unwholesome waters (Isidore of Seville 1964, 57, 66).

The Islamicate medical tradition likewise built on the older Greco-Roman medical tradition, pointing to "a pestilential corruption of the natural environment" as the cause of *wabā'* (epidemics) (Fancy 2022). Swampy regions were deemed more prone to corruption – and thus disease – because vapours arising from their stagnant waters mixed with and corrupted the air. The eleventh-century Latin translation of medical works by Avicenna (Ibn Sīnā) and Haly Abbas (Ali ibn Abbas al-Majusi), among others, then both carried the Hippocratic *On Airs, Waters, and Places* tradition into the European late-medieval medical corpus and reinforced the association between the environments of specific places and disease (Aberth 2013, 13–18; Rawcliffe 2013, 121). The particular features of rural landscapes – marshes, sluggish waterways, and damp and dark valleys – and of urban environments – slaughterhouses, tanneries, garbage heaps, and slow moving canal networks – were all accepted as potential local sources of disease because of their propensity to generate foul-smelling, corrupted, and disease-generating air.

In response, popular regimens of health – a genre of medical advice literature concerned with the preservation and maintenance of physical, mental, and spiritual health – discussed the environmental factors that negatively affected well-being and advised readers to avoid unwholesome outdoor spaces, disagreeable climates, and foul air (Jones 2022b; Nicoud 2007). Civic regulations, policies, and rebuilding efforts were likewise enacted repeatedly across

Europe to manage environments of health and disease, both to improve the perceived unhealthiness of cities (Ciecieznski 2013; Coomans 2021; Fay 2015; Geltner 2013; 2019; Rawcliffe 2013; Rawcliffe and Weeda 2019; Zaneri and Geltner 2020; see also in this volume Peterson and Krolikowski; Agresta; and Barnhouse) and to mitigate the harms found in rural landscapes (Dobson 1997). The arrival of the Black Death (or threat thereof) added urgency to such individual and collective efforts.

Plague in the Domestic Environment

When plague appeared in the Mediterranean region in 1348, physicians believed that the epidemic could be logically explained and rationally treated. They trusted this even though the disease's signs, symptoms, and progression – both through people's bodies and across kingdoms and empires – did not fit neatly within traditional medical classifications and theories. Confidence in their ability to characterize and treat the disease was manifested in a new genre of medical literature: the plague treatise or tract. To a large extent, these works were formulaic in both structure and layout, presenting medical theories and practices in 3 distinct sections: causes and signs of the disease, recommendations for preventing infection through personal and environmental prophylaxis, and remedial therapies for those who fell ill. As devastating outbreaks recurred frequently over the following centuries, these treatises circulated in large numbers throughout Europe and the Middle East (Jones 2022a).

Yet experience with plague challenged medical thinking that was predicated on dealing with individuals or, at most, localized groups of people, and with familiar diseases. In these cases, disease typically was explained as the result of imbalanced humours, poor lifestyle habits, and/or some local environmental disturbance. Plague, however, did not behave as more familiar diseases did. As such, existing explanations needed to be reworked to clarify how this widespread, high-mortality disease with seemingly unique symptoms had been generated and spread.

Medieval physicians typically pointed to two sets of causes. Christian scholastic philosophy dictated that even though God ruled everything on earth (that is, was the prime cause), natural laws could be understood as secondary causes. As a result, although plague was ultimately generated by a supernatural power, it was also part of a natural order that encompassed causes both remote and universal, and near, particular, and terrestrial. Universal and remote causes embodied either natural or supernatural agents, such as earthquakes and adverse astrological conjunctions that affected geographically distant places. Some writers invoked the devastating earthquake of 25 January 1348 (centred in the eastern Alpine Friuli-Venezia Giulia region of modern Italy) as the pandemic's cause because it, following traditional theory, had produced evil vapours capable of corrupting the air that were then spread widely by the wind. Most authors, however, turned to the conjunction of Saturn, Jupiter, and Mars that took place on 20 March 1345. Astrologers had predicted this particular conjunction long before it happened and studied it intensely thereafter for its anticipated malignant effects. Such nefarious impacts included great disease outbreaks (Goldstein and Pingree 1990, 7). As the French physician and astrologer Geoffrey de Meaux explained at the time, this particular conjunction could have generated a global disease since it "affected the whole inhabited world between east and north ... because all parts of the world ... shared in the effect of the configuration" (Meaux 1349, in Horrox 1994, 170). The same conjunction continued to be blamed for subsequent epidemic waves of plague in the fourteenth century, and similar planetary alignments were still being cited as a cause of plague centuries later.

Some early plague tract authors also pointed to insalubrious environments as the cause of plague. Although it strongly promoted the astrological conjunction as the main cause of corrupted air and plague, the Paris Medical Faculty noted "[another] possible cause of the corruption, which needs to be borne in mind, is the escape of the rottenness trapped in the centre of the earth as a result of earthquakes" (Paris Medical Faculty 1348, in Horrox 1994, 161). Furthermore, the Faculty argued, southerly winds had brought "bad, rotten, and poisonous vapours from elsewhere: from swamps, lakes and chasms, for instance." Jacme d'Agramont, a physician in Lérida, argued that "pestilence can come from the earth" and that "every plague begins in one region. But then it sometimes moves to others" (Agramont 1949, 67, 62–3). He elaborated that pestilences could erupt in individual towns if undrained pools, irrigation ditches, and basins full of water surrounded it; if it was located in a deep valley (the locals called such towns "smothered" places, he said); or if hills or tall trees blocked sunlight. Pointing, in particular, to Paris, Avignon, and Lérida, Agramont castigated the filthy streams and streets associated with butcheries and tanneries that contributed to local outbreaks, if not to the wider pandemic (Agramont 1949, 68–9).

Some decades later, the papal physician Raymond Chalin de Vinario pointed to the swamps and stagnant waters of Sardinia as a source of plague and reiterated Agramont's assessment of Paris and Avignon's uncleanliness. Many authors also commented on the southerly winds that invariably spread hot and humid – and therefore unhealthy – air from locations that were already diseased. The prophylactic advice they offered to avoid harmful miasma included moving one's house away from putrefied air, such as that found near "marshy, muddy, and stinking places, stagnant waters and ditches," and increasing ventilation through windows open to the north – to avoid the pestilence-ridden southerly winds – "as long as these [northern exposures] did not pass through putrid and infected places" (Arrizabalaga 1994, 275; see also Dumas 2003, 157–65).

Emerging recognition that plague had become a recurrent local problem – rather than a single widespread universal one – gave the landscape-as-cause argument greater prominence in plague treatises written after the 1360s. Johannes Jacobi, a Montpellier university chancellor and physician, was one of the first authors to explicitly propose that features of local environments better explained the recurrent nature of outbreaks than did a universal, celestial cause (Chase 1985, 157). The terminology he used to describe these disease-producing environments was much the same as that used previously; indeed, he echoed the claims made earlier by Agramont – and by Hippocrates and others centuries before – that pestilences particular to one town or region occurred, in part, because of the nature of the local environment. But now, rather than suggesting as the Paris Medical Faculty had done that plague was caused by corrupted air blown in from diseased environments located "elsewhere," Jacobi argued that it was local causes of plague that should be avoided, notably corpses and corrupted, foul watery places (Wickersheimer 1925, 107). He also believed that the sick emitted poisonous fumes, which then passed the disease on to others (Chase 1985, 157), but the corrupted air that made them ill arose first in the local environment. Jacobi further warned that people living in healthy environments would face greater harm from plague than would those who were already habituated to living in disease-producing environments.

Many later authors adopted Jacobi's explanatory framework and pointed to aspects of their own environments that might be responsible for recurrent outbreaks. A fifteenth-century adaptation of Jacobi's treatise, for example, remarked that local corruption arose from "every foule stynche ... of stabyl, stynkyng feldys, wayes or stretes ... and most of stynkyng waters" (Bisshop of Arusiens 1485, 4v). Sixteenth- and seventeenth-century tract writers continued to blame plague on the same environmental and topographical problems: in 1625, the physician Stephen Bradwell blamed London's outbreaks on corrupted air that arose from "filthy sincks, stincking sewers, channells, gutters, privies, sluttish corners, dunghils, and uncast ditches; as also the mists and fogs that commonly arise out of fens, moores, mines, and standing lakes" (Bradwell 1625, 4). Rotting corpses – whether from London's butchers, street animals, or abandoned pets – that ended up in the city's waterways were likewise problematic. In attempting to understand "why doth the plague haunt one place more than another?" the physician Gideon Harvey suggested that "one place is closer, nastier and more putrid than others ... houses built upon a clay and foggy ground are more subject to conceive pestilent Seminaries" (Harvey 1665, 9).

The stinking ditches and foul streets that authors blamed for plague were familiar in all late medieval and early modern countrysides and towns. At the same time, the tract writers' focus on the disease-generating problems particular to urban landscapes mirrored contemporary observations that after the fourteenth-century high mortality outbreaks were increasingly concentrated in the kingdom's crowded cities and towns. Much like they had been for earlier cleansing efforts, amelioration and prophylactic measures against plague were largely local. Each time plague returned, there were renewed ordinances calls for regular street cleaning, bans on the emptying of cesspools and on the disposal of refuse and carrion in the streets, the relocation of butchers and tanners outside urban residential areas, and tighter regulations concerning livestock and other animals (Rawcliffe 2013; Sloane 2011). Officials lit fires in the streets and householders were advised to scent their homes with vinegar, perfumes, and sweet-smelling herbs and woods. Many preventive measures, thus, aimed to correct or purify the local, potentially diseased environment – both within towns and in individual homes (Slack 1985, 30). Official publications such as *Orders thought meet by her Majesty and her Privy Council*, which was re-issued repeatedly between 1578 and 1625, likewise sought to impose social and sanitary policies to preserve the health of the urban landscape.

While the environment–disease relationship remained largely intact well into the seventeenth and eighteenth centuries, however, by the sixteenth century, a shift can be discerned in where tract writers located corrupted and diseased neighbourhoods. Accounts of the earliest outbreaks had made little socio-economic distinction between plague's victims, noting that it killed indiscriminately. However, prominent citizens who were able to flee during outbreaks increasingly noticed upon their return that the poorer districts had faced particularly heavy burdens of mortality. Legislators in northern Italian city-states early on enacted sanitary legislation that intrinsically linked plague with the poor, and in particular poor migrants and beggars. Segregation, isolation, denial of movement/passage/entry, and similar plague-prevention measures were applied disproportionately to the poor (Carmichael 1986; Cohn 2010; Pullan 1995). Comparable measures appeared in England and France shortly afterwards, as ideas about localized sources of corruption and contamination narrowed to areas that the poor inhabited or that they could infect.

In England, the sheer amount of poverty, coupled with the significant increase in population, became an especially noticeable and growing political, economic, and social concern to the property-owning and governing classes during the sixteenth and seventeenth centuries. Here, the closing of the monasteries also had an immediate and visible effect on poverty rates. The number of beggars on the streets rose, as did the level of their hardship, especially in London where people flocked in search of work (Jones 2022a). A plague outbreak in Windsor Castle in 1517 was blamed, in part, on poor beggars (Roger 2020, 3). Deserving of charity or otherwise, in most early modern English cities and towns, the overcrowded and filthy living conditions occupied by the poor became closely correlated with plague outbreaks. It was easy to link plague to the poor: plague was generated by corrupt or putrefied air and corrupted the bodies of its victims in turn; the poor were believed to be predisposed or susceptible to this putrefaction – or, indeed, capable of even producing and magnifying it – because they were already corrupted on account of their inferior living and moral conditions (Siena 2019, 1–2).

England's national and municipal plague orders included not only direct references to the poor and the spaces they inhabited but also the College of Physicians' prophylactic and treatment advice that, by 1630, went beyond prescribing plague remedies to include overt descriptions of the disease-generating conditions in which the poor lived. Such conditions, the college proclaimed, endangered public health and had to be rectified. The same idea already appeared in contemporary plague treatises, which sometimes blamed epidemics directly on the living conditions of the poor. Clergyman and medical writer Thomas Brasbridge combined local geography and poverty to blame plague on corrupted air that arose "in a fewe houses, or streetes, through the stenche of chanels, of filthie doung, of carion, of standing pudles and stincking waters, of seeges, or stincking privies … of common pissing places, and such like … [and in] a gret company dwelling or lyving in a small room especially if those roomes be not verie clenlie kept" (Brasbridge 1592, A8).

Other late sixteenth- and early seventeenth-century writers warned against the dangers that arose from poor people and from vagabonds who came from (suspected) infected parishes. The physician William Bullein linked plague to "slotishe beastlie people, that kepe their houses and lodginges unclene, their meate, drincke, and clothyng, moste noisome, their labour and travell immoderate" (Bullein 1578, 28). Stephen Bradwell contended that the poor were more subject to plague because of their "living sluttishly, and feeding nastily on offals, or the worst & unholsomest meates … their bodies much corrupted [and] most subject to this Sicknesse" (Bradwell 1625, 46). Indeed, he continued, "we see the *Plague* sweeps up such people in greatest heapes." Bradwell complained not just of the culinary choices and homes of the poor but also their clothing, furniture, habits, and uncleanliness, all of which he contended made them carriers, if not generators, of plague. These writers more charitably offered specific directions for the poor to preserve themselves from plague but, at the same time, perceived that the very spaces that the poor occupied were both actually and metaphorically diseased.

Complementing the plague tracts, weekly broadsheets available for a small cost and later John Graunt's (1665a, 1665b) collected Bills of Mortality reproduced mortality figures by parish for London's major outbreaks between 1592 and 1665. In so doing, they pointed visibly and starkly to which areas of the city and its suburbs had the unhealthiest and deadliest environments (Jenner 2012). Since the poorest parishes were often hit first, and worst, during epidemics, the broadsheets further emphasized the perceived link between the poor and plagued environments. Neighbourhoods already associated with poverty, social unrest, and criminality faced still greater stigmatization when they were also characterized as diseased spaces (Griffiths 2000; Pelling 2000; Siena 2019). Londoners actively used these bills to determine which parishes to avoid. For their part, merchants and shop owners petitioned to have the death figures further delineated since being associated with or working near to infected parishes was bad for business (Sullivan 2010, 81). With well-known physicians also writing that poor parishes were diseased environments, it was difficult to avoid the assumption that poorer, marginalized areas of cities were plague-ridden. Indeed, by the mid-seventeenth century, plague had become so associated with the poor that the physician Nathaniel Hodges wrote "it is incredible to think how the Plague [of 1665] raged amongst the common People, insomuch that it came by some to be called the *Poors Plague*" (Hodges 1720, 15).

French Royal Acts and Orders on plague, in contrast to those produced in England, had little to say explicitly about the poor and their injunctions to limit the movement of goods and people during outbreaks and enact sanitary measures ostensibly applied to everyone. However, municipal councils passed ordinances designed to combat the disease locally that included, among other measures, temporary bans on begging and the exclusion of poor strangers. In many southern French cities, the poor – and the itinerant poor in particular – became especially associated with filth and illness; as such, they were both targeted for coercive isolation measures and blamed for the spread of disease.

Only a very small number of French treatise writers associated plague with "the putrid exhalations that customarily arise from places that are crowded by the poor" (Courcelles 1595, 34)[4], or with "common people" who "live in dirty places and who live dirty lives" (Joubert 1581, 61).[5] Those who did tended to be Protestant, and their views on the poor reflected sixteenth-century Protestant views that unemployment, poverty, and disease were signs of moral failure. The language of plague also entered French discourse about the poor: the broad movement to institutionalize the poor was predicated, in part, on an assumption that they were "as contagious as a plague victim" (Jones 1996, 48). By the Plague of Provence in 1720, more French tract writers pointed to the local slums, especially those near the port, as the location where the outbreak had started.[6] The public prosecutor Pichatty de Croissainte, for example, provided a detailed itinerary of the epidemic's movement, beginning in "the Street of *Lescalle*, a Part of the old Town inhabited only by poor People" (Siena 2019, 58). Few French writers, though, emphasized the specific environment inhabited by the poor as a generator of plague, as their English counterparts were doing. Instead, as I discuss elsewhere (Jones 2022a), they turned their attention to their religious enemies.

But if plague began among the poor or in a particular parish or town, tract writers also needed to explain how it got there. For some, the urban environment itself was the problem. Antoine Davin, a French physician and royal councillor, noted in 1629 that plague began in large and dense cities "such as Grand Cairo, Constantinople, Paris, Toulouse, and Lyons ... where the nature of the place has something to do" with generating the disease (Davin 1629, 45).[7] For others, environmental explanations of plague shifted almost entirely to foreign places. Nathaniel Hodges noted that because "plague affects many regions together at the same time," it was necessary to distinguish it from "Endemick diseases, that is, such that are appropriate to one place only" (Hodges 1720, 36). Recognizing that plague was widespread, Hodge's primary concern was to understand how it flourished in climates that were so different and located so distant from each other. Since from "Reason [it] is very obvious [that] there is so much Difference between the

Diseases of different Climates," Hodges pondered, "how much Alteration [must plague] undergo in such a Travel, from a hot and dry Climate, into a moist and cold one" (Hodges 1720, 64). Such alteration did not and could not, he contended, make plague endemic in England, not even amongst its poor. Although Hodges believed that plague could re-emerge in the same place over a period of time, he argued that its continued reappearance relied entirely on "external Circumstances" (Hodges 1720, 142). Plague was not, in other words, a disease linked to England's environment: it came from elsewhere and then first affected the most susceptible and corrupted parts of a town before engulfing neighbouring districts. It did not take long for this idea to become entrenched.

Plague in the Foreign Environment

Writing in 1722 as the outbreak in Marseille came to an end, former military physician Jean-Baptiste Goiffon sought to distinguish between plague – which he considered to be epidemic, contagious, and of a "moderate and small origin" (Goiffon 1722, 41) – and other non-contagious malignant fevers and common maladies.[8] "These types of diseases," he said, referring to the latter, "always have a vast source and rely [for their eruption] on a vast quantity of spoiled and corrupted matter ... and not on being transferred" from one person or object to another (Goiffon 1722, 43).[9] In other words, outbreaks of non-contagious epidemic diseases in a new country or location relied on the source of the disease having been there all along. Plague, by contrast, began in one specific environment and then spread through contagion. "There can be no doubt," he stated, "that the origin [of plague] is very limited" (Goiffon 1720, 42).[10] Unlike many of the earlier treatise writers who had identified a plethora of local spaces capable of generating the disease, however, Goiffon insisted that plague's primary and original environment was foreign.

Goiffon was not the only writer to make such a claim. George Thomson, an anti-Galenic physician, was one of the earliest English tract writers to point a suspicious finger to the importation of plague from foreign environments whose airs "are observed to produce the Pest Periodically (as in *Gran Cairo* in *Aegypt*) where the beginning and end of raging Plagues may punctually be foretold" (Thomson 1666, 20). Hodges, an equally staunch supporter of the traditional Galenic medical model, traced the arrival of plague into London "from Africa or Asia to Holland and then to England" (Hodges 1720, 64). Another writer similarly noted that the 1665 outbreak "came out of Turky into Germany, out of Germany into Italy, out of Italy into Holland and out of Holland into England" (Gadbury 1665, 10). Although they still acknowledged that plague arose from unhealthy environments replete with "Pools and standing waters ... Lakes that do not run ... stinking sinks, and ditches that are not cleaned" (Kemp 1665, 13), however, what sets these seventeenth-century writers apart from their predecessors is their assumption that such corrupted environments were foreign, not domestic.

Devastating plague outbreaks still impacted seventeenth-century England and France. Before London's great outbreak of 1665, English cities had been hit hard in 1602–5, 1608–11, 1625–7, 1630–1, 1636–9, and throughout the 1640s (Slack 1985, 62). The French kingdom was not free from plague in any year between 1600 and 1700; during the late 1620s–30s, the greatest number of localities was hit, and harder, than at any time in centuries. Lyon, for example, lost half of its population in 1628–30 (Jones 1996, 99). Even so, the incidence or frequency of plague outbreaks was visibly declining in both kingdoms before the mid-seventeenth century, and this decline picked up speed thereafter. Across the Ottoman Empire and especially in Constantinople, by contrast, plague outbreaks had become "a permanent … presence" (Varlık 2015, 186). Coinciding with a significant increase in European travel for diplomacy, commerce, pilgrimage, and pleasure (Borromeo 2007; Brentjes 2010; MacLean 2004), these regular outbreaks must have given travellers with less plague experience at home the sense that the entire eastern Mediterranean was disease-ridden.

Travel writers like Peter Mundy noted the unhealthiness of Scanderone (İskenderun), which "is very unwholesome by reason of the hugh high hills hindringe the approach of the Sunne Beames … [and the] great Marshe full of boggs, foggs and Froggs" (quoted in MacLean 2004, 229). Particularly problematic were the urban streets, which European writers invariably described as filthy, stench-ridden, and pestilential. Writers also pointed to the region's local graveyards and flea markets as sources of disease (Varlık 2015, 78–9). Since they had purportedly personally witnessed the unhealthy foreign landscapes about which they wrote, travel writers were believed to be authorities on the subject, even more so when they were also physicians.[11] Their references to the Ottoman Empire's rural swamps, bogs, fens, and stagnant waters; its crowded and filthy urban streets and ditches; and its foul smelling airs reinforced contemporary European beliefs that such places were, indeed, unhealthy; everyone knew, for example, that similar landscapes at home were unhealthy and to be avoided. These domestic sources of disease had purportedly been cleaned up, however, according to tract writers.

While observing that "the Contagion [is] now spreading it self in Foreign Parts," that is, in Marseille in 1720, the English physician Richard Bradley considered whether the "destruction of the City [of London] by fire in 1666" had forestalled any further outbreaks there (Bradley 1721, 11–12). During London's outbreak in 1665, he noted, the city had been full of the kind of crowded, narrow, unpaved, and suffocating streets that generated plague. Now, however, it was much airier and more salubrious, unlike the plague-ridden cities that travellers described in the Ottoman Empire. The physician John Quincy suggested that unhealthy places, such as those containing stagnant rivers, could be improved by redirecting cleaner waters to flush out the sluggish ones. Such efforts, he noted, had already been made in Oxford and, along with enlarging the city boundaries to ease overcrowding and keeping the streets clean and empty of dung and offal, had freed the city from further outbreaks. The implication was that foreign places where this had not been done, such as "*Grand Cairo* in *Egypt* ... are [therefore] hardly ever free from *Pestilential Disease*" (Quincy 1720, 255).

Further contributing to this transference, contemporary physicians, geographers, and chorographers (who blended geographic, climatic, and cultural descriptions of local places) were expanding their application of the Hippocratic *On Airs, Waters, and Places* tradition and examining why some local places were healthier than others. Although some mentioned unhealthy features of local regions, such as William Lambarde's description of Romney Marsh as "Evill in winter, grevious in Sommer and never good," or William Camden's observation that parts of Essex suffered from "unwholesome vapours [which] very much impair the health of the adjacent inhabitants," more often these writers did *not* discuss disease-generating places in their descriptions of their homeland (Wear 2008, 447; see also Dobson 1997; Peter 1975; Wear 1992). Instead, they painted a picture of overall healthiness. If travel and medical writers often portrayed the Ottoman Empire as a plagued landscape, the fact that outbreaks continued there long after they had slowed down and ended in Western Europe only served to validate the idea that the region was, in both popular and medical terms, the ultimate source of the disease (Varlık 2015, 2017).

The seventeenth-century travel writer Fynes Moryson's (1907, 2:89–90) description of the "pestilent aire," "Fenny Plaine," "most unwholesome" waters, "ill vapours," "boggy earth," and "pailefills" of rain in the eastern Mediterranean – which he said made the region "infamous for the death of Christians" – helped writers of different ilks to direct attention away from local sites and reinforce biases against foreign places, especially those deemed exotic in landscape, custom, and religion. So too did Moryson's contention that the "streetes of this Citie [Constantinople] are narrow ... In many places of the streetes lye carcases, yea sometimes the bodies of dead men, even till they be putrified, and I thinke this uncleanlinesse of the Turks is the chiefe cause that this Citie ... is continually more or lesse infected with the plague" (Moryson 1907, 2:100–101). Other writers made similar claims, and their works helped to foster a growing perception of a West-East geographical and health divide (Jones 2022a). Richard Mead's early eighteenth-century comparison of England's "*Northern Air*" (Mead 1744, 72) and changing seasons with the sultry heats and stagnant waters of Egypt, Turkey, and other southern regions was simply another step in this process. Indeed, Mead argued that "*Northern* Nations ... were not wasted with Plagues" until they had started communicating and trading with these diseased regions of the world, all of which were now part of the Ottoman Empire (Mead 1744, 27).

Curiously, perhaps, such claims were rarely made against the regions and territories incorporated into the imperial domains of European powers. Although some were deemed unhealthy for a variety of reasons (see chapters by Linte and Chouin in this volume), colonial promoters typically found it necessary to assess and market new settlements in terms of their environmental healthiness, and to do so in a familiar way that reflected "an Old World framework of medical and environmental knowledge" (Wear 2008, 451). Overwhelmed by malaria, smallpox, dysentery, and, later, yellow fever, for example, the American colonies were nevertheless considered to be, and continuously promoted as, healthy places to live because their physical environments were much like, or even better than, what potential colonists experienced in England or France (Jones 2022a, 2016, 118). Although plague was an ongoing concern in India, where European ambassadors and traders had established diplomatic and profitable commercial relations with the Mughal Empire, here too Europeans did not discuss it as openly as they did other diseases.

As a result, even though Europeans often viewed foreign spaces and foreign bodies as sites of disease, it made sense to locate the origins of plague in a place that would remain foreign, not in one that they inhabited. If their colonial and imperialist projects required the English and the French to find a place outside of their control in which to situate plague, the economic and political decline of the Ottoman Empire over the seventeenth century provided them with a suitable location. By turns Western Europe's most visible competitor, military threat, and cultural and religious Other, the empire was, until about the mid-seventeenth century, also an important economic and diplomatic partner, a paradox that initially generated a complex image of the Turks among Europeans. But relocating plague among them helped bolster suggestions that outbreaks in Europe were imported from or carried by peoples who were themselves diseased or, otherwise, undesirable (Jones 2022a; Varlık 2017).

Locating the origin of plague in the Ottoman Empire became increasingly easier to do as early modern tract writers began to contemplate the history of the disease as they contextualized current outbreaks. An anonymous commentary on London's weekly Bills of Mortality in 1665, for example, began a discussion of "Forreign Visitations by the Plague" in the mid-fourteenth century, with the disease first emerging, according to the writer, "in the East Indies, among the Tartarians, Saracens and Turks" (Anonymous 1665, 1). While many earlier writers had placed the origins of the Black Death in the lands of the Tartars and Saracens, the specific addition of "Turks" was a uniquely early modern interpolation. The anonymous writer of 1665 continued his commentary by deliberately situating plague in "the city called the Grand Caire ... [where] the plague cometh with such fierceness" because of the vapours and great heat which cometh from the ground (Anonymous 1665, 1). In fact, the writer claimed, "the most part of the people there do die" of plague.

In the 1720s, as the major outbreak in Marseille spread through southern France, these ideas took on greater significance. English writers, such as Richard Mead, often argued that trade and commerce with already-diseased environments was problematic: "in these latter Ages, since our Trade with Turkey has been pretty constant, the Plagues in these Parts of Europe have evidently been brought from thence ... [and] the late *Plague* in *France* came indisputably from Turkey" (Mead 1744, 24). The physician Philip Rose concurred, arguing that plague spread through the importation of goods "especially from ... *Turkish* Dominions" (Rose 1721, 19). There were only a small number of dissenting voices, both to the idea of contagion and to the Ottoman Empire being the source of plague.

French authors soon began to make similar arguments about the origin of the Marseille outbreak at the same time that they idealized the city and its purported cleanliness (Gordon 1997, 69–70), which they contrasted to the filthy cities of the Eastern Mediterranean. The Abbé Martin Gaudereau claimed, based on almost 30 years of personal observation while travelling on diplomatic business throughout the Ottoman region, that "an infinite number of places in Asia are infected by the plague" (Gauderau 1721, 18).[12] The physician and medical writer Jean-Jacques Manget agreed, pointing out that plague had become relatively rare in Europe but was brought in from time to time from "oriental" countries where it occurred regularly, "particularly among the Turks" (Manget 1722, 17).[13] Many pointed to a specific ship – the *Grand-Saint-Antoine* – that had recently arrived from "the countries of the Levant that are often wasted by the plague" (Bertrand 1723, 25).[14] Marseille, by contrast, could not have possibly been an original site in which plague arose because neither the city nor its surrounding countryside had the kind of environment that generated corrupted air; simply put, in Jean-Baptiste Bertrand's words, "Marseille is exempt from all these infections" (Bertrand 1723, 18).[15] By the early eighteenth century, then, both English and French writers almost uniformly portrayed plague as a disease that arose naturally in the environments of some other parts of the world and then spread through various means, including commerce, the winds, or the movement of sick travellers. Europeans already perceived the Ottoman Empire to be in decline; being labelled as a plague environment, as the source of all plagues, was just one further sign of its stagnation and brutishness.

Conclusion

Before the late fourteenth century, plague tract authors were already pointing to domestic environments to explain local outbreaks, including ubiquitous swamps, marshes, and foul-smelling urban industries. Mitigation efforts focused on cleaning up these local sites of disease. English and French writers diverged by the early sixteenth century, however, when it came to assigning blame to the peopled environments that they considered to be disease generating: in England, plague became directly associated with the neighbourhoods of the poor while in France religious tensions spilled over into discourses about the places that generate plague. In the seventeenth and eighteenth centuries, local explanations were increasingly displaced by a foreign pathogenization that allowed writers to contrast their own purportedly salubrious environments with those in other regions of the world that, they argued, were natural habitats for plague. For many tract writers, the Ottoman Empire became the "plaguescape *par excellence*" (Jones 2016, 119) because of the reportedly insalubrious nature of its rural and urban spaces.

As Nathaniel Hodges pondered so many centuries ago, *Yersinia pestis*, and hence plague, moved across and not only survived in but adapted to a wide variety of climates and environments to cause massive human mortality. How it did so, and whether it did become endemic in some parts of Europe and the Middle East – an issue that Richard Mead and others vehemently denied in the early eighteenth century – are questions that are now being asked of the scientific and historical evidence (Bos et al. 2016; Carmichael 2014; Seifert et al. 2016; Varlık 2014). Although these modern studies are unlikely to find evidence that specific stagnant waters, marshes and swamps, or some cities' tanneries and butcheries, or southerly winds from hot climates, are to blame, it is probable that local environments will figure prominently. Since which animal acts as *Y. pestis*'s host varies by location, different species act as host in different areas of the globe. Diverse local ecologies and climates, in turn, can generate altered epidemiological manifestations of the disease – and even variant strains of the bacterium as it moves into and adapts to new local environments (Gage and Kosoy 2005; Green 2018, 14; Poinar 2022).

Modern studies reveal the complexity and multi-layered nature of the relationships between natural and manmade environments, pathogens, vectors, hosts, and disease outbreaks. Medical writers of the past did not, of course, have the benefit of microscopic analysis, climate science, or archaeology to inform their understanding of plague. Nor did their theoretical conceptions of human health and illness leave room to consider the possibility that rodent-borne pathogens had moved into new environments and crossed the species boundary to infect human bodies, transmitted by ever-present fleas. Instead, to explain this strange and highly lethal disease, they drew on what they witnessed, blended it with longstanding medical tradition, and offered their thoughts and advice to those who would listen. As Hippocrates and Galen contended, and as medical writers repeated in their discussions of the plague, it was obvious that particular environments generated particular diseases. For centuries, medical writers could locate the source of plague within the corrupt vapours that arose from stagnant and foul-smelling local environments and unseasonable climates. Just as plague outbreaks were receding in Britain and France, these diseased environments had become notably foreign, not only to explain current outbreaks but also those of the historical past. For Richard Mead and many other tract writers, "the History of the most terrible of all the Plagues, that ever were in these Parts of the World, which was that in the Year 1349, gives a manifest Proof from whence all *Europe* may trace the Origine of these Evils, viz. from *Asia*" (Mead 1720, 10). Even the mysterious sweating sickness, "commonly thought to have taken its Rise here [i.e., in England]," was, Mead suggested, "most probably of a foreign Original ... very probably from a Turkish Infection" (Mead 1720, 6–7).

Such ideas cast the dice: in his contribution to Diderot and d'Alembert's mid-eighteenth-century *Encyclopédie, ou dictionnaire raisonné des sciences, des arts et des métiers,* Louis de Jaucourt wrote the following entry: "the plague comes from Asia, and for two thousand years all the plagues that have appeared in Europe have been transmitted to us by the Saracens, Arabs, Moors, or Turks; all of our plagues had no other source" (Jaucourt 1751–2, 12:452).[16] European environments might have become plagued, temporarily, but the Ottoman environment was especially and permanently plaguey.

Notes

1 I would like to thank Nükhet Varlık for her suggestions that improved an earlier version of this chapter. Longer discussions of several of the arguments made here can be found in Jones (2022a).

2 In fact, plague is caused by *Yersinia pestis,* a naturally occurring coccobacillus bacterium that affects many species of wild ground-burrowing rodents and is spread by their fleas (and sometimes ticks). Other animals and their predators can also carry it.

3 The Black Death is typically dated to c.1346–53, but it has been argued recently that it actually began a century earlier, in the thirteenth century, perhaps tied to the Mongol invasion of western Asia. See Fancy and Green (2021) and Green (2020).

4 "les exhalations putrides qui s'eslevent coustumierent es lieux ou il y-a affluence de povres gens."

5 "le menu peuple ... qui habitent en lieux fort sales et ords, & qui en tout temps vivent salement."

6 On naming the outbreak Plague of Provence, rather than the conventional Plague of Marseille, see Ermus's chapter in this volume.

7 "mon opinion sur ce que dessus, est, qu'on voit ordinairement, que la peste se met aux Villes grandes & fort peuplées: comme au grand Caire, à Constantinople, à Paris, à Tholouse, à Lyon, (à quoy la nature du lieu fait quelque chose)."

8 "il paroit que les Maladies épidémiques contagieuses, & les épidémiques non contagieuses différent par la nature de leurs causes dont l'une n'a qu'une modique & petite origine."

9 "Ces sortes de maladies ont toujours une source vaste & dépendent d'une grande quantité de matière gâtée & corrompuë ... & nullement qu'elle y ait été transférée."

10 "je pense qu'on n'ôsera pas douter que la cause ne soit trés-limitée."

11 Of course, we must also recognise that even if "witnessed," such characterizations played into broader European discourses about and stereotypes of the Ottoman Empire as a despotic, violent, terror-inducing regime, and its people as immoral and religiously suspect. Overall, Europeans passed moral judgment on Oriental ways, ranging from their social practices to their institutions and ideas, and this may well have provided some further context in which their associations with disease were made. See Varlık (2015, 76–88).

12 "On trouve en Asie une infinité de lieux qui en sont infectez."

13 "Mais nous observons seulement que nôtre Europe a souffert peu de Pestes qu'elle ne doive aux levains qui lui en ont été aportés des pays Orientaux, où elle régne ordinairement (particuliérement chés les Turcs, tantôt dans un lieu, tantôt dans un autre)."

14 "les contrées du Levant [qui] sont souvent désolées par la peste." Although the *Grand-Saint-Antoine* has loomed large in scholarship about the Plague of Provence, buttressed by numerous contemporary European accounts blaming the ship, its

crew, and its cargo for importing plague, there are almost no records of outbreaks in the eastern Mediterranean at this time. Ancient DNA evidence also does not support a Levantine origin for the outbreak (Varlık 2020, 287–9).

15 "L'air de Marseille est exempt de toutes ces infections."
16 "La peste nous vient de l'Asie, & depuis deux mille ans toutes les pestes qui ont paru en Europe y ont été transmises par la communication des Sarrasins, des Arabes, des Maures, ou des Turcs avec nous, & toutes les pestes n'ont pas eu chez nous d'autre source."

References

Agramont, Jacme d'. 1949. "Jacme d'Agramont: Regiment de preservacio a epidimia o pestilencia e mortaldats." Translated by M. L. Duran-Reynals and C.E.A Winslow. *Bulletin of the History of Medicine* 23: 57–89.

Anonymous. 1665. *The Weekly Bill of Mortality: With a Lamentable Relation of Many Visitations by the Plague in Times Past.* London: Tho Milbourn.

Arrizabalaga, Jon. 1994. "Facing the Black Death: Perceptions and Reactions of University Medical Practitioners." In *Practical Medicine from Salerno to the Black Death*, edited by Luis García-Ballester, Roger French, Jon Arrizabalaga, and Andrew Cunningham, 237–88. Cambridge: Cambridge University Press.

Bertrand, Jean-Baptiste. 1723. *Relation historique de tout ce qui s'est passé à Marseille pendant la dernière peste.* Cologne: Pierre Marteau.

Bisshop of Arusiens. 1485. *Here begynneth a litill boke necessarye & behouefull agenst the Pestilence.* London: William Machlinia.

Borromeo, Elisabetta. 2007. *Voyageurs occidentaux dans l'Empire ottoman (1600–1644).* 2 Volumes. Paris: Maissoneuve & Larose.

Bos, Kristin I., Alexander Herbig, Jason Sahl, Nicholas Waglechner, Mathieu Fourment, Stephen A Forrest, Jennifer Klunk, Verena J Schuenemann, Debi Poinar, Melanie Kuch, G. Brian Golding, Olivier Dutour, Paul Keim, David M. Wagner, Edward C Holmes, Johannes Krause, and Hendrik N. Poinar. 2016. "Eighteenth Century *Yersinia pestis* Genomes Reveal the Long-Term Persistence of an Historical Plague Focus." *eLife* 5: e12994.

Bradley, Richard. 1720. *The Plague at Marseilles Consider'd.* London: for W. Mears.

Bradwell, Stephen. 1625. *A Watch-Man for the Pest.* London: John Dawson.

Brasbridge, Thomas. 1592. *The Poore Mans Jewell.* London: George Bishop.

Brentjes, Sonja. 2010. *Travellers from Europe in the Ottoman and Safavid Empires, 16th–17th Centuries: Seeking, Transforming, Discarding Knowledge.* New York: Routledge.

Bullein, William. 1578. *A Dialogue Bothe Pleasant and Pitifull, Wherein is a Godlie Regimente Against the Feuer Pestile[n]ce.* London: Ihon Kyngston.

Carmichael, Ann G. 1986. *Plague and the Poor in Renaissance Florence.* Cambridge: Cambridge University Press.

Carmichael, Ann G. 2014. "Plague Persistence in Western Europe: A Hypothesis." *The Medieval Globe* 1, no. 1: 157–92.

Chase, Melissa P. 1985. "Fevers, Poisons, and Apostemes: Authority and Experience in Montpellier Plague Treatises." *Annals of the New York Academy of Sciences* 441, no. 1: 153–70.

Ciecieznski, N. J. 2013. "The Stench of Disease: Public Health and the Environment in Late-Medieval English Towns and Cities." *Health, Culture and Society* 4, no. 1: 92–104.

Cohn, Samuel K. Jr. 2010. *Cultures of Plague: Medical Thinking at the End of the Renaissance.* Oxford: Oxford University Press, 2010.

Coomans, Janna. 2021. *Community, Urban Health and Environment in the Late Medieval Low Countries.* Cambridge: Cambridge University Press.

Courcelles, François de. 1595. *Traite de la peste clair et tres-utile.* Sedan: Abel Riuery.

Cummins, Neil, Morgan Kelly, and Cormac Ó Gráda. 2016. "Living Standards and Plague in London, 1560–1665." *Economic History Review*, 69, no. 1: 3–34.

Davin, Antoine. 1629. *Tres singulier traité de la generale et particuliere preservation, & de la vraye & asseurée curation de la Peste.* Grenoble: Richard Cocson.

Dobson, Mary J. 1997. *Contours of Death and Disease in Early Modern England.* Cambridge: Cambridge University Press.

Dumas, Geneviève. 2003. "La fenêtre en temps d'épidémie : air et miasmes à Montpellier aux XIVe et XVe siècles." In *Par la fenêtre; études de littérature et de civilisations médiévales*, Actes du colloque du CUERMA, 157–65. Aix-en-Provence: Presses universitaires de Provence.

Fancy, Nahyan and Monica H. Green. 2021. "Plague and the Fall of Baghdad (1258)." *Medical History* 65, no. 2: 157–77.

Fay, Isla. 2015. *Health and the City: Disease, Environment and Government in Norwich, 1200–1575.* Woodbridge: Boydell Press.

Freeman, Kathleen. 1948. *Ancilla to the Pre-Socratic Philosophers.* Cambridge, MA: Harvard University Press.

Gadbury, John. 1665. *London's Deliverance Predicted: In a Short Discourse Showing Causes of Plague in General.* London: J. C. for E. Calvert.

Gage, Kenneth L. and Michael Y. Kosoy. 2005. "Natural History of Plague: Perspectives from More than a Century of Research." *Annual Review of Entomology* 50: 505–28.

Gaudereau, Martin. 1721. *Relation des differentes especes de peste que reconnoissent les Orientaux.* Paris: Jacques Quillau.

Gelter, Guy. 2013. "Healthscaping a Medieval City: Lucca's *Curia viarum* and the Future of Public Health History." *Urban History* 40, no. 3: 395–415.

Geltner, Guy. 2019. *Roads to Health: Infrastructure and Urban Wellbeing in Later Medieval Italy.* Philadelphia: University of Pennsylvania Press.

Goiffon, Jean-Baptiste. 1722. *Relations et dissertation sur la peste du Gévaudan.* Lyon: P. Valfray.

Goldstein, Bernard R. and David Pingree. 1990. "Levi ben Gerson's Prognostication for the Conjunction of 1345." *Transactions of the American Philosophical Association* 80, no. 6: 1–60.

Gordon, Daniel. 1997. "The City and the Plague in the Age of Enlightenment." *Yale French Studies* 92: 67–87.

Graunt, John. 1665a. *London's Dreadful Visitation: Or, A Collection of all the Bills of Mortality for the Present Year...* London: E. Cotes.

Graunt, John. 1665b. *Reflections on the Weekly Bills of Mortality for the cities of London and Westminster.* London: Samuel Speed.

Green, Monica H. 2018. "Climate and Disease in Medieval Eurasia." In *Oxford Research Encyclopedia of Asian History.* Oxford: Oxford University Press.

Green, Monica H. 2020. "The Four Black Deaths." *The American Historical Review* 125, no. 5: 1601–31.

Griffiths, Paul. 2000. "Overlapping Circles: Imagining Criminal Communities in London, 1545–1645." In *Communities in Early Modern England: Networks, Place,*

Rhetoric, edited by Alexandra Shepard and Phil Withington, 115–133. Manchester: Manchester University Press.

Hippocrates. 1886. "On Airs, Waters and Places." In *The Genuine Works of Hippocrates: Translated from the Greek with a Preliminary Discourse and Annotations*, trans. Francis Adams, vol. 1. New York: William Wood. https://archive.org/details/genuineworksofhi00tran

Hodges, Nathaniel. 1720. *Loimologia, or an Historical Account of the Plague in London in 1665*. Translated by John Quincy. London: E. Bell.

Horrox, Rosemary, trans. and ed. 1994. *The Black Death*. Manchester: Manchester University Press.

Jaucourt, Louis de. 1751–72. "Peste." In *Encyclopédie, ou dictionnaire raisonné des sciences, des arts et des métiers*, edited by Denis Diderot and Jean le Rond d'Alembert, 12:-452–59. Paris: Sociétés Typographiques.

Jones, Colin. 1996. "Plague and Its Metaphors in Early Modern France." *Representations* 53: 97–127.

Jones, Lori. 2016. "The Diseased Landscape: Medieval and Early Modern Plague-Scapes." *Landscapes* 17, no. 2: 108–23.

Jones, Lori. 2022a. *Patterns of Plague: Changing Ideas about Plague in England and France, 1348–1750*. Montreal: McGill-Queen's University Press.

Jones, Lori. 2022b. "Early Modern Renewal of John Mirfield's Fourteenth-Century *Gouernayl of Helþe* in Wellcome Collection MS 674." In *Genre in Medical English: Sociocultural Contexts of Production and Use 1500–1820*, edited by Irma Taavitsainen, Turo Hiltunen, Jeremy Smith and Carla Suhr. Cambridge: Cambridge University Press.

Jouanna, Jacques. 2001. "Air, miasme et contagion au temps d'Hippocrate et survivance des miasmes dans la médecine posthippocratique (Rufus d'Éphèse, Galien et Palladios)." In *Air, miasmes et contagion: les épidémies dans l'Antiquité et au Moyen Age*, edited by Sylvie Bazin-Tacchella, Danielle Quéruel, and Evelyne Samama, 9–28. Langres: Dominique Guéniot.

Jouanna, Jacques. 2012. *Greek Medicine from Hippocrates to Galen: Selected Papers*. Leiden: Brill.

Joubert, Laurent. 1581. *Traitté de la peste*. Translated by Guillaume des Innocens. Lyon: Jean Lertout.

Kemp, William. 1665. *A Brief Treatise of the Nature, Causes, Signs, Preservation From, and Cure of the Pestilence, Collected by W. Kemp, Mr. of Arts*. London: D. Kemp.

MacLean, Gerald. 2004. *The Rise of Oriental Travel*. Houndmills: Palgrave.

Manget, Jean-Jacques. 1722. *Traité de la peste et des moyens de s'en préserver*. Lyon, FR: Frères Bruyset.

Mead, Richard. 1720. *A Short Discourse Concerning Pestilential Contagion and the Methods to be Used to Prevent It*. London: Printed for Sam. Buckley and Ralph Smith.

Mead, Richard. 1744. *Discourse on the Plague, The Nineth Edition Corrected & Enlarged*. London: Printed for A. Millar & J. Brindly.

Moryson, Fynes. 1907. *An Itinerary Containing His Ten Yeeres Travell*. 2 Volumes. Glasgow: MacLehose and Sons.

Mulhall, John. 2021. "Confronting Pandemic in Late Antiquity: The Medical Response to the Justinianic Plague." *Journal of Late Antiquity* 14, no. 2: 498–528.

Nicoud, Marilyn. 2007. *Les régimes de santé au Moyen Âge*. Rome: Publications de l'École française de Rome.

Pelling, Margaret. 2000. "Skirting the City? Disease, Social Change and Divided Households in the Seventeenth Century." In *Londinopolis, c.1500–c.1750: Essays in the Cultural and Social History of Early Modern London*, edited by Paul Griffiths and Mark S.R. Jenner, 154–75. Manchester: Manchester University Press.

Peter, Jean-Pierre. 1975. "Disease and the Sick at the End of the Eighteenth Century." In *Biology of Man in History*, edited by Robert Forster and Orest Ranum, translated by Elborg Forster and Patricia M. Ranum, 81–124. Baltimore, MD: The Johns Hopkins University Press.

Poinar, Hendrik. 2022. "Synergies of Genetic and Historical Interpretations of Infectious Disease." In *Death and Disease in the Medieval and Early Modern World: Perspectives from Across the Mediterranean and Beyond*, edited by Lori Jones and Nükhet Varlık. York: York Medieval Press.

Pullan, Brian. 1995. "Plague and Perceptions of the Poor in Early Modern Italy." In *Epidemics and Ideas: Essays on the Historical Perception of Pestilence*, edited by Terence Ranger and Paul Slack, 101–23. Cambridge: Cambridge University Press.

Quincy, John. 1720. *An Essay on the Different Causes of Pestilential Diseases, and How They Become Contagious*. London: Printed for E. Bell and J. Osborn.

Rawcliffe, Carole. 2013. *Urban Bodies: Communal Health in Late Medieval English Towns and Cities*. Woodbridge: Boydell Press.

Rawcliffe, Carole and Claire Weeda, eds. 2019. *Policing the Urban Environment in Premodern Europe*. Amsterdam: Amsterdam University Press.

Roger, Euan. 2020. "'To Be Shut Up': New Evidence for the Development of Quarantine Regulations in Early-Tudor England." *Social History of Medicine* 33, no. 4: 1077–96.

Rose, Philip. 1721. *A Theorico-practical, Miscellaneous, and Succinct Treatise of the Plague*. London: T. Jauncy.

Seifert, Lisa, Ingrid Wiechmann, Michaela Harbeck, Astrid Thomas, Gisela Grupe, Michaela Projahn, Holger C. Scholz, and Julia M. Riehm. 2016. Genotyping *Yersinia Pestis* in Historical Plague: Evidence for Long-term Persistence of *Y. Pestis* in Europe from the 14th to the 17th Century." *PLoS ONE* 11, no.1: e0145194.

Siena, Kevin. 2019. *Rotten Bodies: Class and Contagion in Eighteenth-Century Britain*. New Haven CT: Yale University Press.

Slack, Paul. 1985. *The Impact of Plague in Tudor and Stuart England*. London: Routledge and Kegan Paul.

Sloane, Barney. 2011. *The Black Death in London*. London: The History Trust.

Sullivan, Erin. 2010. "Physical and Spiritual Illness: Narrative Appropriations of the Bills of Mortality." In *Representing the Plague in Early Modern England*, edited by Rebecca Totaro and Ernest B. Gilman, 76–94. New York: Routledge.

Thomson, George. 1666. *Loimotomia, or the Pest Anatomized*. London: Nath. Crouch.

Varlık, Nükhet. 2014. "New Science and Old Sources: Why the Ottoman Experience of Plague Matters." *The Medieval Globe* 1, no. 1: 193–228.

Varlık, Nükhet. 2015. *Plague and Empire in the Early Modern Mediterranean World: The Ottoman Experience, 1347–1600*. Cambridge: Cambridge University Press.

Varlık, Nükhet. 2017. "'Oriental Plague' or Epidemiological Orientalism?: Revisiting the Plague Episteme of the Early Modern Mediterranean." In *Plague and Contagion in the Islamic Mediterranean*, edited by Nükhet Varlık, 57–87. Kalamazoo, MI: ARC Humanities Press.

Varlık, Nükhet. 2020. "Rethinking the History of Plague in the Time of COVID-19." *Centaurus* 62: 285–93.

Wear, Andrew. 1992. "Making Sense of Health and the Environment in Early Modern England." In *Medicine in Society: Historical Essays*, 119–47. Cambridge: Cambridge University Press.

Wear, Andrew. 2008. "Place, Health, and Disease: The *Airs, Waters, Places* Tradition in Early Modern England and North America." *Journal of Medieval and Early Modern Studies* 38, no. 3: 443–65.

Wickersheimer, Ernest. 1925. "Jean Jacme et les régimes de pestilence qui porte son nom." *Archivio di storia della scienza* 6: 105–112.

Zaneri, Taylor and Geltner, Guy. 2020. "The Dynamics of Healthscaping: Mapping Communal Hygiene in Bologna, 1287–1383." *Urban History*, 1–26.

5 Managing Disaster and Understanding Disease and the Environment in the Early Eighteenth Century

Cindy Ermus

Introduction

The Great Lisbon Earthquake of 1755 is often credited with spawning new understandings of the nature of disasters and the environment.[1] The shaking began at 9:45 on the morning of 1 November 1755 – All Saints' Day – as thousands gathered in churches across the city for mass. Estimated to have measured at least 8.5 on the moment magnitude scale (M_w), but possibly above 9.1, it was a disaster of biblical proportions (Molesky 2015, 6). The incident quickly evolved into a triple catastrophe: a megathrust earthquake followed by a tsunami and a firestorm. In the end, the combined disasters took as many as 43,000 lives in Portugal and shocked much of the contemporary world.

Some of the most celebrated thinkers of the eighteenth century, including Voltaire, Jean-Jacques Rousseau, Immanuel Kant, among many others, took to their pens to comment on the disaster. They ultimately generated hundreds of texts and commentaries that questioned every aspect of the tragedy: What caused the disaster? Could it have been avoided? Perhaps most notably, how could a just and benevolent God allow such a thing to happen?[2] Such questions informed the conversations of the day and, over time, contributed to this particular disaster being characterized as a monumental event that helped usher in the modern world. Yet the intellectual reshuffling and interrogation of nearly all aspects of life that help define the Enlightenment of the long eighteenth century were not new; instead, they predate the Lisbon Earthquake and are discernible in the aftermath of earlier disasters.

The era known as the "Age of Enlightenment," lasting roughly from the late seventeenth through eighteenth centuries, represents a critical time in the history of disaster, one that saw major shifts in how people understood the environment, especially extreme events and their causes.[3] Where previously disasters were almost universally perceived as acts of God, some contemporary thinkers now increasingly came to perceive them as naturally occurring phenomena. The very origins of the word "disaster" – which comes to us from the Greek *ástro,* or the Latin *astrum,* and *dis* – which expresses negation, i.e., "bad star" or "ill-starred event" – point to its divine and astrological associations

DOI: 10.4324/9780429055478-8

and the ways in which events perceived as disastrous had been understood. Yet, by the eighteenth century, writers such as Rousseau, Kant, and Harvard professor John Winthrop, among others, questioned these understandings and even expressed an awareness of the central *human* element in disaster causation. Which is to say, they focused on the idea that human decisions could determine the extent to which a natural hazard – a naturally occurring environmental phenomenon with the potential to harm or destroy – adversely affects a human population. In 1756, for example, Rousseau responded to Voltaire's "Poème sur le désastre de Lisbonne" with a letter in which he points to the idea that disasters result not strictly from divine retribution, nor even solely from natural processes, but rather from human decisions:

> I think I have shown that most of our physical pains, except for death ... are also our own work. Without leaving your Lisbon subject, concede, for example, that it was hardly nature who assembled there twenty-thousand houses of six or seven stories. If the residents of this large city had been more evenly dispersed and less densely housed, the losses would have been fewer or perhaps none at all ... You would have liked—and who would not have liked—the earthquake to have happened in the middle of some desert, rather than in Lisbon. Can we doubt that they also happen in deserts? But no one talks about those, because they have no ill effects for city gentlemen (the only men about whom anyone cares anything) (Rousseau 1967, 37–50).

And this, we can say, is how many, particularly those of us in disaster studies, understand disaster today.[4] In the words of Shakespeare, "The fault...is not in our stars, but in ourselves, that we are underlings" (Shakespeare 1992, 1.2. 147–8). Attempts to understand the environment and all that transpires in it, whether positive or negative and whether natural or manmade, must include humans and human action.

Drawing from the history of the Great Plague of Provence of 1720 (traditionally known as the Great Plague of Marseille),[5] this chapter explores developments and changes in early-eighteenth-century approaches to disaster management. These new ways of thinking included debates around, and shifts in understandings of, contagion and the place of disease in the environment. Long before the Lisbon Earthquake shook the intellectual foundations of Europe, the Plague of Provence similarly agitated contemporaries and contributed to the development of new methods for handling disasters. It also triggered waves of inquiry about the relationship between disaster, the environment, and disease.

The Centralization of Disaster Management in the Early Eighteenth Century

The Plague of Provence was one of the last major plague epidemics in Western Europe. Caused by the bacillus *Yersinia pestis*, a bacterium discovered by

Alexandre Yersin and Kitasato Shibasaburō in 1894, the disease reappeared in the port city of Marseille in May 1720. According to the traditional narrative, the infection arrived on a ship called the *Grand-Saint-Antoine* that had spent a year in the Levant gathering goods for a major annual trade fair in the south of France known as the *Foire de Beaucaire*.[6] Rather than undergo the usual quarantine, the vessel was rushed through so that its lucrative cargo could be unloaded in time for the fair. Almost immediately, several porters who had handled the ship's merchandise fell ill; they perished within days. From there, the number of cases began to mount, accelerating rapidly by July. By some accounts, as many as 1,000 people perished each day in Marseille alone at the height of the outbreak. Over the next 2 years, numerous "waves" of the epidemic took the lives of more than 126,000 people in the French provinces of Provence, Languedoc, Auvergne, le Comtat, and the Dauphiné (in modern-day Rhône-Alpes).[7] Despite its virulence, however, the outbreak was ultimately contained to southern France, at least partly as a result of stringent measures put in place not only in France but also across Europe and the Atlantic and Mediterranean worlds.

The centralization of disaster management was a major part of state formation, and the Plague of Provence represents one of the earliest, if not the earliest, most pronounced instance of a rigorous, centralized response to disaster. Despite the fact that the infection never spread beyond southeastern France, reactions to the threat of plague came from the capitals of emerging nation-states across Europe, including Spain, England, and Portugal. Each directed extraordinary effort towards plague prevention measures both to fend off the infection and to impose a variety of measures that would advance the very processes of administrative centralization and control that were already underway. When it became clear in Paris that municipal responses in Marseille (or lack thereof) had failed to prevent the infection from spreading outwards into Provence,[8] the administration of the regent, Philippe d'Orléans, deployed military commanders, bestowed them with unlimited authority to manage the crisis, and imposed martial law; these efforts, unlike those attempted at the municipal level, were deemed a success. At least until well into the nineteenth century, numerous texts pertaining to the subjects of contagion and/or public health management made reference to the perceived success of these centralized responses to the Plague of Provence.

In August 1720, the State Council of the King issued one of several comprehensive *arrêts* (decisions or orders) "au sujet de la maladie contagieuse de la ville de Marseille" ("on the subject of the contagious disease in the city of Marseille") that suspended all commerce between Marseille and the rest of Provence, under pain of death, until January 1723. This greatly vexed local officials, although the suspension was eased before January. It expanded on an earlier, initial blockade of Marseille issued on 31 July 1720 by the *parlement* of Aix, which itself soon dissolved temporarily in the face of the spreading infection. Through various *arrêts* issued in August and September, the movement of people out of Provence beyond the natural boundaries of the rivers Rhône, Verdon, and Durance was severely constrained through the use of strict quarantines and *certificats de santé* (health certificates) and enforced through the use of military cordons or barriers (National Archives of the UK, hereafter TNA, SP 78/166).

This military *cordon sanitaire* involved not only city bourgeois militias and provincial levies but also one-quarter of the regular army. Ordinances issued by the royal government in September laid out the manner in which troops guarding the lines should behave; they emphasized that no persons whatsoever were "to stir out of the said places under pain of death" and that these sanitary lines and regulations were to be strictly enforced (TNA SP 78/170). One contemporary source, Claude Isnard, hebdomadary of Saint Agricol and prior of Roquemartine, reported in his diary years later that whatever the "great ravages" caused by the epidemic, things would have been much worse had the royal government not put all precautions in place, "[For] the King even sent troops to surround each location that was infected and prevent any communications" (Archives départementales des Bouches-du-Rhône, Marseille, 24 E 11, 35–6).[9] In fact, about half the total correspondence between 1720 and 1723 of Claude Le Blanc, the *Secrétaire d'État de la Guerre* (minister of war) during much of the Regency, concerned this plague barrier (Brockliss and Jones 1997, 352; Panzac 1986, 61; Takeda 2011, 214). Notably, the military cordon eventually resulted in the building of a *mur de la peste*, or plague wall, that one can still see in parts of Provence today.

On 5 September 1720, the Crown appointed Charles Claude Andrault de Langeron, *Chef d'escadre des galères et maréchal des camps et armées du Roy* (marshal in the king's army), as *commandant en chef* (Commander in Chief) of the city of Marseille and its territory (Biraben 1975, 238). Along with the local *échevins* (municipal magistrates) of Marseille, he was responsible for overseeing the massive endeavour of municipal plague management on behalf of the king. Although Langeron faced opposition from local magistrates who resented what they perceived to be an overreach of the centralized government in violation of Marseille's local liberties (Ermus 2021, 780–1; Takeda 2011, 153–7), the *commandant* saw to it that food and relief were distributed, that dogs and cats were slaughtered (thus, unbeknownst to him, eliminating the rat vector's most prominent predators), that cannons were fired often (to dispel miasmas)[10] (*Daily Courant*, 2 Nov. 1720), and that merchandise and other properties suspected of infection were burned. Streets, homes, and merchandise likewise underwent ritual disinfection and perfuming with vinegar or herbs including rosemary and lavender.[11]

With local authorities, Langeron designated prayer days and organized religious processions while cancelling social events of all kinds and closing or regulating markets, taverns, inns, and houses of ill repute in infected areas. The Regent in Paris even sent orders, as English member of Parliament Daniel Pulteney wrote to the English Secretary of State James Craggs on 3 September, to "banish out of that city forever such of the orders of monks there who decline to attend the people on this occasion" (TNA,

SP 78/166) – including tending to the sick and offering them the last rites. Apparently, the Capucins, Jesuits, and Recolets had not failed in their duties and were allowed to stay. Essentially, Langeron was charged with executing martial law and held absolute power in matters pertaining to the policing and administration of the city (Takeda 2011, 132, 140). In his "Paris Circular" of September 1720, Sir Robert Sutton noted that "They write from Marseilles that Monsieur de Langeron, commandant of that place, continues to take all possible precautions to prevent the spreading of the plague, as well by causing the dead bodys [sic] to be burned [and] by daily watering the streets which is found to be of great service" (TNA, SP 78/166).

Crown control was further expressed through the creation of new *bureaux* of health in Provence and, most notably in the spring of 1721, a new *Conseil de Santé* (Health Council) in Paris that was to "meet twice a week at the Louvre," and that consisted "of the Princes of the Blood, the Chancellour [sic], the Marshal de Villeroy, the Comptroller General, the Secretaries of the State, and the King's First Physician, before whom all the Letters relating to the infected or suspected places are to be laid, [so] they [could] give the necessary Directions upon them" (*London Gazette*, 20–23 May 1721). Both the new and previously established health bureaus in Provence were now to operate under the *Conseil* that was located almost 800 km away in the capital. This council was tasked with keeping careful record of, and control over, all aspects of crisis management in southern France during the plague outbreak; it directed, for example, the distribution of food and aid from the royal treasury, the quarantining of infected towns, and other measures taken in cities suspected of being plagued. In La Canourgue, for example, it shut two of the city's four gates in 1721 to more easily control traffic.

Together, Langeron and the *Conseil* served as integral links in a tight network that connected southeastern France with the capital and allowed for centralized management and supervision. Moreover, the absence of the *parlement* at Aix and the temporary closure of institutions such as the Chamber of Commerce in Marseille served only to further augment the central government's administrative powers (Takeda 2011, 143). The circulation of information was brought under increased royal regulation during the outbreak, and all individual *bureaux de la santé* in Provence were ordered to submit monthly registers to Paris. These consisted of information on a variety of health-related points and included such details as the number of staff employed at hospitals to dispose of bodies, updated mortality rates and number of patients, and the number and quality of beds, sheets, drugs, aromatics, provisions, and personnel – both religious and secular – available at each hospital (Takeda 2011, 127).

The Regent's handling of the crisis in Provence seemed to be an effort to gain the support of the people – the very people who had greeted him in throngs in 1715 when he moved the royal court and seat of administration from Versailles to the Palais-Royal in Paris (until 1722). Daniel Pulteney, who resided in Paris throughout the epidemic, reported in his letter of 18

November 1720 to Secretary of State Craggs that "Paris itself is not thought out of danger. [But] the Regent said on this occasion that he would [nevertheless] remain here, as the Emperour [sic] did at Vienna when the plague was there [in 1679]" (TNA, SP 78/166). Moreover, since the "freethinking duke" (Israel 2001, 103) had eased censorship upon assuming the Regency, letters from Provence relating the horrifying news during the height of the outbreak were being published in Paris (TNA, SP 78/166). Already aware of public sentiment, the Regent wished to appear as though he was doing all he could both to contain the epidemic in Provence and to protect and inform all the people of France. Indeed, in April 1721, English newspapers reported from Paris, "The Duke Regent ha[d] given orders to Messieurs Paris [the famous Pâris brothers, financiers] to send two Millions of Livres in Specie into Provence, for the Relief of such places as are yet infected with the Plague; and Directions are likewise given to the Intendents [sic] of the neighbouring Provinces, to furnish them with all sorts of Provisions" (*London Gazette*, 4–8 April 1721).[12] By June, the Pâris brothers along with Samuel Bernard, who according to the duc de Saint-Simon was the richest and most famous financier in Europe, had, indeed, advanced 2 million livres "towards the Relief of the miserable Provençals (which Sum is to be repaid them in two year's time)" (*Daily Courant*, 1 June 1721).

Many of the actions that Langeron and the others took would have been familiar to those who had faced plague in the past. Much like previous outbreaks, the epidemic of 1720 saw the issuing of strict quarantines, the use of sanitary cordons to restrict travel, and traditional methods of disinfection, including the use of vinegar, smoke, and loud sounds. Officials regulated the movement of people, issued curfews, and required certificates of health for mobility. Smuggling practices also came under tighter scrutiny and control. The difference, however, was that these standard practices, which previously had rested in the hands of municipal officials, were now decided, controlled, and overseen by the central government and its newly established *Conseil de la Santé* in Paris. The royal government placed its men on the ground in Provence, issued all necessary *arrêts*, and demanded to be kept aware of any and all developments throughout plague years. The Crown was more heavily involved in the management of this crisis than ever before, signifying an increasing concentration of state oversight that continued through the eighteenth century and survived the French Revolution.

Such responses to the threat of infection took place not only in France but across Europe and the colonies, as neighbouring states also issued restrictions to prevent the spread of plague into their own territories. Even before it was confirmed as plague, news of the outbreak quickly spread across Europe to cities such as London, Genoa, Venice, Cádiz, Barcelona, Lisbon, and from there to colonial towns overseas. All of these port cities and many more across the globe were instructed to mobilize against the threat of plague from France. For European and colonial cities alike, this meant quarantines, controversial vessel searches, the use of health certificates, and the prohibition of any French ships into port, in many cases even if they had not stopped in Provence. But in some cities, most notably in Spain and parts of Italy, protection against infection in 1720 also meant curfews, restricted movement (through the use of quarantine lines and certificates of health), mandatory participation in religious processions, the suspension of festivals or other celebrations, the closure of brothels, and so on – all of this despite the fact that the outbreak never spread beyond France (Ermus 2016, 167–93). And these new policies were mostly enforced under pain of death, incarceration, and/or the confiscation of goods. In the end, this style of comprehensive, centralized plague governance, supervision, and control during the 1720 outbreak served as a model for the prevention and management of epidemics in many parts of the world for decades, as Europe and its colonies battled outbreaks of yellow fever and other diseases into the nineteenth century.

Like other environmental disasters, infectious disease outbreaks can be as revealing as they are destructive, "laying bare underlying power structures; the strengths or vulnerabilities of existing resources and infrastructures; and the values, prejudices, and belief systems of an affected population" (Ermus 2021, 778). The epidemic of 1720–22 symbolized a break from the past, marked, in part, by a more involved central government and augmented communication between the Crown and city officials that represents an early example of the more modern, state-centralized response system to disasters that we see all over the globe today. It also inspired new inquiries and debates about the nature of contagion and its relationship to the environment. Taking place not only in France but also across the English Channel and beyond, these debates remind us that, as I have emphasized elsewhere, infectious disease outbreaks are fundamentally environmental from their origins to their transport to their transmission and have been understood as such for centuries (Ermus 2021, 778). Ultimately, the Plague of Provence very much represented both the last chapter in the book of medieval plagues and the first chapter in the book of environmental management of modern disease outbreaks and disasters.

Shifting Understandings of Disease and Contagion

Perhaps the most fundamental medical doctrine in Western medicine prior to the twentieth century was the theory of humourism (or humoural theory), based on the ideas of Greek and Roman physicians such as Hippocrates (c. 460–370 B.C.E.) and Galen (129 C.E.–c. 216), and then expanded upon by the Islamicate physician Avicenna (Ibn Sīnā, c. 980–1037) (Hammond 2020, 29, 64).[13] In this context, the words "humoural" or "humour" mean "moisture" or "fluid." According to the theory as it developed over many centuries, the human body contains four bodily humours that determine all aspects of a person's health and personality. Each of the humours corresponds with one of the four elements and is characterized by its own sensations or qualities: blood (air; hot and moist); black bile, also known as melancholy (earth; cold and dry); yellow bile, also known as choler (fire; hot and dry); and phlegm (water; cold and moist) (Hammond 2020, 63). Diseases, ailments, and disabilities of all kinds reflected an imbalance in an individual's unique humoural makeup. An overabundance or deficiency of any of the four humours was known as *dyscrasia*, while the balance of the humours – associated with good health – was known as *eukrasia*.

In humoural theory, then, the cause of disease was not understood as external to the body, like a virus or a bacterium, but rather as a state of humoural imbalance. *Dyscrasia* could result from a number of different causes or disturbances, either internal (tied, for example, to menstruation or the onset of puberty) or external. Exposure to cold air, for instance, could cause an overabundance of black bile or phlegm, which could lead to respiratory illness (Brunton 2014, 105). Perhaps most notably, disease could result from the inhalation or absorption of miasmas through the pores.[14] These were disease-causing foul odours or noxious vapours in the air that could be released from a variety of sources, including corpses, stagnant water or swamps, astrological events like the position of the stars or the arrival of a comet, or even God's desire to punish a human population for its sins.[15] Because people believed that many illnesses resulted from exposure to miasmas, treatments or regimens often emphasized the elimination of these corrupt vapours and the rebalancing of humours through practices such as bloodletting, purging via emesis (vomiting) or with laxatives or enemas, as well as the practice of prayer and/or the use of stones, talismans, minerals, and brews or concoctions. Such understandings and practices persisted in Europe, largely unchanged, for centuries.

Beginning in the sixteenth century and especially in the seventeenth and early eighteenth centuries, however, questions and ideas about the nature of disease and contagion saw important shifts, and the Plague of Provence of 1720 marks a significant moment in this process. The outbreak of plague in Marseille appeared at a time when understandings of disaster and contagion, and ideas about how to best manage them, were very much in flux. The so-called Scientific Revolution and subsequent Enlightenment Era ushered in new empirical and mechanistic ways of understanding disease and the environment. These new ideas arose against traditional humoural theories and offered in their place chemical, mechanical, and corpuscular explanations of the human body and of the environment, slowly diminishing the sway of earlier religious or astrological explanations.

These epistemological developments laid the groundwork for an outpouring of writing and debate in 1720, inspired by the epidemic in France, that sought to explain contagion and its place in the environment in new, more rational ways. The ideas that characterized these debates were not new, however. Discussions about the nature of disease and contagion had existed in one form or another for centuries. Yet in 1720, the number of publications on such questions surged in direct response to the Plague of Provence. Plague tracts (or treatises), plague sermons, and other epidemic-inspired writings were published across Europe and in some overseas colonies as intellectuals, physicians, clerics, and others sought to understand the public health disaster and/or to cope with the threat it posed. In France, the epidemic inspired new experiments and numerous texts by scholars and physicians such as Anton Deidier, Jean-Baptiste Goiffon, and Jean Astruc who supported the view that plague was, in fact, contagious (transmissible from person to person) rather than resulting from corrupted air (miasmas) (DeLacy 2016, 147–170).[16] The city of Marseille, in particular, "was a site of intensive reflection on the causes of the plague and on the relationship of epidemic disease to commercialization" (Gordon 1999, 5).

However, the largest number of such writings came out of London. It is here that debates between contagionists and anti-contagionists about the efficacy of quarantining and the nature of contagion re-emerged with particular force. The debate centred on very different conceptions of how diseases were transmitted or acquired, and therefore which preventative and therapeutic measures were best (DeLacy 2016; Mullet 1936; 1956; Santer 2015; Slack 1985; Zuckerman 2004). In a word, anti-contagionists were miasmists (or miasmatists), meaning that they accepted the traditional, Galenic understandings of miasma theory. Basing their opinions on the idea that poisonous vapours in the air cause illnesses, they challenged the utility of practices like quarantines and trade embargoes that served only to interrupt commerce and cause economic ruin.

Contagionists, by contrast, held that the practice of quarantine was integral for preventing the arrival of diseases like plague. Although such ideas were longstanding (albeit marginalized in the historiography), a belief that there exists some type of infectious material gained traction by the late seventeenth to early eighteenth century. Some writers thought it could be a sort of chemical; others speculated that it could be a living entity, what the Dutch researcher Antoni van Leeuwenhoek had called an "animalcule" (from the Latin "animalculum" or "small animal") in 1676.[17] This "microscopic animal," they postulated, would be transmitted in some manner – perhaps person to person or through the pores; perhaps by contact with a sick person or with objects that had been in contact with a sick person. For at least some contagionists, then, one major cause of disease outbreaks was commerce and the interchange of peoples and commodities that accompanied it. Measures such as trade embargoes, sanitary lines, and quarantines were, thus, integral for the preservation of public health.

Among the more notable of the eighteenth-century English contagionists were the physician Richard Mead (1673–1754) and the botanist Richard Bradley (c. 1688–1732). Both had written previously about the question of contagion, but each was inspired by the Plague of Provence to take up the issue anew. Despite their shared view that certain diseases are spread by *something* in the air, each had unique ideas about what that something was (Santer 2015, 142). For some like Goiffon in France or Bradley in England, it was a living agent, while for others like Mead, an inanimate agent was at work (Santer 2009, 567).

In *A Short Discourse Concerning Pestilential Contagion and the Methods to be Used to Prevent it*, published in 1720, Mead proposed that the corrupted air could not spread or cause disease by itself; if it could, the disease would have spread much farther and faster beyond the confines of Marseille. Instead, he argued, the illness was spread through "contagious particles" inhaled and spread throughout the body via the saliva and the blood:

> It is evident, that Infection is not received from the Air itself, however predisposed, without the Concurrence of something emitted from *Infected* Persons ... Of this we have had a fresh Proof in the present unhappy *Plague* in *France*, which, by keeping careful Guard, was confined for a considerable Time within the Walls of Marseilles; so that none of the adjacent Villages suffered any thing by it; till at length some Persons finding Means to escape carried the Infection along with them ... The Way, by which a sound Person receives the Injury [is infected], I suppose most commonly to be this. These *Contagious* Particles being drawn in with the Air we breath [sic], they taint in their Passage the *Salival* Juices, which being swallowed down into the Stomach presently fix their Malignity there; as appears from the *Nausea* and *Vomiting*, with which the Distemper often begins its first Attacks. Though I make no Question but the *Blood* is also more immediately affected by hurtful Particles being mixed through Inspiration with it in the Lungs.
>
> (Mead 1720, 15–16).

Over the decades that followed, Mead revisited and expanded his argument. In 1744, for example, he cited the experiments undertaken by Dr. Anton Deidier in the wake of the Plague of Provence to revise his theory:

> Now it appears by the Experiments [of Deidier] mentioned in the *Preface*, of giving the *Plague* to *Dogs* by putting the *Bile*, *Blood* or *Urine* from infected Persons, into their Veins, that the whole mass of the animal Fluids in this Disease is highly corrupted and putrefied. It is therefore easy to conceive how the *Effluvia* or Fumes from Liquors so affected may taint the ambient Air ... From these [secretions of "active particles"] therefore the Air will be impregnated with *pestiferous Atoms*: which being taken into the Body of a sound Person will, in the Nature of a *Ferment*, put the Fluids there into the like Agitation and Disorder. The Body, I suppose, receives them these two ways, by the *Breath*, and by the *Skin*; but chiefly by the former.
>
> (Mead 1744, 44–5).

Such ideas had many opponents. Numerous anti-contagionists took to their pens to refute Dr. Mead's findings, including a series of anonymous authors whose titles made clear where they stood on the matter (Anonymous 1722; DeLacy 2016, 159; Pringle 1722). However, Mead's suggestions were broadly representative of the kind of theories put forth by a number of other "contagionists" at the time of the Provençal plague, even if they differed in detail.

In *The Plague of Marseilles Consider'd*, published in 1721, Richard Bradley drew heavily from his observations of plant diseases to determine that illnesses affecting animals and humans were caused by what he called "poisonous insects" (Bradley 1721, 20; DeLacy 2016, 160). Once these insects invaded a body, the infected person or animal then communicated the disease to others by spreading the eggs of these insects in the air while breathing:

> [S]o in Animals it may be … that their very Breath may entice those poisonous Insects to follow their way, 'till they can lodge themselves in the Stomach of the Animal, and thereby occasion Death. We may likewise suppose that [these insects] will certainly lay their Eggs there, which the Breath of the diseased Person will *fling* out in Parcels, as he has occasion to Respire; so that the Infection may be communication to a stander by, or else, through their extraordinary smallness, may be convey'd by the Air to some Distance.
>
> (Bradley 1721, 20–1).

Such ideas reflect what we today refer to as airborne transmission. Given the authority and influence of traditional, Galenic understandings of disease in the eighteenth century, these theories did not revolutionize medical thinking overnight, yet they were nevertheless remarkable. In the following century, the contagionist argument that diseases are caused by organisms that existed in the environment – some living, like bacteria, and some non-living infectious agents, like viruses – and that these can be transmitted from person to person, was proven correct with one of the biggest breakthroughs in the history of science and medicine: the development of the germ theory of disease that most famously took form with the work of Louis Pasteur in the 1850s and Robert Koch in the 1880s.[18]

Conclusion

The Plague of Provence has often been seen as the closing of a chapter in Europe, one of the last of a long series of medieval outbreaks of plague. Yet it signified a beginning in many ways. It marked a major shift in Europe from local or municipal-level disaster management, towards more centralized methods for handling crises – developments that would have lasting global ramifications. It also inspired new inquiries into the nature of contagion. Plague tracts at this time were published not only in France and Britain but across the Atlantic world, including the Holy Roman Empire, Italy, Spain, and the North American British colonies. Plague prevention methods during the 1720 epidemic – based, in part, upon these new ideas of how disease erupted and spread in the environment – were considered such a success that they continued to be referenced in disease- and commerce-related manuals on both sides of the Atlantic well into the nineteenth century. In 1793, for example, as a yellow fever outbreak raged in Philadelphia, responses to plague in Provence were still being referenced and studied (Assalini and Pinckard 1806, 85; Carey 1794; College of Physicians of Philadelphia 1798). In these ways and more, the early eighteenth century was a transformative time both for the management and for our understandings, of disaster, disease, and the environment.

Notes

1 I would like to thank Junko Thérèse Takeda for reading an earlier draft of this article and for her invaluable suggestions.
2 In 1756, the *philosophe* Voltaire famously wrote his "Poème sur le désastre de Lisbonne" (Poem on the Disaster in Lisbon) in which he began to lay out his arguments against Leibnizian optimism (as delineated by Gottfried Wilhelm Leibniz in his *Essais de Théodicée sur la bonté de Dieu, la liberté de l'homme et l'origine du mal*, or *Essays of Theodicy on the goodness of God, the freedom of man, and the origin of evil*, published in 1710), which is to say, the tenet that "All is best in the best of all possible worlds," or that everything that unfolds in the world is for the best, since it was by God's design. In doing so, Voltaire attacked the age-old conviction that catastrophes are fundamentally caused by God's vengeful wrath. He later expanded upon his criticism of Leibnizian optimism in his satirical novel *Candide, or Optimism*, published in 1759. It is worth noting that Leibnizian optimism never really goes away, neither in the eighteenth century nor today. Then as now, there are those who argue that even the worst disaster can only lead to renewal. Catastrophe, for the opportunist, is a gift.
3 For our purposes, "disaster" may be broadly defined as "a serious disruption of the functioning of a community or a society involving widespread human, material, economic, or environmental losses and impacts, which exceeds the ability of the affected community or society to cope using its own resources" (United Nations Office for Disaster Risk Reduction). Such disruptions can result from natural hazards such as earthquakes, floods, large storms, pathogens, and others, or from more directly human-made causes (for example, war related violence or nuclear accidents).
4 By referring to an "extreme event" or a "natural hazard" rather than a "natural disaster," I mean to highlight the fact that natural occurrences with the potential to harm are not, in and of themselves, disasters. Naturally occurring phenomena, such as hurricanes or volcanic eruptions, only *become* disasters when they adversely affect a human population, and the extent to which this happens is largely determined *not* by nature, but by human decisions (for example, building along vulnerable coasts; weak infrastructure; government negligence). For this reason, a general understanding among many in disaster studies is that there is no such thing as a *natural* disaster; disasters are human made.
5 The outbreak began in the port city of Marseille and quickly spread throughout the French region of Provence and neighboring areas, including Aix, Toulon, Avignon, Arles, and many other towns. For this reason, I find it more appropriate to refer to the epidemic as the Plague of Provence.
6 Archival documents across the Atlantic world pertaining to the epidemic's origins agree that plague was transported into France on the doomed vessel.

More recent genetic studies, by contrast, have proposed that the 1720 outbreak had its origins not on the *Grand Saint-Antoine*, but in possible plague foci, or reservoirs, in or near Europe itself. Although none have yet been conclusive, these studies have raised important questions about the influence of modern science and technology on the practice of history and vice versa. Examples of recent genetic studies include Bramanti et al. (2021); Guellil et al. (2020); Spyrou et al. (2019); Namouchi et al. (2018); and Bos et al. (2016). For historians' perspectives, see Varlık (2020) and Carmichael (2014). For a discussion of the recent research, see Slack (2021) and chapter one of Ermus (2023).

7 For reference, the population of Provence in 1700 was roughly 658,000 (Bourde 1987, 316).

8 Jean-Baptiste Estelle, Marseille's *premier échevin* (chief municipal magistrate), had used his influence to arrange for the premature unloading of his cargo of infected silks and bales of cotton into the city's warehouses.

9 "Il y avoient meme des troupes que le Roy envoya pour investir tous les endroits qui étoient infectes, et empêchés toute communications[;] chaque ville et villages prenvient des tres grandes precautions pour ne pas s'infectes."

10 For more on miasmas, see the later section on "Shifting Understandings of Disease and Contagion."

11 "Paris, 1 October: Directions for the Precautions to be observ'd in the Provinces where there are Places infected with the Plague, and in the neighbouring Provinces, have been printed here by Royal Authority, the Substance of which is as follows." (*Evening Post*, 25-28 Sep. 1721)

12 The Pâris brothers were Antoine Pâris, sometimes known as Grand Pâris (b. 1668), Claude Pâris known as Pâris *La Montagne* (b. 1670), Joseph Pâris known as Pâris-Duverney (b. 1684), and Jean Pâris known as Pâris-Montmartel (b. 1690).

13 The development of humoural theory is largely associated with the ancient Greek physician Hippocrates. Known as the "Father of Medicine," Hippocrates based his findings primarily on empirical observation rather than on religion, superstition, or magic. Roughly sixty medical treatises make up what is known as the *Hippocratic Corpus* (while based on his teachings, the texts' actual authorship remain unknown). Six centuries later, the Roman physician Galen of Pergamon adapted and built upon the work of Hippocrates. Then, in the early eleventh century, Avicenna synthesized the medical work of Galen and the philosophical work of Aristotle in his *Canon on Medicine*.

14 "Miasma" comes to us from the Greek word μίασμα, meaning contagion or contamination.

15 These understandings are epitomized, as noted above, in the religio-astrological origins of the word "disaster," from the Greek and Latin terms for "bad omen" (literally, "bad star"). From ancient times through very recent history, there was a fine line between the astrological and the divine.

16 Whereas the pneumonic form of plague can be transmitted from person to person, the notorious bubonic form is communicated from rodents to humans through the bites of infected fleas. That said, contemporary evidence suggests that pneumonic plague was widespread during the Plague of Provence.

17 Along with the English polymath Robert Hooke (1635–1703), and Jesuit scholar Athanasius Kircher (1602–1680) before him, Antoni Philips van Leeuwenhoek (1632–1723), at times called the "Father of Microbiology," was among the first to observe microorganisms (specifically, bacteria, which he called "animalcules") under a microscope.

18 Important predecessors include, among others, Girolamo Fracastoro (ca. 1478–1553) and Marcus von Plenciz (1705–86).

References

Archival Sources

Archives départementales des Bouches-du-Rhône, 24 E 11
National Archives of the UK, SP 78/166
National Archives of the UK, SP 78/170

Newspapers

Daily Courant (London), 1 June 1721; Issue 6119.
Daily Courant (London), 2 Nov. 1720; Issue 5939.
Evening Post (London), 25–28 Sep. 1721; Issue 1898.
London Gazette, 4–8 April 1721; Issue 5944.
London Gazette, 20–23 May 1721; Issue 5957.

Printed Sources

Anonymous. 1722. *Doctor Mead's Short Discourse Explain'd. Or, His Account of Pestilential Contagion, and Preventing, Exploded.* London: J. Peele.
Assalini, Paolo and George Pinckard. 1806. *Observations on the Disease called the Plague, on the Dysentery, the Ophthalmy of Egypt, and on the Means of Prevention; with Some Remarks on the Yellow Fever of Cadiz, and the Description and Plan of an Hospital for the Reception of Patients Affected with Epidemic and Contagious Diseases,* translated by Adam Neale. New York: Printed and sold by T. & J. Swords.
Biraben, Jean-Noël. 1975. *Les hommes et la peste en France et dans les pays européens et méditerranéens, tome 1.* Paris: Mouton & Co.
Bos, Kirsten I., Alexander Herbig, Jason Sahl, Nicholas Waglechner, Mathieu Fourment, Stephen A. Forrest, Jennifer Klunk, Verena J. Schuenemann, Debi Poinar, Melanie Kuch, G. Brian Golding, Olivier Dutour, Paul Keim, David M. Wagner, Edward C. Holmes, Johannes Krause, and Hendrik N. Poinar. 2016. "Eighteenth-Century *Yersinia pestis* Genomes Reveal the Long-Term Persistence of an Historical Plague Focus." *eLife* 5: e12994. https://doi.org/10.7554/eLife.12994.
Bourde, André. 1987. "La Provence au grand siècle." In *Histoire de la Provence,* edited by Édouard Baratier, 305–41. Paris: Privat.
Bradley, Richard. 1721. *The Plague of Marseilles Consider'd: With Remarks upon the Plague in General, shewing its Cause and Nature of Infection, with necessary Precautions to prevent the spreading of that Direful Distemper...* London: W. Mears.
Bramanti, Barbara, Yarong Wu, Ruifu Yang, Yujun Cui, and Nils Chr. Stenseth. 2021. "Assessing the Origins of the European Plagues Following the Black Death: A Synthesis of Genomic, Historical, and Ecological Information." *PNAS* 118, no. 36: 1–6.
Brockliss, Laurence and Colin Jones. 1997. *The Medical World of Early Modern France.* Oxford: Clarendon Press.
Brunton, Deborah. 2014. *Health and Wellness in the 19th Century.* Santa Barbara, CA: ABC-CLIO.
Carey, Mathew. 1794. *A Short Account of the Malignant Fever, Lately Prevalent in Philadelphia: With a Statement of the Proceedings That Took Place on the Subject, in Different*

Parts of the United States, To which are added Accounts of the Plague in London and Marseilles... Philadelphia, PA: Printed by the Author.

Carmichael, Ann G. 2014. "Plague Persistence in Western Europe: A Hypothesis." *The Medieval Globe* 1: 157–91.

College of Physicians of Philadelphia. 1798. *Facts and Observations Relative to the Nature and Origin of the Pestilential Fever, which Prevailed in this City in 1793, 1797, and 1798.* Philadelphia, PA: Printed for Thomas Dobson.

DeLacy, Margaret. 2016. *The Germ of an Idea: Contagionism, Religion, and Society in Britain, 1660–1730.* London: Palgrave.

Ermus, Cindy. 2016. "The Spanish Plague That Never Was: Crisis and Exploitation in Cádiz During the *Peste* of Provence." Special issue on Humans and the Environment in the Long Eighteenth Century. *Eighteenth-Century Studies* 49, no. 2: 167–93.

Ermus, Cindy. 2021. "Memory and the Representation of Public Health Crises: Remembering the Plague of Provence in the Tricentennial." *Environmental History* 26, no. 4: 776–88.

Ermus, Cindy. 2023. *The Great Plague Scare of 1720: Disaster and Society in the Eighteenth-Century Atlantic World.* Cambridge: Cambridge University Press.

Gordon, Daniel. 1999. "Confrontations with the Plague in Eighteenth-Century France." In *Dreadful Visitations: Confronting Natural Catastrophe in the Age of Enlightenment,* edited by Alessa Johns, 3–30. New York: Routledge.

Guellil, Meriam, Oliver Kersten, Amine Namouchi, Stefania Luciani, Isolina Marota, Caroline A. Arcini, Elisabeth Iregren, Robert A. Lindemann, Gunnar Warfvinge, Lela Bakanidze, Lia Bitadze, Mauro Rubini, Paola Zaio, Monica Zaio, Damiano Neri, N. C. Stenseth, and Barbara Bramanti. 2020. "A Genomic and Historical Synthesis of Plague in 18th Century Eurasia." *PNAS* 117, no. 45: 28328–35.

Hammond, Mitchell L. 2020. *Epidemics and the Modern World.* Toronto: University of Toronto Press.

Israel, Jonathan I. 2001. *Radical Enlightenment: Philosophy and the Making of Modernity 1650–1750.* Oxford: Oxford University Press.

Mead, Richard. 1720. *A Short Discourse Concerning Pestilential Contagion and the Methods to be Used to Prevent it.* London: Sam. Buckley and Ralph Smith.

Mead, Richard. 1744. *A Discourse on the Plague.* London: A. Millar and J. Brindley.

Molesky, Mark. 2015. *This Gulf of Fire: The Great Lisbon Earthquake, or Apocalypse in the Age of Science and Reason.* New York: Vintage.

Mullett, Charles. 1936. "The English Plague Scare of 1720–23." *Osiris* 2: 484–516.

Mullett, Charles. 1956. *The Bubonic Plague and England: An Essay in the History of Preventive Medicine.* Lexington: University of Kentucky Press.

Namouchi, Amine, Meriam Guellil, Oliver Kersten, Stephanie Hänsch, Claudio Ottoni, Boris V. Schmid, Elsa Pacciani, Luisa Quaglia, Marco Vermunt, Egil L. Bauer, Michael Derrick, Anne Ø. Jensen, Sacha Kacki, Samuel K. Cohn Jr., Nils C. Stenseth, and Barbara Bramanti. 2018. "Integrative Approach Using *Yersinia pestis* Genomes to Revisit the Historical Landscape of Plague during the Medieval Period." *PNAS* 115, no. 50: E11790–E11797.

Panzac, Daniel. 1986. *Quarantaines et lazarets: l'Europe et la peste d'Orient, XVIIe-XXe siècles.* Aix-en-Provence: Édisud.

Pringle, Dr. John. 1722. *A Rational Inquiry into the Nature of the Plague. Shewing That as the Air Only is Capable of Producing, or Communicating It; the Method of Prevention Now*

Practis'd in France, Is Not Only Inhumane, but Useless, and Even Pernicious. London: J. Peele.

Rousseau, Jean-Jacques. 1967. "Lettre à Voltaire, 18 August 1756." In *Correspondance complète de Jean-Jacques Rousseau, Tome IV,* edited by R.A. Leigh, translated by R. Spang, 37–50. Geneva: Institut et musée Voltaire.

Santer, Melvin. 2009. "Richard Bradley: A Unified, Living Agent Theory of the Cause of Infectious Diseases of Plants, Animals, and Humans in the First Decades of the 18th Century." *Perspectives in Biology and Medicine* 52, No. 4: 566–78.

Santer, Melvin. 2015. *Confronting Contagion: Our Evolving Understanding of Disease.* Oxford: Oxford University Press.

Shakespeare, William. 1992. *The Tragedy of Julius Caesar,* edited by Barbara A. Mowat and Paul Werstine. New York: Folger Shakespeare Library.

Slack, Paul. 1985. *The Impact of Plague in Tudor and Stuart England.* London: Routledge & Kegan Paul.

Slack, Paul. 2021. "Perceptions of Plague in Eighteenth-Century Europe." *Economic History Review.* https://doi.org/10.1111/ehr.13080

Spyrou, Maria A., Marcel Keller, Rezeda I. Tukhbatova, Christiana L. Scheib, Elizabeth A. Nelson, Aida Andrades Valtueña, Gunnar U. Neumann, Don Walker, Amelie Alterauge, Niamh Carty, Craig Cessford, Hermann Fetz, Michaël Gourvennec, Robert Hartle, Michael Henderson, Kristin von Heyking, Sarah A. Inskip, Sacha Kacki, Felix M. Key, Elizabeth L. Knox, Christian Later, Prishita Maheshwari-Aplin, Joris Peters, John E. Robb, Jürgen Schreiber, Toomas Kivisild, Dominique Castex, Sandra Lösch, Michaela Harbeck, Alexander Herbig, Kirsten I. Bos, and Johannes Krause. 2019. "A Phylogeography of the Second Plague Pandemic Revealed Through the Analysis of Historical *Y. pestis* Genomes." *Nature Communications* 10, no. 4470: doi: 10.1038/s41467-019-12154-0.

Takeda, Junko. 2011. *Between Crown and Commerce: Marseille and the Early Modern Mediterranean.* Baltimore, MD: Johns Hopkins University Press.

United Nations International Strategy for Disaster Reduction. https://www.undrr.org/terminology.

Varlık, Nükhet. 2020. "Rethinking the History of Plague in the Time of COVID-19." *Centaurus* 62, no. 2: 285–93.

Voltaire. 1756. "Poème sur le désastre de Lisbonne." *Gallica. https://gallica.bnf.fr/essentiels/anthologie/poeme-desastre-lisbonne.*

Voltaire. 1991. *Candide, ou l'Optimisme.* Paris: Larousse.

Zuckerman, Arnold. 2004. "Plague and Contagionism in Eighteenth-Century England: The Role of Richard Mead." *Bulletin of the History of Medicine* 78, no. 2: 273–308.

6 "Hot Climates" and Disease

Early Modern European Views of Tropical Environments

Guillaume Linte

Introduction

In the fifteenth century, Europeans' geographical horizons began to broaden considerably.[1] In the wake of the first Portuguese explorations along the coasts of West Africa, which ultimately led to the opening of a maritime route to the Indian Ocean, and of the discovery of a New World across the Atlantic, representations of the inhabited terrestrial space took on unprecedented dimensions. The most important point was the new opening to the largest part of the world, widely ignored until then: the region located south of the Tropic of Cancer, which generally marked, more or less, the southern limit reached by European sailors in the Middle Ages. Cape Bojador, located on the north-western coast of Africa (directly below the Canary Islands), had posed a barrier, more symbolic than physical, that fell definitively only in 1434 when the Portuguese navigator Gil Eanes passed by it.[2] From the fifteenth century onwards, overseas voyages to the south and east required travelling through a particular geographical space that represented a significant climatic alterity for Europeans: the part of the world located between the Tropic of Cancer and the Tropic of Capricorn.[3] Not only did explorers pass through the region, but colonies and trading posts, meant for the spice and slave trades, were also established within it. A variety of geographies – the West African coasts, the Caribbean islands, the Indian peninsula – then witnessed a growing European presence during the early modern period.

In sixteenth-, seventeenth-, and eighteenth-century geographical thought, this space between the tropics, which since Ancient times had been called the Torrid Zone, acquired a distinctive meaning. By the end of the Middle Ages, the world was perceived through two, sometimes contradictory, systems that divided the globe into zones and climates, respectively (Gautier Dalché 2017). The zone system, formulated by Aristotle in *Meteorology*, traced a series of symmetrical parallel bands that accorded with celestial circles (Cosgrove 2005). It divided the Earth into five latitudinal strips, each represented by its own climate conditions: two polar zones at the antipodes, a torrid zone between the two tropics, and two temperate zones, located north and south of the torrid zone. The climate system, by contrast, limited itself to defining

DOI: 10.4324/9780429055478-9

the climates of the oecumene, meaning the known, inhabited part of the northern hemisphere: Europe, Africa, and Asia.[4]

The oecumene was traditionally divided into seven horizontal parallel strips that did not extend directly from the Equator to the Arctic, but rather from the borders of the inhabitable world. They represented the seven *climata* in which humans lived, each distinguished by its specific climate conditions and different lengths of the summer solstice day (Gautier Dalché 2017). In this system, the beginning of the inhabitable area was located further south than it was in the zone system. The first climate in the south, acting as a reference point, centred on the city of Meroe (Sudan), located at 16°55′ north; the second was Syrene, in Egypt, located just below the Tropic of Cancer. The images in Figure 6.1 appeared in the *Cosmography* of Peter Apian, first printed in Paris in 1524. They represent the system of zones (left) and the system of climates (right), at this point adapted to the entire globe by assuming symmetry between the northern and southern hemispheres. In his version of the climate system, Apian distinguished not seven, but nine parallel stripes above and below the equator, demonstrating that even the conception of climate zones had not been perfectly fixed since antiquity (Besse 2003).

The complexity of this system prevented a consensus from emerging with regards to the habitability of the torrid zone. Since the thirteenth century, academics had discussed the subject extensively: Johannes de Sacrobosco's *De Sphaera Mundi*, written in the early thirteenth century, posited that the torrid zone was uninhabitable, but others disputed his assumption. These contrary scholars included Albertus Magnus, who, shortly after Sacrobosco, defended the existence of a burning hot region where life was difficult and unpleasant (*indelectabilis*) but not impossible (Gautier Dalché 2017). In the early modern period, oceanic expansion led by the Portuguese and the wider European colonial experience definitively disproved the contention that the region was either burning hot or uninhabitable (Besse 2003). Still, as the image of an *indelectabilis* space located between the tropics lingered, so too did the question

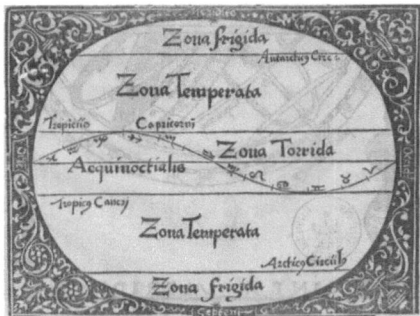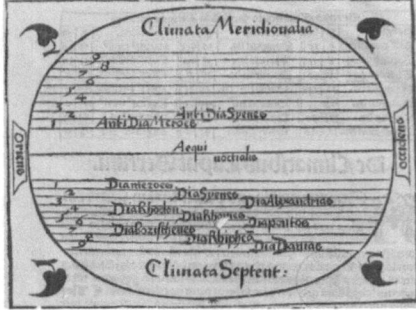

Figure 6.1 Peter Apian. 1524. *Cosmographicus liber Petri Apiani Mathematici studiose collectus* (Landshut) 10, 14. Bibliothèque nationale de France, département Cartes et plans, GE FF-9356 (RES), Public Domain.

of its inhabitability for Europeans used to living in a temperate climate. This same question was subsequently – and naturally – appropriated by medicine and medical writers as the region began to pose a real health concern for Europeans.

Building a Representation of the Tropics in Early Modern Medicine

Between the fifteenth and seventeenth centuries, descriptions of the regions of the world located between the tropics came mostly from travellers and naturalists. In the aftermath of the first voyages to Africa and the Indies, Europeans became increasingly infatuated with exploring botany and publishing their knowledge about nature. The Portuguese physician Garcia de Orta, for instance, published his famous *Colóquios dos simples e drogas da India* (Colloquies on the Simples and Drugs of India) in 1563, nearly 30 years after moving to Goa. The book, which provided an ordered introduction to the botanical knowledge of his day, was quickly and extensively circulated in Europe. Gardens were deeply reshaped by the introduction of exotic plants from all over the world. The first university botany chairs emerged, while lavishly illustrated books presented the fauna and the flora of the West and beyond (Egmond 2010). The observation and study of nature elicited a surge of interest among sixteenth-century European elites, arousing the curiosity of scholars and the appetite of collectors of curiosities. In addition to becoming respectable pursuits, botany and the cultivation of exotic plants came to serve as tools for social representation and prestige. As Brian W. Ogilvie (2006) has shown, by the eighteenth century, natural history was a collective undertaking, nourished by intense exchanges of knowledge and practices within and among the community of naturalists. In that context, knowledge about the plants and spices found in the Eastern and Western Indies contributed to the construction of a representation of their natural living environments.

From the mid-seventeenth century onwards, and to a greater extent in the eighteenth century, a specialized body of medical literature on exotic diseases also developed. A key concern pertained to the health of European populations living in hot countries or climates. The torrid zone created difficult living conditions, and it logically ensued that the health of those who travelled or settled there would be affected. As the first European colonial empires were being built, questions about the torrid zone's habitability assumed even greater prominence. At the crossroads of medicine and geography, this literature on exotic diseases – produced primarily by physicians and surgeons who served aboard ships or in the colonies – provided key inputs for contemporary understanding of the intertropical environments. Books on the sicknesses encountered in overseas places where Europeans lived, mainly in the West Indies, were published with increasing frequency during the last century of the early modern period. For example, Portuguese physicians who had experience in the colonies, especially Brazil, wrote treatises on their health conditions and diseases. In 1694, João Ferreira da Rosa published a treatise on "the pestilential constitution of Pernambuco," while in 1707, Miguel Dias Pimenta, a doctor at the University of Coimbra, presented a book on "*bicho*," a common disease in both Brazil and Angola.

At the same time that it was establishing itself as the greatest European maritime power, Great Britain quickly became the leading source of scholarship on health in the tropics. Richard Towne, a physician who had practised medicine on the island of Barbados, prepared a *Treatise of the Diseases Most Frequent in the West-Indies, and Herein More Particularly of those which Occur in Barbadoes* in the 1720s. Four decades later, the famous Scottish doctor James Lind offered his seminal *Essay on Diseases Incidental to Europeans in Hot Climates*. In the late eighteenth century, another flurry of books on this new area of research appeared in Great Britain. In 1773, John Clark released *Observations on the Diseases in Long Voyages to Hot Countries*, while Benjamin Moseley, a member of London's Royal College of Physicians, penned a *Treatise on Tropical Diseases; And on the Climate of the West-Indies*. The 1787 book marked a shift in the terminology used for this subject: Moseley abandoned the idea of diseases from hot countries or hot climates, referring instead to "tropical diseases," which thereby implied the diseases found between the tropics. French physicians also wrote many medical texts based on their Caribbean experience. The colonial population's health in Saint-Domingue was their primary concern (Lafosse 1787; Poissonnier-Desperrières 1763), but other contributions involved less significant possessions, such as Guiana (Bajon 1777).

For each colonial physician, the first task at hand was to become familiar with the nature of the climate in his place of practice. Following the Hippocratic tenet, the latter's influence was considered key to understanding the men and women who lived there and to adopting relevant therapeutic strategies. Clinical experience was obviously required, but so too was knowledge of the natural resources in the new environment. The two weighty volumes of Bertrand Bajon's *Mémoires pour servir à l'histoire de Cayenne et de la Guiane Françoise* (Memoirs to Serve the History of Cayenne and French Guiana) (1777) drew on his 12-year experience as surgeon in the colonial city of Cayenne, in French Guiana. The book comprised twenty-eight essays, only half of which pertained to medicine. The remaining fourteen touched on the natural history of French Guiana – birds, in particular, were the subject of five essays, but quadrupeds, fish, and fruit trees were also addressed – and on land cultivation. The relative lack of organization and hierarchization of information in the book reflected the fact that medicine in the colonies was not fully emancipated from natural history. Still, there is a palpable sense that the author believed he was helping to bring about the emergence of a new field. His medical writing was, in his view, his main contribution to knowledge about the country:

> The history of diseases will probably be the most comprehensive, as they have been the main subject of my occupations. I did the utmost to

provide an exact History of diseases in these parts, especially as to date no one has appeared to have properly fulfilled this task; and as the temperature of this climate and the diseases prevailing there appeared to a great many people to be the main obstacles to the growth of this Colony.

(Bajon 1777, vol. 1, II)[5]

Bajon's work not only offered improved knowledge about Guiana's diseases but also gave insights into the diseases of hot countries in general, meaning those located in the torrid zone. The climate, meaning its nature or temperature, became the main concern of this burgeoning field of the medicine of hot countries – or hot climates. In France, a body of literature emerged that followed the blueprint of James Lind's *Essay on Diseases Incidental to Europeans in Hot Climates*. Like Bertrand Bajon's work, the French literature presented itself generally as colonial medicine, often limiting its scope to a given geographical area (Saint-Domingue, the French West Indies, French Guiana, etc.). Nonetheless, it partook in a broader reflection on tropical regions. Jean-Barthélemy Dazille's 1785 *Observations générales sur les maladies des climats chauds* (General Observations on Diseases in Hot Climates) drew essentially on his time as a royal physician in Saint-Domingue. His book was intended to "instruct Physicians who plan to travel to the Colonies," and his remarks were meant to apply to all climates similar to the one he described, regardless of where in the world they were located (Dazille 1785).

Hot, Wet, and Unhealthy: Defining the "Torrid Zone"

During the Portuguese explorations of the fifteenth century, the West African coast south of the Sahara initially appeared healthy due to its lush nature. Travellers soon realized, however, that anyone visiting this region was plagued by endemic fevers.[6] At the beginning of the following century, the unhealthy nature of the region was widely acknowledged by Portuguese authors (Cagle 2015). Hugh Cagle considers that the chronicler João de Barros "articulated a definitive rejection of the Edenic vision" of the West African regions, referring to the words of the Lusitanian in his *Décadas da Ásia* (1552): "God [...] has placed [here] a striking angel with a flaming sword of deadly fevers, who prevents us from penetrating into the interior [and on] to the springs of this garden" (Cagle 2015, 202). From the first half of the early modern period, in particular during the sixteenth and seventeenth centuries, travel literature also contributed to the dissemination of knowledge about diseases contracted in hot climates. The spaces between the tropics were usually considered to be detrimental to human health because, it was believed, their hot and wet nature induced putrefaction of all sorts. However, the burning heat of the torrid zone did not singlehandedly define the living conditions of all the regions that it encompassed since there were environmental variations.

One particular region came to embody the apex of the putridity and morbidity associated with the torrid zone: the African coast of Guinea. In the sixteenth and seventeenth centuries, Guinea was far from being a well-defined territory or population. The term referred to a vast area with flexible borders, extending roughly from Senegal to the south of the Gulf of Guinea. Europeans were more afraid of that area than any other place in the world. A 1558 book written by French cosmographer André Thevet claimed that Europeans visiting Guinea could not stay long; otherwise, they would contract a serious disease (Thevet 1558, 32). As a rule, "Guinea" was presented as being utterly detrimental to the health of Europeans in the sixteenth and seventeenth centuries. The image of this region in travel literature was not only that of a place where life was unpleasant, since the very health of Europeans travelling on the West African coast seemed to be tenuous.

In medical thought, the conditions imposed by the climate and the specificities of the seasons were disease-inducing. The deadly character conferred on the Guinean coast took on a particular face: that of rot. In contemporary medical thought, many diseases were explained by the "corruption of humours." Following a medical tradition that dated back to the fifth century BCE, the prevailing conception of the body was based on humourism. This theory held that four fluids coexisted within each individual: blood, yellow bile, black bile, and phlegm (or pituitary secretion). The balance and quality of these fluids in a person's body determined his or her health and temperament, with one or more humours prevailing over others. The mix was not equivalent in all individuals; instead, each individual had their own humoural balance – their complexion – and temperament.[7] Living in a place where environmental conditions appeared to be conducive to putrefaction and rot meant that it was inevitable that one's humours would become corrupted. Illness would follow. The onset of diseases in individuals living under those conditions was, thus, a logical development for a physician in the early modern period, and they regularly reported witnessing and treating – if not personally experiencing – fevers of all kinds (Cagle 2018).

The pathological character of the West African coastal regions was also explained by precepts drawn from a foundational text of Western medicine: the treatise *On Airs, Waters, and Places* from the Hippocratic corpus.[8] This work counted winds and waters among the most important parameters for ascertaining the health risk a place posed to its inhabitants. Its author(s) wrote that one should "consider, with respect to the seasons of the year, the effects that each is capable of producing," "then, warm or cold winds," and "additionally, consider the properties of waters." The treatise also called on readers to consider the nature of soils, as well as the inhabitants' lifestyles. According to that reasoning, this information would determine the health conditions of a place. Applied to the context of European oceanic expansion in the early modern period, these recommendations provided a structured intellectual framework for interpreting the features of new environments.

These recommendations did not, of course, apply only to West Africa. The most frequented and colonized places, such as the East Indies (i.e., South and Southeast Asia), were also the subject of growing interest by the seventeenth century. A medical treatise on health in these regions, entitled *De medicina Indorum*, was published in Leiden in 1642. Its author, the Dutch physician Jakob de Bondt, offered through it a commentary on Garçia de Orta's *Colóquios dos Simples* and an inventory of the diseases encountered in East Indies. Using a dialogue with a fictional physician at the hospital in Batavia,[9] a man named Andreas Duræus, de Bondt describes the climate on the island of Java, where he had practised medicine for several years before his death in 1631. As a fictional character, Duræus represented a European who assumed that tropical regions were particularly dry as a result of their overwhelming heat. His staged naivety reflects an awareness of the limitations inherent in representations of the world based on climate zones:

DURÆUS.

Very well: but as the heat of the air in this country is extremely great all the year over, I should imagine that this climate was very dry.

BONTIUS.

Not at all. Nay the air here, as well as in the adjacent islands and continent, is exceeding moist. Many arguments might be adduced to confirm this fact, but I shall mention only one; which is, that even in the driest season of the year in these places, iron, steel, brass, and silver, contract rust, and verdegris much sooner here, than in Europe in the most rainy autumns.

DURÆUS.

You say very right: and we know likewise, that if cloaths are laid up in chests here they soon contract mouldiness, and, if not sometimes exposed to the sun and winds, easily become rotten. (Bondt 1769, 109).

In this excerpt from the dialogue between Andreas Duræus and Jakob de Bondt, the author emphasizes the great humidity of the region in which he practises medicine. He cites as evidence physical phenomena such as year-long fast corrosion. The ideas of rot and decay are central in the representation of the environment with which humans must contend in Java.

In early modern medicine, the air was considered to be one of the main carriers of disease. The healthiness of a place depended on its qualities, and these could be influenced by climate or environmental factors. In his treatise, de Bondt painted a particularly pessimistic picture of Java. In addition to the excessive heat and humidity, considered to be "the efficient causes of putrefaction," Batavia was surrounded by stagnant waters and swamplands (Bondt 1769). This type of landscape, in European medical conceptions, was also identified as particularly conducive to the development of the worst diseases, such as plague (Jones 2016). The wetlands emitted "fetid" vapours, which would poison the air when carried by winds towards inhabited areas. According to de Bondt, this infection of the air was accompanied by insect infestations. Not only was breathing the air detrimental to health, according to seventeenth-century medicine, but living in such a pestilential atmosphere made things even worse. At the time, indeed, the skin was perceived as a porous envelope that could be harmed by penetration from air whose qualities were adverse to good health. As heat was believed to open and loosen skin pores, the risks appeared greater in hot climates. Still, de Bondt noted that Batavia's atmosphere was not always this dangerous: when winds brought ventilation from the sea, they chased away the noxious vapours and purified the air, making it healthy once again.

Unlike in Western Europe, where the year was divided into four seasons characterized by temperature changes, seasons in the torrid zone were defined by the intensity of rainfall – or rather the variation in rainfall. Europeans living there quickly internalized this seasonality, and it is this point that is essential for understanding how early modern writers conceived the relationship between hot climates, environment, and disease. Guinea's and Java's climates were characterized by alternating dry and wet seasons. During the dialogue that runs through part of *De medicina Indorum*, Andres Duræus asks de Bondt: "At what time then do you reckon the summer here to commence?" The latter answers without hesitation: "When continual rains begin to fall" (Bondt 1769, 113). The Dutch physician considered this rainy season, from November to May, to be the disease season. By contrast, the dry season (from May to October), he believed to be perfectly healthy, as long as cool winds blew: "in the dry season, and during a clear state of the air, the people here are healthy. For then, too, the winds blowing with greater coolness, ventilate and purify the atmosphere still more" (Bondt 1769, 114).

This concept of wetness was an important component of the representation of hot climates and the health of the populations living in them. During the early modern era, tropical regions were represented in more complex ways than they had been in the Middle Ages when they were essentially perceived as being burned by the effect of a blazing sun. The understanding of the climate phenomena that characterized such places – the alternating dry and wet seasons – suggested that these environments *were* healthy, but only for part of the year. The representation of an *indelectabilis* torrid zone, where life was difficult, thus endured but was crystallized within this new model. The periods when hot and putrid rains came pouring down made these regions particularly unhealthy since hot wetness meant that these places were conducive to the corruption of humours and the generation of disease and death.

The "Deadly" Rain of the Tropics: West Africa and Its Coasts

Alternating rainy and dry seasons, which characterized many regions located in the torrid zone, those with monsoon or tropical climates, were a new phenomenon for Europeans. Together with intense heat, these conditions were perceived as conducive to swift and inevitable rot. In his account of his journey to Senegal, printed in 1643, the French traveller Claude Jannequin wrote of a "deadly" season that spanned the months of August to November.

During that period, rain fell continually, and a particularly oppressive, stifling heat prevailed, to the extent that "one finds it quite difficult to breathe." These meteorological conditions were believed to be directly responsible for health hazards:

> The rains are so dangerous, that if someone is wet while wearing clothes, and does not change fully before the heat has them dry on his skin, he sees himself reduced to falling to pieces, to bits, by the worms that appear between leather and skin and cause an entire corruption through all parts of the body, to a few animals and to man alike.
>
> (Jannequin 1643, 182–3).

Jannequin's description exemplifies the extent to which rain – or at least tropical rain – was perceived to be dangerous. To Europeans, the seasons during which large amounts of rain fell daily were manifestations of the intemperance that marked the climate of regions located in the torrid zone. To the seventeenth-century traveller, water only had to come into contact with an individual's skin to make him rot away. This conception is perfectly consistent with the Hippocratic tradition, on which early modern medicine drew, since it too considered rainwater to be the most susceptible to corruption. The author(s) of *On Airs, Waters, and Places* claimed that "of all waters, the quickest to putrefy and smell bad is rainwater, because it is formed by a convergence and blend of very many waters, meaning that it putrefies very quickly" (Jouanna and Magdelaine 1999, 115–16). Therefore, rainwater was not only a climatic phenomenon that contributed to the humidity of the tropics, but was itself directly involved in producing the pathogenic properties of intertropical environments.

Even if they were only passed by, the coasts of West Africa remained particularly hostile to life in European minds, especially because of the rains that fell at sea. In his travel account, *Some Yeares Travels into Divers parts of Asia and Afrique* (1638), the English traveller Thomas Herbert described an entry into the torrid zone, experienced when he was sailing towards the East Indies in 1626:

> In changing so many parallels, the weather increast from warme to raging hot, the Sunne flaming all day, insomuch that *Calentures* begun to vexe us. [...] The infectious raines most damnifying the poore saylers, who must be upon the decks to hand in their sailes, abiding the brunt, and (which is worse) commonly get forthwith into their beds (hamackoes) resting their tyred bodies in wet nasty clothes, thereby breeding many furious and mortall diseases, as burning Feavers, Calentures, Fluxes, Aches, Scurvy, and the like (Herbert 1638, 7).

More than the sun, the rain appeared to be the greatest health hazard for European travellers in Thomas Herbert's account. This is an important point to understand how the representation of tropical environments was reshaped as unhealthy. Even if it contributed to the global humidity of such places, rain constituted a specific parameter that significantly affected the health of human beings during at least part of the year. On 20 November 1556, three ships left Honfleur, in France, to establish a colony in Brazil. A member of the expedition named Jean de Léry published an account of his years of adventure following his return to Europe and the failure of the French attempt to settle in Brazil. In his *Histoire d'un voyage fait en la terre de Brésil* (History of a Travel Made in the Land of Brazil), printed in 1578, de Léry devoted an entire chapter to the hardships suffered by the crew as the ships crossed the equator. He described a rain that "not only stinks and smells quite foul, but is also so contagious that if it falls on the flesh, pustules and large bladders will rise; and it even stains and spoils clothes" (Léry 1994, 138). Food supplies and freshwater were affected just like men. De Léry deplored that biscuits, which were the sailors' daily nourishment, were "spoiled and mouldy" due to rainwater seeping into the ship's hold. The damage was evidenced by the presence of worms in the food. Even freshwater was so smelly that "when you drank it, you had to hold the cup with one hand, and hold your nose with the other" (Léry 1994, 139). Although it did not come from a doctor's observation, this description is very representative of sixteenth-century accounts of tropical journeys. *Corruption* and *rot* were the notions primarily used to represent and make sense of this experience in the early modern period. Under the action of a "burning" sun and putrid rains, everything spoiled and putrefied. In Jean de Léry's writing, this was materialized in rotten food, the ubiquity of worms, and especially nauseating smells. The stench was the most glaring sign of rot, for biscuits and men alike. The morbidity of the situation soon appeared obvious to all sixteenth- and seventeenth-century Europeans.

A few years later, another French traveller, Jean Mocquet, published an account of his journey on a Portuguese ship of the *Carreira da Índia* – an annual maritime expedition between Lisbon and the East Indies. In the spring of 1608, this apothecary, who contributed to the King of France's cabinet of curiosities, arrived in Lisbon to satisfy his yearning to travel to the East Indies. Having submitted his plans to the *Casa da Índia*, the institution in charge of Indian trade, he was given the authorization to embark on a Portuguese ship. In his account of crossing the Indian Ocean, the most interesting passage is undoubtedly the one in which he describes the state of travellers as they crossed the intertropical space. In addition to the "excessive heat," Mocquet described the "hot rains of the coast of Guinea" as being so putrid that worms would appear on everything that did not dry quickly. "These rains," the Frenchman wrote, "emit such a stench that they rot and spoil not only the body, but also clothes, chests, utensils and other things." Without a single dry item of clothing left, the traveller had to sleep covered in wet clothes on a worm-infested mattress. According to Mocquet, these conditions had dire consequences for his health, as he experienced fever and kidney pains that ceased only shortly before he arrived at his destination. He established a direct connection between the climatic conditions of the coast of Guinea and the onset of disease – "fever."

In the sixteenth and seventeenth centuries, the intertropical zone was characterized by excessive heat and humidity. Yet, some regions of the world were considered even more unhealthy, such as West Africa, where heavy "stinky" rains fell for several months during the year. This was an important insight concerning European expansion history. While West Africa was popular with Europeans for the slave trade, many other travellers and seamen crossing the Atlantic first passed close by the continent. Ships on their way to the Indian Ocean sailed along the coast for some time and then moved away, thanks to the favourable *Volta* winds. These travellers' accounts exude a sense of dankness. The tropical journey plunged all those who ventured into a state of deliquescence that applied not only to humans but also to most of the constituent elements of their environment.

The Medical Exploration of "Hot Climates" in the Eighteenth Century

From the last decades of the seventeenth century, climate and environment held central roles in the theory and practice of medicine in various colonized areas (Barrett 2000; Harrison 2010). With an ever-growing contingent of physicians and surgeons moving to and living in the Americas (including its islands), the East Indies, and the African trading posts, descriptions of these potentially diseased places abounded. Representations of them became more refined, as did meteorological observations. The latter sometimes came with regular records of temperature and atmospheric pressure. Some authors made observations of the medical constitution of seasons during several consecutive years. The practice consisted of noting which diseases had manifested themselves more often over a given period, as well as the meteorological conditions or significant events recorded during that time.

On 22 October 1732, French physician Jean-Baptiste-René Pouppé-Desportes arrived in Saint-Domingue, where he then settled permanently. He recorded the epidemic constitution of all the seasons for some 15 years. As in West Africa or in Java, life on the island was regulated by the succession of two annual periods: the winter (November–April) was the rainy season, while the summer (April–November) was the dry season. Unsurprisingly, Pouppé-Desportes considered the former to be the least conducive to the health of its inhabitants. He reported on the influence of winds, temperatures, and humidity, the diseases most often observed, and the frequency of their occurrence. He concluded with a few narrative disease stories. In the summer of 1735, for instance, he noted that "the months of March, April and May were neither too dry nor too rainy," a balance that proved "very beneficial to health" (Pouppé-Desportes 1770, 1: 61). Eleven years later, regarding the summer of 1746, Pouppé-Desportes reported "frequent and almost always stormy rains in April and May," during which time "acute diseases struck ship crews in the harbour, especially those of the King's vessels" (Pouppé- Desportes 1770, 1: 158–9). The physician did not just give descriptions but also proposed an analysis based on his study of the constitutions he had observed during the course of his practice. He noted that during the 2 years that followed his arrival, 1732 and 1733, constitutions were largely similar to those of 1745, 1746, and 1747. Based on this conclusion, he began to ponder the possibility of there being a climatic cycle in Saint-Domingue. With this meteorological medicine, Pouppé-Desportes opened perspectives for an unprecedented mastering of the colonial environment, allowing one to plan for the constitution of seasons and to anticipate their risks: "Knowledge of a periodical order in the constitutions would be all the more useful as we would have a sound method for anticipating the good and bad effects resulting from them" (Pouppé-Desportes 1770, 1: 188).

While he did not describe it as such, the approach proposed by Pouppé-Desportes was essentially medical topography, based on the observation of the environment, climate, and landscape in order to identify the origin of diseases. He gave a detailed description of the island of Saint-Domingue, "bisected across its entire length by a mountain range," from which "plenty of rivers or streams descend, which, as rain falls abundantly, form torrents that carry soil and substances of various natures, which they spread over all the *Esteres*" (Pouppé-Desportes 1770, 1: 15–16). These *Esteres*, which in America referred to "coastline areas uncovered during the low tide, and covered by the high tide," were an important part of the author's description.

Spreading over two-thirds of the island, they formed "highly muddy and swampy salt pans." According to the physician, these soils affected the health of populations, purportedly emitting nauseating vapours that corrupted and poisoned the air. Their stagnant waters also caused the proliferation of mosquitoes on the island. These insects, which "only hatch in corrupted waters," were responsible for a "continual inconvenience" due to their "burning sting," which "left considerable burns" (Pouppé-Desportes 1770, 1: 17).

This description is reminiscent of Dutch physician Jakob de Bondt's writings on Batavia and its surroundings, especially as he added that insect proliferation was a nearly universal sign of a putrid air constitution. Already from the seventeenth century, this representation of mosquito-infested environments as a symbol of morbidity was widespread in the discourse concerning the Caribbean world (McNeill 2010), West Africa, and the East Indies. In line with sixteenth- and seventeenth-century representations of the torrid zone, Pouppé-Desportes wrote that the island was characterized by a prevailing sense of putridity, the result of excessive humidity, heat, and foul vapours. He argued that these conditions caused humours to be corrupted in all humans, thus making them prone to disease. In his view, this intuition was confirmed by the fact that corpses rotted more quickly and that meats could not be kept as long as in Europe. He also viewed the great number of insects as evidence that the air was corrupted (Pouppé-Desportes 1770).

During the second half of the century, James Lind tried his hand at synthetizing knowledge on human health in the torrid zone. In *An Essay on Diseases Incidental to Europeans in Hot Climates*, first printed in 1768, the Scottish physician proposed a general characterization of human health in tropical countries depending on the season:

> Most tropical countries have, properly speaking, only two seasons, the wet and the dry; the former being commonly of about four months continuance, and the season of sickness; whereas, for many months in the dry season, most parts of this country are equally healthy and pleasant with any in the world.
>
> (Lind 1777, 46).

Lind argued that outside the rainy season, tropical regions were no less healthy than others. This claim evidently involved a comparison with Europe and its temperate climate. In stating that the "season of sickness" generally lasted only 4 months, he depicted the torrid zone in a less scary light, as a place that posed no risk for most of the year, meaning during the dry season. Still, when the rainy season came, some tropical regions saw Europeans dropping like flies. In Guinea, they were struck with fevers that killed them in a matter of days.

James Lind's ideas were inspired, in part, by the writings of the previous centuries that gave an important role to the rain. Using the example of Senegal, where he claimed that as much precipitation would fall within 4 months as it did in England over 4 years, the physician confirmed the putrid character of the rainwater that fell there. He presented the first rains as the most dangerous: those that fell during the first few days were believed to make leather shoes rot in less than 2 days and to stain clothes. More significantly yet, according to eighteenth-century medical conceptions of putridity, worms would develop with prodigious rapidity:

> At this time skins, part of the traffic at Senegal, quickly generate large worms, and it is remarked that the fowls, which greedily prey on other insects, refuse to feed on these. It has been farther observed, that woollen cloths, wet in those rains, and afterwards hung up to dry in the sun, have sometimes become full of maggots in a few hours.
>
> (Lind 1777, 51).

This idea that the first days of the rainy season were the worst, while concurring with previous representations of the putrid rain that fell on Guinea, paved the way for the development of a new theory. Without denying the rain's corrupted character, Lind believed that the adverse fate that befell the place had its roots in the soil. As it dried up excessively during the arid season, the soil was thought to trap vapours that then became extremely putrid during the course of their long captivity in the ground. When the first rains fell, according to

Lind, they would rise and spread their poison and stench into the atmosphere. While partly exonerating the rain itself, this nevertheless tied in with the belief that the first weeks of the rainy season were the deadliest (Lind 1777).

At the end of the early modern period, representations of tropical environments became even more complex. The atmospheric conditions of places were systematically investigated. More than heat, humidity and rains increasingly appear as the main origin of the torrid zone's pathogenic character. In a manuscript medical treatise written around 1790, another French physician named Du Cassan denounced the inadequacies of the discourse then taking place in Europe concerning the nature of intertropical climates (Du Cassan c. 1790). According to him, the idea that heat was the most influential factor that affected the body was a prejudice. Taking readings with a mercury barometer in St. Lucia, where he lived, the physician noticed only tiny variations in the atmospheric pressure despite greater variations in climate. This "phenomenon" was, in his opinion, proof "that humidity continuously affects organisms." According to Du Cassan, three factors were involved in the formation of such conditions: (1) evaporation from the sea; (2) mountainous relief; and (3) the presence of forests. Du Cassan believed that seawater evaporated every day in large quantities under the action of heat. The atmosphere, in his own words, "must be regarded as constantly soaking and saturating itself with rising vapours." Du Cassan's text provides an example of a sophisticated understanding of an environment located between the tropics. Based on new methods of investigation, medicine greatly contributed to reshaping the image of the torrid zone in the eighteenth century.

Conclusion

During the early modern period, representations of tropical climates in the Western world became more detailed and complex. Their experience of hot climates led Europeans to rethink the inhabitability of these places, focusing on their potential risks for health. In West Africa especially, the supposedly putrid rains that fell on both sea and land explained the coexistence of a lush, green nature and the idea of a region where life was hard and riddled with pathogenic threat. This meant that life in the torrid zone was no longer merely perceived as difficult because of the warm climate but also as harmful due to the influence of a pathogenic environment. The medicine of hot climates developed, mainly in the eighteenth century, as greater attention was paid to tropical environments and their characteristics. As illustrated by the works of Lind, Pouppé-Desportes, or Du Cassan, doctors sought to determine features that were observable across the entire torrid zone but also specific to local environments. In his discussion of Guinea's insalubrity in the early days of the rainy season, which he attributed to vapours trapped in arid soils, Lind opened key prospects for the colonial project, as risks could now be conceivably reduced using land planning and cultivation (Lind 1777). Transforming the environment was not a new idea, as it had existed from the beginning of European oceanic expansion (Fressoz and Locher 2020), but it was now taking on a new significance with the development of medicine of hot climates. Changing colonial environments from unhealthy to healthy was then to become a central issue in the nineteenth and twentieth centuries (Anderson 2003; Carey 2011).

Notes

1 This chapter was translated from French by Jean-Yves Bart, with support from the Maison des Sciences de l'Homme d'Alsace (MISHA) and the Excellence Initiative of the University of Strasbourg. I would like to express my sincere gratitude to the colleagues who have greatly contributed to improve the quality of this paper with their valuable comments and ideas. Special thanks to Hugh Cagle and Paul-Arthur Tortosa for their careful review, and to Lori Jones for her support and advice throughout the writing process.
2 Until that point, European trade with Africa south of the Sahara was conducted through North African and cross-Saharan middlemen. One of the key the motivations of the European sailors was precisely to obtain direct access to African trade goods.
3 The Tropics correspond to 23°27′ North and South latitude circles. Taking their name from the constellations to which they refer, they reflect an idealized cosmographic representation of earth and heaven. As Denis Cosgrove noted, "The originating tropics are celestial rather than terrestrial markers within a geocentric cosmos − in ontological terms, idealist spaces" (Cosgrove 2005, 199).
4 Also inherited from the Greeks, the climate system gained traction in the West only in the tenth century as Arabic cosmographic treatises were translated into Latin (Cattaneo 2009).
5 All translations have been made by Jean-Yves Bart.
6 For a detailed examination of early modern travel writing and its influence on ideas about the unhealthiness of Africa, please see Gérard Chouin's chapter in this volume.
7 The main temperaments were sanguine, choleric, melancholic, and phlegmatic. This is a very rough presentation; although defined by their dominant humour, each individual possessed a unique temperament, determined by an infinity of possible balances.
8 The Hippocratic corpus is a collection of around sixty books from the fifth and fourth centuries BCE. These texts were for a long time wrongly attributed to Hippocrates himself. Twentieth-century philological research showed that the corpus was not the work of one man, but of multiple authors, most of whom have not been identified but are associated with the Hippocratic school of Kos (Jouanna and Magdelaine 1999).
9 Founded in 1619 on Java, Batavia − present-day Jakarta − was the main Dutch settlement in the East Indies in the seventeenth and eighteenth centuries.

References

Anderson, Warwick. 2003. "Environment and Race in the Colonial Tropics". In *Nature in the Global South: Environmental Projects in South and Southeast Asia*, edited by Paul Greenough and Anna Lowenhaupt, 29–46. Durham, NC: Duke University Press.

Arnold, David. 1996. "Introduction: Tropical Medicine before Manson." In *Warm Climates and Western Medicine (1500–1900)*, edited by David Arnold, 1–19. Amsterdam: Editions Rodopi.

Bajon, Bertrand. 1777. *Mémoires pour servir à l'histoire de Cayenne et de la Guiane françoise*. Paris: Grangé.

Barrett, Frank A. 2000. *Disease & Geography. The History of an Idea.* Toronto: Geographical Monographs.

Besse, Jean-Marc. 2003. *Les grandeurs de la Terre. Aspects du savoir géographique à la Renaissance.* Lyon: ENS Éditions.

Bondt, Jakob de. 1642. *De medicina Indorum.* Leiden: Franciscum Hackium.

Bondt, Jakob de. 1769. *An Account of the Diseases, Natural History, and Medicines of the East Indies.* London: T. Noteman.

Cagle, Hugh. 2015. "Beyond the Senegal: Inventing the Tropics in the Late Middle Ages." *Journal of Medieval Iberian Studies* 7, no. 2: 197–217.

Cagle, Hugh. 2018. *Assembling the Tropics. Science and Medicine in Portugal's Empire, 1450–1700.* Cambridge: Cambridge University Press.

Carey, Mark. 2011. "Inventing Caribbean Climates: How Science, Medicine, and Tourism Changed Tropical Weather from Deadly to Healthy." *Osiris*, 26, no. 1: 129–41.

Cattaneo, Angelo. 2009. "Réflexion sur les climats et les zones face à l'expansion des XVᵉ et XVIᵉ siècles." *Le Monde des cartes : revue du Comité français de cartographie*, 199: 7–21.

Chakrabarti, Pratik. 2013. *Medicine and Empire: 1600–1960.* Houndmills: Palgrave Macmillan.

Cosgrove, Denis. 2005. "Tropics and Tropicality." In *Tropical Visions in an Age of Empire*, edited by Felix Driver and Luciana Martins, 196–216. Chicago, IL: University of Chicago Press.

Dazille, Jean-Barthélemy. 1785. *Observations générales sur les maladies des climats chauds, leurs causes, leur traitement, et les moyens de les prévenir.* Paris: Pierre-François Didot le Jeune.

Du Cassan, C. 1790. *Traité de l'influence des climats chauds sur les corps animés. Suivi d'un tableau des maladies particulières à la zone torride.* Archives of the French "Royal Society of Medicine" (Paris), SRM 179, no. 7.

Egmond, Florike. 2010. *World of Carolus Clusius: Natural History in The Making (1550–1610).* London: Pickering & Chatto.

Fressoz, Jean-Baptiste and Fabien Locher. 2020. *Les révoltes du ciel. Une histoire du changement climatique XVᵉ-XXᵉ siècle.* Paris: Editions du Seuil.

Gautier Dalché, Pierre. 2017. "Un débat scientifique au Moyen Âge : l'habitation de la zone torride (jusqu'au XIIIᵉ siècle)." *Topoi Supplément* 15: 145–81.

Herbert, Thomas. 1638. *Some Yeares Travels into Divers parts of Asia and Afrique.* London: J. Blome and R. Bishop.

Harrison, Mark. 2010. *Medicine in an Age of Commerce and Empire: Britain and Its Tropical Colonies, 1660–1830.* Oxford: Oxford University Press.

Jones, Lori. 2016. "The Diseased Landscape: Medieval and Early Modern Plague-Scapes." *Landscapes* 17, no. 2: 108–23.

Jannequin, Claude. 1643. *Voyage de Lybie au royaume de Senegal.* Paris: Charles Roüillard.

Jouanna, Jacques and Caroline Magdelaine. 1999. *Hippocrate. L'Art de la médecine.* Paris: Flammarion.

Lafosse, Jean-François. 1787. *Avis aux habitans des colonies, particulièrement à ceux de l'isle de S. Domingue, sur les principales causes des maladies qu'on y éprouve le plus communément, & sur les moyens de les prévenir.* Paris: Royez.

Léry, Jean de. 1578. *Histoire d'un voyage fait en la terre du Brésil: autrement dite Amérique...*, La Rochelle: Antoine Chuppin.

Léry, Jean de. 1994. *Histoire d'un voyage faict en la terre de Brésil (1578)*, edited by Frank Lestringant. Paris: Classiques Garnier.

Lind, James. 1768. *An Essay on Diseases Incidental to Europeans in Hot Climates.* London: T. Becket and P. A. de Hondt.

Lind, James. 1777. *An Essay on Diseases Incidental to Europeans in Hot Climates.* London: T. Becket.

Merrens, H. Roy. and George D. Terry. 1984. "Dying in Paradise: Malaria, Mortality, and the Perceptual Environment in Colonial South Carolina." *The Journal of Southern History* 50, no. 4: 533–50.

McNeill, John. R. 2010. *Mosquito Empires: Ecology and War in the Greater Caribbean, 1620–1914.* New York: Cambridge University Press.

Mocquet, Jean. 1617. *Voyages en Afrique, Asie, Indes Orientales et Occidentales.* Paris: Jean de Heuqueville.

Ogilvie, Brian W. 2006. *The Science of Describing: Natural History in Renaissance Europe.* Chicago, IL: University of Chicago Press.

Orta, Garçia de. 1563. *Colóquios dos simples.* Goa: Joannes de Endem.

Poissonnier-Desperrières, Antoine. 1763. *Traité des fièvres de l'isle de S. Domingue.* Paris: P. G. Cavelier.

Pouppé-Desportes, Jean-Baptiste-René. 1770. *Histoire des maladies des S. Domingue [Tomes I & II]; Traité ou abrégé des plantes usuelles de S. Domingue [Tome III].* Paris: Lejay.

Thevet, André. 1558. *Les singularitez de la France antarctique.* Paris: héritiers de Maurice de la Porte.

Section III

Science Meets Historical Disease Environments

7 Environments of Health and Disease in Tropical Africa before the Colonial Era

Gérard Chouin

Introduction

Marine engineer Louis Ancelin de Gémozac was a decent artist and an efficient spy.[1] Crisscrossing the Atlantic from West Africa to La Martinique, and then back to the port at Rochefort (in south-western France) aboard the French man-of-war *Le Tourbillon* in early 1671, he spent a great deal of time in his quarters, drawing and writing. A few weeks earlier, he had taken advantage of his visits to the Dutch fortified trade posts on the African Gold Coast to sketch their layouts; he was now putting the finishing touches on an impressive series of confidential plans intended for Jean-Baptiste Colbert, Louis XIV's all-powerful Secretary of State of the Navy.[2] De Gémozac probably kept a private journal of his voyage in which he documented his experiences, and which he later used to produce a short travel account published anonymously in 1674 (Chouin 2011). Like many other early modern European travellers to West Africa, he recorded gruesome details of the health hazards to which sailors were exposed in this part of the world. For instance, he mentioned a mysterious illness that affected some crewmen after the ship had left São Tomé, an island he described as being "the most unhealthy in the world" (Chouin 2011, 142). Some died within three weeks, he wrote, while it took others four months to recover from what he described as extreme fatigue. Because the men affected by this illness also bled profusely from the penis, he blamed the condition on an excessive "dissipation of spirit" that occurred during intercourse with the native island women, whom he considered randy and dangerous.

De Gémozac's report fits into an entrenched western perception of Africa as a diseased continent and Africans as vectors of deadly diseases. In nineteenth- and early-twentieth-century Great Britain, this notion was epitomized by the widespread use of the phrase "the White Man's Grave," an expression made popular by traveller F. Harrison Rankin's 1836 book *The White Man's Grave: A Visit to Sierra Leone, in 1834* (Curtin 1961; 1992; Skotnes-Brown 2019). This metaphor for tropical West Africa, however, contradicted synchronous colonial propaganda that sought to present Africa as a new "White Man's Opportunity." In the twenty-first century, after many decades of advances in tropical western medicine, the old scares have evolved but remain firmly embedded

DOI: 10.4324/9780429055478-11

in global health discourses about Africa. Even though the idea of the "White Man's Grave" has disappeared, Africa remains perceived as a reservoir of global bio-threats to western nations. The HIV/AIDS pandemic and the more recent 2013–16 West African Ebola virus epidemic provide ample evidence that the "backward" and "diseased continent" narrative endures, alongside the stigmatization and structural violence that accompanies it (Joffe 2011, 449–51; Jones 2011; Leach 2010; Wilkinson and Leach 2015). In the same vein, Western media that loudly predicted mayhem in Africa in the wake of the Covid-19 has been much less vocal since the continent eventually proved to be less severely impacted by the virus than many parts of the Western world.

We need to critically examine this long-term narrative about the deadly entwining of Africa and diseased environments. Detailed histories of various diseases and epidemiological patterns have taken into account both environmental and global factors, but most focus on relatively recent case studies (Echenberg 2011; Pépin 2021; Webel 2019). In contrast, there is limited published research on Africa's disease landscapes before the nineteenth century, including those parts of the continent engaged in pre-modern Atlantic trade (Cagle 2018). In the face of a ghostly historiography and scattered sources, the task of writing a chapter on the history of diseased environments in pre-modern Africa is more than a challenge; it is an act of intellectual tightrope walking on a dotted line. I, therefore, address the topic by providing impressionistic, fragmented, and, sometimes, provocative answers to three primary questions.

First, was pre-modern tropical Africa as dangerous a diseased environment as is often suggested in the western scholarly literature? One way to respond to this question is to revisit European travelogues about the early modern Atlantic world. We need to probe them as historical sources and reflect critically on their contribution to the deeply rooted and enduring perception of tropical Africa as a metaphor of the world's darkest unwholesomeness. From this emerges a second question: how did Africans themselves conceptualize their environment and its diseases before the nineteenth century? In other words, is the modern concept of diseased landscape useful in a pre-modern Africa-centred perspective? Finally, how might we historicise the intersections between human activity, diseases, and environments in Africa? To engage with these critical questions, I will investigate how pre-modern connections between the Old and New Worlds contributed both to the emergence of specific African diseased landscapes and their projection beyond the continent's shores.

Sickening Sources? Early Modern European Travelogues and the Construction of Disease in Tropical Africa

Walking a Fine Line: Early Modern European Writings as a Source for the History of Disease in Tropical Africa

Early modern travellers' accounts of their visits to Atlantic Africa are replete with horrendous stories about the deadly or debilitating illnesses that awaited

European crewmen. Authors noted three main origins of such diseases: sexual intercourse with African women, miasmas generated by abundant rains and heat, and freshwater. The latter usually only appeared in connection with the parasitic infection caused by the Guinea worm, from far the most discussed condition.

Like Louis de Gémozac, Johann von Lübelfing and Samuel Brun noted that spending the night with local women in São Tomé and Cape Lopez, respectively, could cost men their lives (Jones 1983, 16,. 72).[3] A barber-surgeon, Brun explained that "the men's sperm or genitals decayed, till blood and finally death itself followed" (Jones 1983, 72). All three men described similar signs leading to death but provided no detailed clinical descriptions and did not attempt to identify a particular disease.[4] Instead, the connections they established between "the Black wenches" and the visible lesions on the men's bodies rested primarily on Christian moral and racial/gendered prejudices, not on what we would call medical evidence today. As such, they foreshadowed eighteenth-century discourses that linked tropical women and venereal diseases (Siena 1998). Of course, the mention of casual intercourse in West African port cities suggests that the men could have already suffered from a range of sexually transmitted conditions and might have contracted new ones. None of these diseases on its own would have offered a short-term death sentence. Reading between the lines of these sources, though, we see that intercourse also meant that the men spent time ashore in local settlements, by day and night, drinking, eating, flirting, bathing, and, as a result, exposing themselves to tropical pathogens and parasites.

Notwithstanding Andrew Cunningham's (2002) now-classic warning against interpreting past diseases in modern terms, we should examine the symptoms reported by the three traveller-writers. De Gémozac's brief description of the men's illness suggests that they suffered from gross haematuria (blood in urine visible to the naked eye). Red-coloured urine and Brun's mention of blood in the men's semen – a condition known as haematospermia – are symptoms consistent with a parasitic, mostly non-lethal infection known in modern medical terms as schistosomiasis, and more specifically its urogenital variant.[5] People become infected with the parasite while bathing, swimming, or wading in waters infested with larvae of trematode worms (*Schistosoma haematobium* or *S. guineensis* in the case of urogenital infection) released by freshwater snails. What we know of its evolutionary history as a human parasite suggests that it was already present in Africa in the premodern period and transmitted to tropical America by the slave trade (Noya et al. 2015; Webster et al. 2006).

Without engaging in further retrospective diagnoses, it is enough to note that a contextual assessment points towards a much more complex picture than that offered by a superficial reading of the socially and culturally constructed seventeenth-century travel narratives. Not only did the illness likely have nothing to do with the sexual behaviour of the victims, but the infection of their urogenital systems – dramatic as it might have looked – would not have caused their deaths.

Most certainly, those men who died after leaving the African shores suffered from several diseases, in the modern sense of this term. The suggestive location of their physical symptoms created a smokescreen behind which less visible life-threatening conditions lurked – malaria, yellow fever, or typhoid (again in modern medical terms) – that were not yet conceptually constructed in the seventeenth century. More than being the result of any single disease, the high mortality rates more likely indicated co-infection by multiple pathogens in short-term travellers who were habituated to radically different epidemiological environments. In the sixteenth and seventeenth centuries, many men serving on the ships that sailed across the southern Atlantic Ocean, or who were posted to fortified European trading posts, suffered from relatively poor health: they were mal- and under-nourished, probably dehydrated, and exposed to numerous wounds and infections (Fury 2012; Watt et al. 1981). In these conditions, it is not all that surprising that their immune systems could not cope when they encountered several new pathogens in unfamiliar tropical environments.

The cases discussed above illustrate the complexity and limitations of using early modern European sources to discuss the pre-modern African epidemiological landscape and to diagnose its diseases. In most cases, the writers of these accounts used concepts they had learned in Europe, not in Africa, and they usually focused on the health of European travellers, not on Africans. Cunningham has already argued that historians should stop trying to make retrospective diagnoses and should focus instead on "how diagnosis happens" (2002, 16). Nevertheless, although our cognitive experiences and interpretations of disease might be radically different from those of past societies, the biological fundamentals that connect us to our environments evolve at a much slower, almost imperceptible pace. For instance, we can justifiably assume that the parasitic blood flukes (flatworms) of *Schistosoma spp.* were present in seventeenth-century western Africa and that the biological processes leading to the infection of human hosts in a variety of freshwater habitats were no different than those of today. From there, we can anticipate that they contributed to the morbidity aboard European ships plying the southern Atlantic. We likewise can expect some signs of their presence in European sources.

Can I know that the men who died on De Gémozac's ship were infected by schistosomiasis? No, I cannot; but I can establish a dialogical relationship between a seventeenth-century written source and a corpus of contemporary medical evidence, which allows me to interpret that source and reconstruct fragments of Africa's past epidemiological state. Despite the inherent risks of over- or misinterpretation, a catalogue of these fragmented pieces of evidence about health conditions mentioned in travel accounts and other written sources about Atlantic Africa before the nineteenth century could help us to map out the myriad ways that illnesses and environments interacted across time and space. This, in turn, might enable us to fully characterize the concept of "diseased landscapes" in pre-modern Africa.

Truth or Hoax: Pre-1800 Tropical West Africa Was a Dangerous Disease Environment

African history books often present the pre-modern continent – and its tropics in particular – as "one of the most dangerous disease environments in the world for human beings to inhabit" (Roberts 2011, 482). They likewise characterize the struggles of Africans as an admirable "defense of civilization against nature" (Iliffe 2017, 1). John Iliffe's *Africans: The History of a Continent* is just one example of an influential textbook in which "abundant insects, and unique prevalence of disease" appear as a particularly heavy and hostile burden on the pre-modern continent and its people (2017, 1).[6] Although the book gives a unique place to diseases as a prime historical factor in the continent's subsequent under-development, many others echo the idea of Africa's long-standing embedded environmental constraints and its unique "disease burden" (Akyeampong 2006, 186–87; Fauvelle 2018, 14; Webb 2006, 37).

Not all scholars agree that Africa's pre-nineteenth-century disease environment "was particularly bad," especially when compared with other parts of the Old World (Thornton 2012, 68; Weil 2014, 98–100). Indeed, many textbooks do not discuss disease at all as a factor in pre-modern African history (Ehret 2016, 2002; Harms 2018; Shillington 2019; Smythe 2015). After all, the fact that European mariners died in tropical Africa had as much to do with their encounters with new pathogens as it did with the generally poor health conditions they had long endured on European soils and ships (Mackenbach 2020, 25–28, 121–216; Steckel 2010, 43; Steckel et al. 2019). Studies on health in pre-industrial Europe show that inhabitants of temperate latitudes, far from enjoying disease-free environments, were constantly battling infections, parasites, oral health issues, nutrition deficiencies, physical stress, and the weather. Diseases such as malaria, sometimes presented as a "fundamental challenge to West African pioneers" (Webb 2006, 37), also infested many parts of contemporary Europe (Boualam et al. 2021; Dobson 1997; Newfield 2017; Packard 2021). In the absence of studies contrasting empirical health data from Europe and Africa over the past 2,000 years, we should not assume that their respective populations were more or less affected by disease.

In this context, we need to go back to the early modern European sources for two main reasons. First, the travellers sometimes provided broad comparative statements that are worth considering. Second, and despite their many limitations and biases, they may encapsulate fragmented, selected, and transformed – yet precious – African voices. European documents about Africa are certainly European in penmanship, language, structure, order, and function, but most are a patchwork of information derived, in part, from African informers. In some circumstances, it is possible to retrieve those voices and look at narrative elements from an African perspective (Chouin 2001).

Pieter de Marees was a trader aboard one of the Dutch vessels that contested the Portuguese monopoly in the Gulf of Guinea in the late sixteenth century. In 1602, he published a *Description and Historical Account of the Gold Kingdom of Guinea* [*Beschrijvinghe ende historische verhael vant gout koninckrijck van Guinea*], which later travel accounts often plagiarized. One short chapter focuses on African attitudes towards rain. The author likely relied on his own observations when noting that the people "fling their arms over their shoulders to shake the rain from them" (De Marees 1987, 115), but there are traces of interactions with anonymous African informants behind his explanation that this gesture was not due to the coolness of the water but rather "because of the unhealthiness of the body they experience from it." De Marees concluded this short chapter by noting that rains in these parts of Africa "may cause great, dangerous diseases." It is quite clear from his tone that both Europeans and Africans acknowledged the morbidity of the rainy season.[7]

Another chapter of the book, entitled "About Their [i.e., Africans'] Injuries and Diseases, and What Remedies They Use," also relied on a blend of the author's direct observations and probably some interaction with a European barber-surgeon on board his ship. Among the six diseases De Marees mentioned, three were explicitly sexually transmitted – poxes ("pocken," i.e., the "Great Pox" or syphilis), chancres ("clapoozen," another reference to syphilis), and gonorrhea ("dzuppaerts") – which may be interpreted as a moral judgement based on his perception of African sexuality (De Marees 1602, 76; 1987, 173).[8] They might also mirror his and other mariners' fear of sexually transmitted diseases. The three other mentioned diseases were headache, worms, and "hot fevers." This chapter is notable in its betrayal of De Marees's limited understanding of medicine and of his bias in favour of European pharmacopeia. Furthermore, his mention of an African remedy against headache – which he describes as "a kind of pap which they make out of leaves and with which they smear the place which hurts them" (De Marees 1987, 173) – is the only possible indication of an African voice. He also mentioned surgical procedures to treat boils and signalled that Africans "do not practice bleeding." But the most interesting practice he mentioned is what we today would call social distancing: healthy people avoided contact with people suffering from "other natural illnesses"[9] and the sick were relocated away from their communities. It is difficult to know what specific knowledge these practices echoed. They might have indicated that his African informants understood a concept of contagion and had developed quarantine-like strategies to limit the propagation of some types of infections.[10] De Marees did not understand the principles guiding this practice, however, and he firmly condemned it on moral grounds:

> When they have some other natural illnesses, they will not help or assist one another; when someone becomes ill or sick, they will avoid him like a Plague and expel the Sick person like a Dog, and they will not aid him with a drop of Oil or water, even if they are able to do something.

Indeed, a Father would let even his own son lie like a Beast and perish of hunger and misery; for they are of such a nature that they do not help sick people.

(De Marees 1987, 173–74).

As a merchant who spent only a few weeks in West Africa, De Marees was not in the ideal position to collect information about African healing practices. However, his narrative, limited as it is, still provides indications that the African society he interacted with did not lack therapeutic resources and conceptual tools against illnesses. Sores, abscesses, and other wounds did not seem to hamper social dynamics, and De Marees praised the physical courage of Africans, who "do not complain much when they have sores and injuries" and "are not squeamish, but quite stout-hearted" (De Marees 1987, 173).

A century after De Marees, Willem Bosman (1705) published his *New and Accurate Description of the Coast of Guinea, divided into the Gold, the Slave, and Ivory Coasts* [*Naawkeurige Beschryving van de Guinese-Goud-Tand-en Slavekust* (1704)].[11] It consisted of 22 letters. Bosman had arrived on the Gold Coast in 1688 as a 16-year-old boy in the employ of the Second Dutch West India Company. By 1698, he had risen to the post of Chief Merchant, the second-highest office in the Gulf of Guinea. In 1702, aged 29, he returned to the Netherlands to retire and successfully face accusations of mishandling the company's affairs. Bosman spent some 13 years in the Gulf of Guinea, holding positions in several Dutch outposts at Axim, Butri, Komenda, and Elmina on the Gold Coast and at Whydah, on the Slave Coast (Delaunay 1994, 97–98, 150–51; Van Dantzig 1975). As a long-term resident in West Africa, Bosman developed a much better understanding of his surroundings than many of the shorter-term travellers, and his writings on disease reflect his empirical knowledge. Letter VIII of the book focused on the "Insalubrity of the Coast," and contains a particular focus on the European experience of disease based on his personal observations. He identified the months between April and September as particularly dangerous – most especially July and August – because of the fog:

A thick, stinking and sulphurous damp or mist riseth, especially near little rivulets or watry-places: which mist so spreads it self, and falls so thick on earth, that it is almost impossible to escape the infection.

(Bosman 1705, 105; Van Dantzig 1976, 108).

One recognizes here the influence of Hippocratic theories of diseased landscapes that were widespread in early modern Europe and North America (Jones 2016; Wear 2008). Bosman, however, was not entirely trapped in the Hippocratic *Airs, Waters, and Places* tradition. He recognized aggravating factors such the absence of "good food," the use of corrupted medicines, the ignorance of barbers, excessive drinking, and unbridled sexuality among the Dutch company's recruits in the Gulf of Guinea (Bosman 1705,

106–107; Van Dantzig 1976, 108). In the same letter, Bosman noted that "how unwholsome soever this Country is we find very few of the Natives afflicted with distempers" because they were born "in the air" and raised "in the stench" (Bosman 1705, 108; Van Dantzig 1976, 109). He did not describe a healthy Eden, far from it. Still, he made it clear that the concept of "unwholesome … country" when applied to the coast of Guinea was a European construct, relevant primarily to the health of Europeans, not the Africans. The only concession to this was his contention that "To two Diseases they [i.e., Africans] are however more subject than the Europeans, which are Small-Pox and [Guinea] Worms" (Bosman 1705, 108; Van Dantzig 1976, 109).[12]

In Letter XIII, Bosman returned to discussing health, this time exclusively of Africans. Here, African voices – although anonymized and reformulated – can be heard. Among them were probably the "Slaves or servants to the Europeans" and the "Mulatto women" whom Europeans often married; Bosman mentions them explicitly in this chapter (1705, 223, 224). The contrast with De Marees's account is striking. Bosman explained that illnesses were taken seriously among Africans and the sick promptly attended to: "they leave no means unessayed which may contribute to the extending of the Thread of Life to as great a length as possible" (Bosman 1705, 221; Van Dantzig 1978, 234). He also noted that Africans looked at illness from a dual therapeutic and spiritual dimension:

> In Sickness (in which they agree with all the rest of the World) they first have recourse to Remedies, although they consider them too impotent to keep their body alive through them alone and to recover their health; therefore, more potent means need to be applied, which they always believe to be the usual exercise of their Idolatry.
> (Bosman 1705, 221; Van Dantzig 1978, 234–35).

We will return below to this fundamental distinction between the European and African pre-modern conceptualization of disease. Despite his disdain for African religions and their practitioners, Bosman did not hide his admiration for African remedies, which he described as including Lime juice, seeds of *Aframomum melegueta*, roots and barks of trees, and "green herbs, of no less than thirty different kinds… and particularly powerful" (Bosman 1705, 224; Van Dantzig 1978, 235). He noted that although the choice and combination of these plants might have seemed unsuitable to the Western eye, they were, in fact, more effective than European remedies:

> I have seen several of our Country Men cured by them, when our own Physicians were at a loss what to do… the strange Efficacy of these Herbs, that I have several times observed the Negroes cure such great and dangerous Wounds with them, that I have stood amazed thereat.
> (Bosman 1705, 225).

De Marees and Bosman are only two of many European travellers who left rich records of their experiences in Guinea. Calling on others would undoubtedly contribute to a more in-depth and thicker understanding of environmental health challenges faced and met by people in tropical West Africa during the early modern era. Already, however, these authors help us dissipate some common misunderstanding on the subject. First, they provide no evidence that the disease environment of pre-modern tropical Africa was any more challenging to its population than was that of Europe or the Americas to their own. The absence of a significant, recurrent threat like plague in the Gulf of Guinea between the fifteenth and nineteenth centuries is one indicator among others that the contrary might have been true. Although malaria is suspected of having been a major burden, its mortality burden fell primarily on "the very young, in whom the society had invested few resources" (Depetris-Chauvin and Weil 2018, 1232), and does not seem to have impaired economic life or population density after the sixteenth century.

Second, these accounts provide no evidence that pre-modern African healthcare systems were any less able to offer appropriate responses to environmental health challenges than their European equivalents. In fact, in some respects, the reliance of African healers on long-standing herbal remedies and spiritual healing might have been more effective than excessive blood-letting or other contemporary European practices.

Thinking about Illness and the Environment in Pre-Modern Africa: Human Ecology Between Pragmatic Knowledge and Spirituality

What Is Health? Conceptualizing Illness and Healing in Pre-Modern Africa

Any attempt to conceptualize, in a few paragraphs, illness and healing in pre-modern Africa is a risky endeavour. The limitations of our sources and issues of conceptual distance mean that every attempt to generalize is suspect. In Africa, as in Europe, the meaning of and practices related to health, medicine, and healing changed through time although these changes are not always well documented and understood. As John Janzen noted in his study of the *Lemba* area of equatorial west-central Africa, "any standardized picture of ... [African] therapeutics is only as good as its depiction of local variance and historical vicissitude" (1982, 15).[13] To cut the proverbial Gordian knot, I will first build on remarks made by European travellers between the sixteenth and eighteenth centuries, alongside other available sources. Then, I will reflect on my own field experience in Ghana with oral traditions and place it in the more general framework provided by discussions of disease in the anthropological and historical literature. Pre-modern Africa, in this case, is limited to the sixteenth to nineteenth centuries although some fundamental ways of looking at the world were no doubt inherited from earlier periods. Archaeology might provide us with sets of evidence for earlier times.

In his description of the coast of Guinea, Willem Bosman made an interesting comment about the knowledge and use of herbs to heal wounds received in warfare:

> The Natives are very much to be pitied, that being shot, cut, or otherwise wounded in their Wars, they neither know nor have any other way of cure than by green Plants, which they boil in water and foment the [wounded] part with them; which proves effectual in some cases, these Vegetables being endowed with a wonderful Sanative Virtue. But others either not knowing the Simples, or being ignorant how to prepare them aright, apply their Fomentations in vain.
>
> (Bosman 1705, 110; Van Dantzig 1976, 110).

In this excerpt, Bosman suggested that knowledge of medicinal plants was not restricted to a few specialists. In his 1714 travelogue account of his visit to Assinie (Ivory Coast), Dominican Father Godefroi Loyer also admired the power of the local herbal medicines used for the treatment of wounds, noting "For the wounds, they press on them the juice and marc of an herb they have, which provides such incredible healing that they do not worry about a wound five fingers deep..." (Loyer 1714 (1935), 209).[14] Although not everyone was equally knowledgeable in recognizing and using them, there was a "shared body of herbal knowledge" that has remained true in Ghanaian rural communities at least until the early twentieth century (Akyeampong 2006, 194). Bosman's comment, however, seems to contradict another observation he made elsewhere, which implied the presence of specialized healers who were also religious actors: "he who here acts the parts of the Doctor, is also a *Feticheer* or Priest" (Bosman 1705, 221–22).

John Janzen (2011, 1982), who worked extensively on pre-modern indigenous health systems in Central Africa and wrote a history of the *Lemba* cult extending from the seventeenth century to the 1930s, suggested dividing "afflictions" into "naturally-caused" and "human-caused"[15] categories (1982, 13). Although this is a view reconstructed by an anthropologist in the second half of the twentieth century in the context of a specific cult, It fits with echoes of the past I recorded in southern Ghana in the 1990s and 2000s, and with other anthropological work across Africa (Chouin 2009).

The first group includes wounds resulting from overt human aggression, guinea worms and other visible parasites such as sand fleas, physical degeneration due to age, and various diseases that were commonly recognized and managed or treated with plants. Although the ill sometimes consulted oracles to verify that the illness indeed belonged to that category, they did not require recourse to a religious specialist (Janzen 1982, 13, 15). Instead, the treatment of "naturally caused" ailments and wounds took place most often within the household, where the most experienced close relatives would have passed knowledge on from one generation to the next.

Doctors, to use Bosman's term, or consecrated healers, were required when attempts to mobilize folk medicinal knowledge failed, suggesting that they intervened in the second group of afflictions, those caused by humans (Janzen 1982, 13). Ludewig Rømer, an employee with the Danish West India and Guinea Company who spent 9 years on the Gold Coast between 1739 and 1749, noted this two-level healing system in Accra:

> When a Black wishes to ask the fetish (oracle) about something ... because his family, a friend, his children, of his wife are ill ... he goes to the fetish maker .... He asks if he may hear the fetish speak .... But the sick person tries first to see if he can be helped with herbs or [other] remedies known to be effective in such an illness.
>
> (Rømer 1760 (2000), 89–90).

The aetiology of "human-caused" afflictions was extensive and included all symptoms that could not be treated by folk remedies, including both ailments that modern medicine would recognize as diseases – such as smallpox[16] – and many others that could be related to witchcraft and violence that took place beyond the physical realm. "Human-related" afflictions thus resulted from humans interacting improperly with each other or with a myriad of powerful entities in the spiritual realm. What they all had in common was that they reflected a disruption of the relationship between humans and their physical, social, and religious environments. The relative polysemy of the words used in many African languages to refer to "human-caused" afflictions and their translation as "disease" or their equivalent in European languages has resulted in much conceptual confusion, stereotyping, and ridicule in past (and recent) perceptions of African health systems and disease environments (see, for instance, Green (1999, 11–20)).

In his 1981 study of *nganga* – healers – in Cameroon, for example, De Rosny spoke of an "annoying and persistent misunderstanding" between his interlocutors and himself about the meaning of the word *diboa* (in the Douala language), translated in French as *maladie* (disease). Bad luck, he noted, was often referred to as a disease, as was measles (De Rosny 1981, 103–105). De Rosny's research in Cameroon led him to interpret the word "disease" – as used in African languages – as encompassing different processes inducing the disruption of harmony and natural order in the interconnected biological, social, and spiritual realms. Disease, therefore, was chaos, and healing a process aimed both at reversing human-driven perversions (as well as their visible somatic or psychological symptoms on patients) and restoring God's "natural" order (De Rosny 1981, 121–22).

However, what our early modern European travellers likely missed was that for the African populations they encountered, healing was not only about applying remedies to eliminate symptoms – as was still common

practice in contemporary Western medicine – but also an attempt to identify the source and nature of the conflicts that threatened to disrupt order.
Ultimately, healing was about the identification, prevention, and containment of conflicts and the restoration of order. Located at the overlap of the
physical, mental, and spiritual realms – including the natural environment
itself – the healing of "human-caused" ailments could only be practised by
individuals who had a strong understanding of the philosophical universe
that gave meaning to these concepts. Only men and women who had received from higher powers the gift of double vision and had fortified themselves spiritually through initiation and ritual enhancement could survive
the dangers of perilous investigations that often led them into unchartered
territories in the invisible realm. The entanglement of medicine and religion comes to create a functional symbiosis, to the point that some scholars
suggest we should look at African religions as inherently therapeutic (De
Rosny 1981, 284–91).

This distinction between "naturally caused" and "human-caused" diseases
is conceptually appropriate to the pre-modern era. It is quite clear, as we read
above in De Marees's travelogue, that Africans had observed the contagious
nature of some diseases and created physical barriers between the sick and the
healthy; as elsewhere in the pre-modern world, however, such beliefs had a
cultural and religious foundation, rather than a scientific one (Ziegler 2016,
102). Furthermore, long before the twentieth century, West African populations also had learned from experience that settling in specific environments
brought excessive deaths; they often responded to such threats through mobility. Yet, these empirical observations were discussed in terms of pollution,
chaos, and spiritual attacks or warnings, not in terms of infection, contagion,
or environmental danger.

The conceptualization of illness translates into specific attitudes towards
space, landscape, and the environment as actors in the dramatic production of
diseases. Lori Jones (Chapter 4 in this volume; 2016) has discussed how ideas
derived from Hippocratic treatises influenced the way medical authorities in
medieval Europe linked pestilence, corrupted air, and unwholesome waters.
The same conceptual corpus informed many of the comments made by early
modern European travellers to tropical Africa. From a Hippocratic perspective, landscapes could be organized from healthy to unhealthy. Much later,
the emergence of germ theory followed by the development of landscape epidemiology also generated their own discourses about landscapes; although on
very different theoretical foundations, landscape epidemiology demonstrated
how diseases and their vectors were integrated into physical and human
landscapes. It was through landscape epidemiology that colonial and post-
colonial authorities throughout Africa shaped their sanitation rhetoric and
other grand schemes to eradicate tropical diseases.[17] The question we ought
to ask at the end of this conceptual exploration of health and healing in pre-
modern Africa is, if and how the "naturally caused" and "human-caused"
categories of diseases integrated the environment (the physical landscape) as

a variable or functional part of the health system as it was perceived from an African standpoint.

Therapeutic Landscapes: Spatial and Environmental Dimensions of Health, Disease, and Healing

Before the late-1800s, Europeans often classified landscapes as healthy or unhealthy according to criteria that echoed miasma theory (Dobson 1997). After 1900, landscapes became even more central as germ theory and "seed and soil" metaphors contextualised diseases in the much broader environment "as a part of the physical, cultural and political landscape" (Ziegler 2016, 100). As an intellectual endeavour, this approach led to remarkable breakthroughs in the development of a holistic understanding of the dynamics of pathogens, their hosts, vectors, and the unfolding of human epidemics/pandemics; it also, however, led to contested practices, especially in the context of colonial and post-colonial health policies in Africa (Mavhunga 2018, 223–88).

This is not the place for a longer discussion of imperial discourses and colonial assumptions about African (lack of) recognition of the concept of diseased landscapes and ways to mitigate them, or of the silent appropriation and integration of local knowledge into colonial medicine (Cooper 2011; Tilley 2011; Wagoner 2003). Yet in the biomedical research archives in colonial Africa lie fragments of a longstanding vernacular science (Tilley 2011, 181, 196) that can help us understand how African societies conceptualized and acted upon diseased landscapes before the 1800s.

The archive of long-standing colonial efforts to control the tsetse fly in Africa is one of the most obvious ones where such fragments of past African systems of knowledge can be located. Tsetse flies are vectors of parasites responsible for trypanosomiasis (also known as sleeping sickness), a deadly disease that affects both humans and cattle. The disease has a long history in Africa, and its complex epidemiological framework and ecological entanglements make it one of the most interesting case studies of diseased landscapes on the continent. Colonial archives provide a clear case of transfers of long-standing indigenous knowledge about the fly and the disease it causes from vernacular science to colonial institutions.

In south-eastern Africa, for instance, people had long recognized the role the fly played in both animal and human trypanosomiasis. They had produced a pragmatic, experimental knowledge of its ecology, and applied this knowledge to define "dirty" – tsetse-fly infested – spaces that should be avoided, and settlement strategies and patterns of mobility to limit exposure (Mavhunga 2018, 4–7, 10–14, 23–37). Sometimes, diseased landscapes became no man's lands, part of defensive strategic efforts to weaken any military incursions by foreigners, such as was used in the Munhumutapa kingdom located between the Zambezi and Limpopo rivers; rulers here "deliberately left an area near the Indian Ocean unsettled because of the presence of *mhesvi* [tsetse fly] and *hutunga* [mosquitoes]" (Mavhunga 2018, 31).[18] The deadly trap is reported to have caused heavy losses of horses and men during a Portuguese incursion in 1569. Similar strategies were employed in the Songhai Empire, in West Africa.

One major difference in the ways pre-modern Africans and Europeans acted on diseased landscapes was that while Europeans preferred to imagine ways to transform and tame the landscapes they perceived as diseased, Africans chose to adapt their own behaviour to minimize exposure to diseases rather than act on the landscape itself. Avoiding riverbanks, building on higher ground, selecting specific moments of the day and night to move across the landscape, taking cattle to riverine grazing pastures only during the dry season – when the tree foliage had dropped and did not offer the fly protection against the sun – were among the many strategies one might call "strategic deployment... the transformation of natural features such as steep mountainsides, swamps, and forests into pest-control infrastructure without even touching them" (Mavhunga 2018, 30). In her exploration of the colonial archive, Tilley (2011) also found material documenting the experience of Charles Swynnerton, a twentieth-century English naturalist interested in indigenous management of tsetse flies in the Mossurize area of western Mozambique. Swynnerton's oral material collected from local communities highlighted long-standing and historical methods implemented to combat the tsetse fly; these included "carefully timed annual grass fires" and the "culling and regulation of game" that served as reservoirs for the parasite (Tilley 2011, 186–88). These well-planned practices enabled the residents to get rid of the fly along with other insect vectors of disease, such as ticks.[19] Later colonial authorities, in contrast, chose to bring the disease under control by eradicating the fly in more drastic and environmentally damaging ways.

Community responses to tsetse fly infestation were not, of course, the same everywhere and throughout history. They ranged from avoidance strategies to the active transformation of diseased landscapes and depended on the nature of the landscape, the level of infestation, the migrations of the fly, the history of the communities in a specific landscape, and a range of other sociopolitical and economic factors. These responses, informed by deep knowledge of the fly's ecology, were pragmatic and aimed at avoiding encounters between humans and insects. They are representative of a dynamic behaviour that shaped anthropic landscapes in pre-modern Africa south of the Sahara in response to therapeutic needs and expectations.

Many other features in the landscape, especially forest islands of various sizes often called "sacred groves," structured what we could call a therapeutic landscape, the conceptual opposite of a diseased landscape. Sacred groves marked either the presence of shrines consecrated to earth spiritual entities that shared the same landscape as people or areas revered because they housed the burial place of ancestors. Together, they formed local and regional networks connected to kin groups and structures of justice and authority. Their primary function, however, was to shield communities from incoming "human-caused" diseases. For that reason, many were strategically located around each settlement, along access routes, or near the gates of fortified towns.

The therapeutic function of sacred groves emerged very strongly in oral historical fieldwork I conducted in Southern Ghana in the mid-to-late 1990s (Chouin 2019). Oral traditions collected in the area refer constantly to the historical threat of disease – especially smallpox and dysentery. In Abrem, a small political unit located in the Komenda–Edina–Eguafo–Abrem district of the Central Region of Ghana, for example, political history is tightly related to smallpox, locally known as *Mpata*. One of Abrem's sacred oaths is *Mpata Ntam* (the smallpox oath), which refers directly to "the visitation in this country of the smallpox epidemic, when the Abirem Oman lost 270 persons" (Central Regional Archives, Cape Coast, ADM 23/1/498, 20).[20] The medicinal therapy they sought is *Tweneboa*, a tree-residing spirit that the founders of the village of Abrem Berase had carried during their migration in the first half of the eighteenth century and installed in a small grove at the centre of the village. The *Tweneboa*, in turn, indicated through an oracle where the local residents could procure anti-smallpox medicine known as *Siw Omanano*. In the early twentieth century, when the village of Abrem Berase was moved less than a kilometre south, *Tweneboa* was moved again and installed in a different sacred grove north of the present settlement, where it still stands.

The story of *Tweneboa* is not all that unique nor is it a solely modern phenomenon. In my survey of about seventy sacred groves, almost all of these shrines were remembered as strategic locations that had prevented diseases and other dangerous forces from reaching local communities. The oral traditions drew on long-standing knowledge and experience going back centuries, and in each case, the epidemic-preventing power attributed to the grove and its resident spirit loomed large. When not used as a shield against diseases, groves could be used as places of quarantine, healing, and burial. I rediscovered one such grove during fieldwork near Eguafo, the ancient capital of a small polity west of Elmina. The place, called Eyipow, is remembered as a burial ground for people who died from smallpox some centuries earlier but also as a place where victims settled temporarily and received a treatment. The presence of bamboo suggests that sheds made of this plant were once built there. I was led to the site in February 2002 by Abusuapanyin Nana Gyefu Mensah, who pointed to the *Kakaedukuva* trees that, he told me, were used to produce medicine (Chouin 2009, 356–57).[21]

Although most of the oral material about diseases I collected during fieldwork probably relate to the nineteenth century, the principle behind these therapeutic landscapes has a very deep history that suggests a sound vernacular knowledge of the relationship between trade routes and the spread of disease. Not only groves but also rock formations and rivers formed a defensive, therapeutic network that translated into the visible landscape both people's anxieties about illness and the epic conflicts taking place in the invisible world between the forces of death and life. It is particularly interesting to note that sacred groves were located along major trade routes that stretched

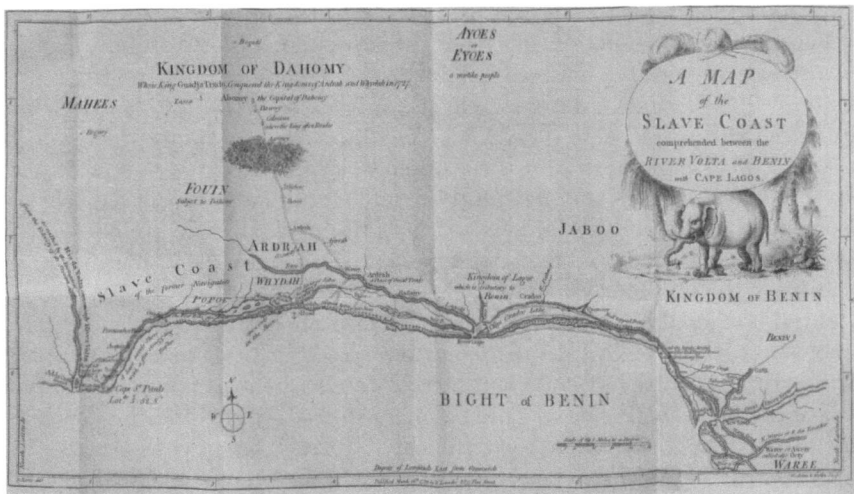

Figure 7.1 Robert Norris. 1789. "A Map of the Slave Coast Comprehended between the River Volta and Benin with Cape Lagos." In *Memoirs of the Reign of Bossa Ahádee, king of Dahomy, an Inland Country of Guiney* (London). The Newberry, Creative Commons Public Domain License.

from the seashore to the interior of Africa. This is wonderfully illustrated in the Map of the Slave Coast included in Robert Norris's *Memoirs of the Reign of Bossa Ahádee, King of Dahomy, an Inland Country of Guiney*, published in 1789 (see Figure 7.1). Along the royal road that linked the seashore to Abomey, the capital of the Dahomey Kingdom, the map's creator included a large forest that seems to serve as a buffer between conquered territories and Dahomey itself. The intent was clear: the spiritual forces at work in the groves filtered away all forms of sickness that circulated along these routes before they could reach settlements where the king resided.

The Making and Demise of Diseased Landscapes in Pre-Modern Western Africa

Because diseased landscapes, everywhere, keep changing through time and space, it is impossible to characterize them at the scale of the African continent, regardless of time period. Some diseases have come, circulated, and gone, leaving elusive traces of their passage that historians, archaeologists, and biologists struggle to describe. Others have deep and continuous histories that fostered complex and evolving relations with local societies. Some global diseases arose on the African continent, often bearing witness to social and environmental changes that took place in one part of the continent or another, under specific circumstances. Many others originated from other parts of the world and diffused to Africa, taking advantage of the movement of people, animals, and things. Writing the history of these brief or durable encounters between mobile pathogens and dynamic societies is particularly challenging because many parts of the many epidemiological and societal puzzles are yet to be identified and contextualized. As a result, there is no constituted historiography of disease in Africa south of the Sahara in the centuries and millennia that preceded the twentieth century, only a scattering of works. Therefore, here I attempt not a history of diseased landscapes in pre-1450 Africa (i.e., before the incorporation of West Africa into the newly developing Atlantic world) but rather an exploration of a few scenarios to illustrate working hypotheses about the making, demise, or subsistence of diseases in selected regions of the continent's environment and their interaction with populations. To this end, I have selected two diseases with very different historical trajectories: malaria as an example of a resilient mosquito-borne disease that originated in Africa and plague as an example of a pathogen with roots outside the continent.

Agrarian Societies and Mosquito-Borne Diseases: Challenges from Within and Resilience

Malaria has a long history in Africa, maybe as long as the genus *Homo* (Packard 2021; Webb 2009). Recent phylogenic studies suggest that the two most widespread malaria parasites, *Plasmodium vivax* (*P. vivax*) and *Plasmodium falciparum* (*P. falciparum*) find their origins in deep time and infected African apes before humans (Liu et al. 2014, 2010). Whereas *P. vivax* "emerged from an ancestral stock of parasites that infected chimpanzees, gorillas and humans," *P. falciparum* "resulted from a [more] recent cross-species transmission of a parasite from a gorilla" to humans (Loy et al. 2017, 87).

P. vivax has the most extended history on the continent, probably emerging much earlier than 60,000 years ago (Loy et al. 2017, 93). The prolonged selection pressure imposed by *P. vivax* on human populations in Africa eventually led to the emergence of the Duffy-negative phenotype[22] that conferred protection from the disease among most African people and brought the relative demise of this parasite. It is suggested that the ancestral lineage of modern human *P. vivax* was transported to Asia before the mutation took place in Africa, with the modern form later reintroduced to parts of Africa (Loy et al. 2017, 93).

P. falciparum has a much more recent history – in the range of 10,000 years. Lesser prolonged selection pressure explains why the parasite is still a major cause of morbidity and mortality in sub-Saharan Africa despite the emergence of selections of genes conferring resistance to the disease (Hedrick 2011; Kariuki and Williams 2020). Because of its connection to gorillas, it is undisputable that the disease first emerged in the forest environment of equatorial Africa, before adapting to other environments, especially those characterized by the presence of dense population and natural/artificial waterways.

Thus, *P. falciparum* was already established in the Nile Valley by Egyptian pre-dynastic times, about 3200 BCE (Bianucci et al. 2008). Initially, the sylvatic vector (i.e., wild transmitter) of the parasite from apes to humans was likely several species of mosquitoes known to bite both gorillas and humans, such as *Anopheles vinckei*, *Anopheles moucheti*, and *Anopheles marshallii* (Loy et al 2017, 95). However, the subsequent dispersal of the human-specialized version of the parasite must have required a parallel adaptation and specialization of various types of Anopheles mosquito species, including *Anopheles gambiae* and *Anopheles coluzzi*, which have since become the principal vectors of malaria. These species are highly anthropophilic (attracted to humans) and heliophilous (attracted to sunlight) and, thus, prosper in anthropogenic (human) landscapes characterized by openings of forest cover (Yasuoka and Levins 2007). This suggests a deep causal link in tropical Africa between human disturbances of the equatorial rainforest, the demographic growth of forest-dwelling communities, and the emergence of *P. falciparum* as a major parasitic health challenge to humans.

Although we can trace human *P. falciparum* evolutionary history back to the early Holocene (i.e., c. 11,000 years before present), when ape *P. falciparum* crossed the species barrier, its successful adaptation to human communities in humid, tropical Africa might have been facilitated by the late-Holocene rainforest crisis and the emergence in some locations of a forest-savannah mosaic. The contributing factors of this crisis during the second half of the first millennium BCE remain debated (Bayon et al. 2019; Giresse et al. 2020). In fact, complex climatic variations might have contributed to the crisis, together with farming communities engaged in the clearing of tropical forests (Bayon et al. 2012; De Saulieu et al. 2021; Garcin et al. 2018). In West Central Africa, it is now established that "population growth (~2500–2000 cal. yr BP [i.e., calendar years before present]) seems coeval with environmental and vegetation changes" (De Saulieu et al. 2021, 24) as the clearing of the forest fostered demographic growth and vice versa.

At the same time, however, environmental transformations and the denser network of human settlements probably silently paved the way to the making of broader pathogenic landscapes. For instance, the opening of the forest's canopy brought the light needed for heliophilous Anopheles to prosper. Also, increased erosion (Bayon et al. 2012) resulting from the deforestation of large expanses of rainforest would have fostered the movement of soils from highlands to lowlands, possibly altering previous drainage patterns and supporting the formation of different types of wetlands. The latter, in turn, would have become breeding-grounds for vectors of diseases such as malaria and yellow fever, which could have affected the demographic dynamics of communities descended from those who had successfully cleared patches of the high forest. Unfortunately, long-term demographics in Africa during the last three millennia remain a grey area. Innovative statistical methods deployed by archaeologists in West Central Africa, however, offer a window into early demographics that fits remarkably well with the prospective scenario described above (Sebag et al. 2016). Although the statistical tools are not precise enough to capture the details of the chronological thread of this decline, we observe significant population growth beginning by the mid-first millennium BCE, succeeded by a brutal decline from the eighth to the eleventh centuries CE, followed by a recovery achieved only by the sixteenth century, just prior to the beginnings of large-scale human trafficking across the Atlantic (De Saulieu et al. 2021).

The tools used to capture this trend are not meant to explain the brutal collapse and drastic reduction of the number of settlement sites and, in the absence of additional data, we can only speculate about what must have happened. Here, I would like to suggest an intriguing hypothesis: that the development of some of the pathogenic landscapes that helped characterize Africa as a disease-ridden continent from a Western perspective emerged from the long process of deforestation and increased human settlement in the tropical forest, which, in turn, allowed a complex array of pathogens and their mosquito vectors to become endemic. These pathogens imposed demographic constraints on early-to-late medieval communities in forested Africa and beyond. By the fifteenth or sixteenth century, however, those communities exposed to a long-lasting selection pressure exerted by tropical diseases – in essence, human biology adapted to the disease threat – had become resistant enough to overcome the threat previously imposed by these pathogenic landscapes. Of course, the latter caused higher mortality among members of the newly connected Euro-American Atlantic communities who had a less significant history of exposure to most of these tropical diseases prior to the fifteenth century. As a result, the unique and long-term history of African communities vis-à-vis tropical diseases – diseases emerging from the local environment – could be a key factor to understand the European perception that Africa was a diseased landscape, the forced and brutal transfer of "disease resistant" Africans across the Atlantic during the early modern age, and the limited impact of European imperialism in sub-Saharan Africa before the nineteenth century.

Death from Far Away? The Problem of the Second Plague Pandemic in Africa

The external view of Africa as a diseased continent is not the only expression of Africa's perceived exceptionalism in matters of global health that I oppose. Indeed, it is not uncommon for Africa to be excluded from historical discussions of pre-modern global health. Although the absence of readily available historical sources is often brought forward to justify the erasing of the massive continent and its populations from such historical narratives, this silence has deep epistemological roots in the fictional trope suggesting that Africa was disconnected from the rest of the Old World before modern times, in terms of both geography and human mobility. This toxic and marginalizing fiction, which was first engineered outside the continent, has since gained some traction in Africa itself among intellectuals who perceive it as a radical pathway to decolonize African history. Admittedly, it could seem paradoxical, on the one hand, to challenge the concept of diseased Africa, while, on the other hand, to suggest that Africa and Africans need to be integrated in broader and deeper historical narratives of global health and pandemics. Both arguments, however, aim at deconstructing discrete categories of discourses about disease and health in Africa that have generated noises or silences in lieu of histories with farfetched consequences on memory and the "pathologizing of Africans" as observed again during the Covid-19 crisis (for instance, Chachage 2020).

Nevertheless, it takes some intellectual audacity to question the invisibility of Africa in many global health narratives and suggest, for example, that the Second Plague Pandemic might also have affected a continent that had remained, until recently, largely outside the focus of historians and other specialists of plague studies. In a series of articles published in 2018, archaeologists and historians examined the hypothesis that the Second Pandemic might have circulated in sub-Saharan Africa. For the first time, this hypothesis escaped from the odd footnotes to which it had been relegated and was instead scrutinized extensively through different sources available in different regions of Africa south of the Sahara.

The idea had emerged from my 2009 dissertation on southern Ghana, and the realization that there had been a rapid and radical shift in the later fourteenth century between a type of settlement pattern attested in the forests of Ghana since the mid-first millennium CE to another that was later encountered, documented, and mapped by European travellers in the Atlantic age (Chouin and DeCorse 2010). The regional nature of the shift called for an exploration of causal factors that went beyond local processes. As I gradually adjusted the lens of my study and zoomed out to wider geographical areas, I came to realize that other parts of Africa had experienced similarly deep transformations of their urban landscapes during the same period of time. Further, these alterations echoed parallel changes documented in the Mediterranean and Northern European worlds in relation to the Second Plague Pandemic (Chouin 2018). When reintegrated into a global historical framework, the events leading to the settlement pattern transformations we had observed in fourteenth-century southern Ghana now compelled us to question the impact of the plague pandemic on Africa south of the Sahara.

The results are two-fold. On the one hand, the 2018 study established that the pathogen responsible for the Second Plague Pandemic had entered and circulated in the eastern part of the continent, sparking a number of crises in the region. In the case of Ethiopia, written sources – especially hagiographies – are compelling (Derat 2018). In eastern Central Africa, a "living archive" of genetic data combined with a new reading of linguistic and documentary evidence from the fourteenth through twentieth centuries led to the conclusion that "plague did have a significant impact on pre-modern East Africa" (Green 2018). In fact, in East and Central Africa, some strains of *Yersinia pestis* that derive from those involved in the Second Plague Pandemic are still active in the modern landscape and provide the ultimate, if derivative, evidence that plague cannot be excluded as a potential factor in pre-modern African historical narratives.

On the other hand, the 2018 study could not unearth definitive evidence that plague also circulated in West Africa despite much circumstantial evidence of change and, sometimes, acute crises that are visible in the archaeological record and possibly echoed in oral traditions (Chouin 2018; Chouin and Lasisi 2019; Gallagher and Dueppen 2018). The limited survival of locally produced written material for this period and their continued rarity until the seventeenth century, combined with the fact that there is no evidence that any strain of *Y. pestis* persisted in the landscape as it did in East Africa, do not help sustain the plague hypothesis in West Africa. Yet, we know this part of Africa was not disconnected from the rest of the continent and, indeed, the wider world. If, as Monica Green encouraged to do, we are to take the word "pandemic" seriously (Green 2014), we need to continue engaging with the plague hypothesis in West Africa, even if, so far, we have not yet unearthed definitive biological evidence that the disease spread to this part of the world.

One way of engaging with the plague hypothesis is to interrogate the difference we observed between East Africa and West Africa, in terms of the presence or absence of the *Y. pestis* pathogen in the modern landscape. Why did *Y. pestis* become endemic in parts of eastern central Africa but not in the west? In eastern Central Africa, the persistence of pathogens belonging to a lineage responsible for the Second Plague Pandemic (1.ANT) suggests not only that plague penetrated the area through the Nile, the Red Sea or, less likely, the Indian Ocean but also that it encountered environmental conditions that enabled it to become endemic.

Unfortunately, the ecology of plague in Africa in relation to vectors, hosts, and landscapes remains largely understudied. Limited evidence suggest that the ecology of plague foci associated with the 1.ANT lineage might be very complex and involve "a complex suite of rodent species" as reservoirs, including native African species such as *Arvicanthis abyssinicus* (Abyssinian grass rat, see Figure 7.2) and invasive species such as the infamous *Rattus rattus* (black rat) (Neerinckx et al. 2008), as well as a complex array of flea species with various efficiency as plague vectors (Makundi et al. 2015). The complexity of plague ecology – or rather plague ecologies as suggested by Anne Laudisoit (2009; Laudisoit et al. 2009) – in East Africa points to a long history of interactions between the pathogen and multiple species of rodents and fleas. Other understudied factors, such as altitude, climate and microclimate, landscape connectivity, and soil biology as illustrated in the hypothetic telluric cycle need to be taken into account. In West Africa, by contrast, the absence of plague reservoirs is evidence that the pathogen did not find the complex set of environmental conditions that enabled endemicity. In particular, it did not find a suitably resistant host among the many existing species of rodents it might have encountered and infected (although, see Nükhet Varlık's chapter in this volume, which considers a similar ecological question in pre-modern Anatolia from a different perspective).

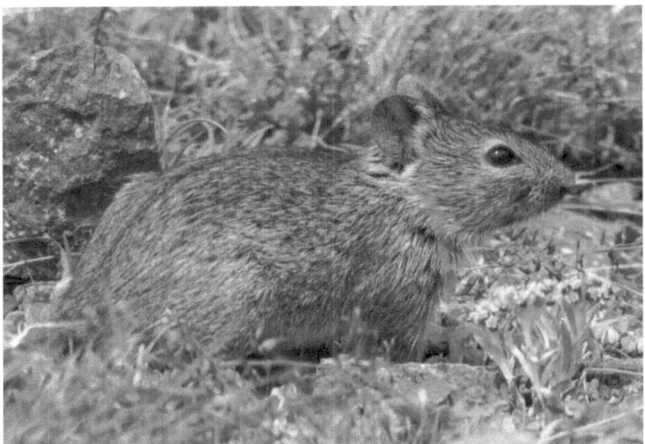

Figure 7.2 Abyssinian Grass Rat. Photo by Forest Jarvis, 2019, Attribution-NonCommercial 4.0 International (CC BY-NC 4.0).

As opposed to East African species that might have been exposed to pathogens circulating in the context of the Justinianic Plague (Green 2018, 13–14), West African rodents had little or no previous interaction with *Y. pestis* and, therefore, would not have been selected against the bacillus. This would have had consequences for the history of plague in West Africa. The arrival and the rapid spread of the pathogen among populations of rodents sensitive to the disease would have caused mass mortality events among them, creating a population bottleneck. This scenario will be confirmed or dismissed by future studies in population genomics of West African rodents. It would also have weakened native rodent infrastructures, opening new opportunities for invasive species such as *Rattus rattus* and *Rattus norvegicus* (Norwegian rat) to take advantage of the opening of the Atlantic trade to occupy new niches in West Africa (Etougbétché et al. 2020; Puckett et al. 2016). In the absence of a long-term reservoir in which the pathogen could subsist until a demographic rebound occurred among rodent populations and enabled a subsequent spillover, the collapse of the original rodent infrastructure would have meant that the circulation of the disease was a brutal but relatively brief experience for West African societies. As such, it might not have been characterized by the multiple, long-term epidemic waves over several centuries that have been documented in other parts of the world. If recurrent waves did occur, they must have had a limited geographical impact, since we only have limited evidence for plague-like diseases during the seventeenth and eighteenth centuries, when internal written sources become more common (Chouin 2018, 22–23).

In short, I believe that much of the future of the history of diseases in pre-modern Africa lies in the historical and interdisciplinary deciphering of the embedded ecologies and biologies of pathogens, reservoirs, hosts, and vectors that structure the landscapes that past societies have exploited, transformed, and experienced. As Monica Green has shown in her reframing of pandemics, there exists a plethora of new sources for the crafty and connected historian of pre-modern Africa that, once explored, will transmute today's historiographical silences into compelling and transformative narratives (for instance Green 2017).

Conclusion

Pre-1800 Africa need not be singled out as a diseased continent when compared with other parts of the Old World. Africa's history cannot be framed around myths, even – or especially – when the latter's veracity seems comforted by common sense. The idea of a continent defined by a hostile and pathogenic nature against which heroic yet sickly African Sisyphi would have fought an everlasting losing battle for progress and health is nothing more than a trope that still feeds from its own historiography. The idea of a continent that was a long-lasting, quasi exclusive source of diseases for the rest of humanity is another myth, born of the previous one. In fact, the exchange of pathogens is a constant in human history, a by-product of connectedness, and all societies, climates, and environments have contributed – and still contribute – to shaping the ever-changing global pathogenic landscape. In Africa, as in every corner of the world, people have long interacted with familiar landscapes and their associated pathogenic risks. They evolved immune defences against some of the most lethal diseases, and they developed social norms and responses to deal with them based on practice, experience, and existing worldviews.

Yet coping with diseases and with the tropical diseased environment does not also mean that societies were successful at keeping illnesses at bay if measured against modern, scientific terms. It would be naïve to overturn the table and imagine pre-modern Africa as the paragon of health. In fact, Africans were as successful or unsuccessful facing their disease burdens as were other pre-industrial societies. Success was often measured in the simple facts of identifying the health issues, constructing a discourse around them, and mitigating their impact through pharmaceutical or spiritual means. Similarly, it would be naïve to believe that Africa was disconnected from global health landscapes, and only faced local, tropical diseases. Using the Second Plague Pandemic as an example, I have shown that Africa was as exposed to past pandemics as it is to modern ones, even though silences in the historiography might suggest otherwise. As in other parts of the world, pandemics that resulted in rapid and excessive mortality could generate deep crises that contributed to the shaping and reshaping of societies.

There is, therefore, nothing radical in stating that the overwhelming pressure exercised by its pathogenic environment cannot define pre-modern Africa historically. Such a statement is the simple outcome of critically reading sources, both old and new, which indicate that Africans struggled, endured, mitigated, disseminated, and adapted to the specific illnesses associated with the diseased environments they inherited, lived in, exploited, and shaped, just as did other populations in other parts of the world. European travel accounts of the seventeenth and eighteenth centuries present compelling evidence that Western travellers found Africa's environment unhealthy – on the basis of their own mortality in the face of tropical diseases – but, paradoxically, praised Africans for their physical strength and overall health condition.

Tragically, the strength and healthiness demonstrated by African populations in tropical climes, compared to the debilitating health faced by most Europeans under the same conditions, were defining factors that led to the trafficking of enslaved Africans across the Atlantic. In essence, the forced migration of millions of enslaved Africans to the Americas is an appalling testimony of the success of African populations in coping with tropical diseases and of the difficulty Europeans faced in adapting to tropical milieux.

In this regard, and as a concluding remark, I need to underline a fundamental gap in the historiography of the Atlantic world. During the sixteenth century, Central and South America suffered a demographic crisis with few parallels in the world's history. The collapse of native populations has been the focus of a long historiographic tradition seeking to explain this catastrophe.[23] The focus has been on the impact of Eurasian germs and European warfare and led to competing scenarios that are only partially able to account for all aspects of the mass mortality. In an effort to "rock" the (historiographical) boat, Monica Green (2021) suggested new, bold directions. Not only does her approach take into account critical advances in the sequencing of pathogens, both ancient and modern, but also calls for a reframing of the Great Dying in a broader, more global history of diseases that takes into account human behaviour and includes Africa – a missing piece in most Great Dying narratives. In fact, taking Africa into account might be particularly relevant if, as I suggest, the demographic crisis that shook Native America – and threatened to annihilate the indigenous labour resources needed to support empire building by Europeans in Central and South America – was, in part, the result of the unsuspected projection across the early Atlantic of the epidemiological complex of tropical Africa that would have adapted easily to similar environmental conditions in tropical America. The transfer of African tropical pathogens, together with their human reservoir and vectors, was facilitated by European vessels sailing from Senegambia, the Gulf of Guinea or Angola to South America and the Caribbean islands with their human cargoes of enslaved West and West-central Africans, starting in the sixteenth century. The transfer to tropical America of fragments of the diseased landscapes of West and West-central Africa might have included Yellow Fever, for example, the modern clinical picture of which echoes some descriptions of the sixteenth-century affection known as *Huey Cocoliztli* that struck Mexico from the mid-sixteenth century onwards (Acuna-Soto et al. 2004; Marr and Kiracofe 2000), or *Salmonella enterica* subsp. *enterica* serovar Paratyphi C, for which genomic evidence was recovered from ten individuals buried at

Teposcolula-Yucundaa, Mexico (Vågene et al. 2018). Overall, the demand for unfree African labour in Spanish America might have been boosted by superior resistance of African settlers to diseases transferred to the New World as part of the Columbian exchange. Such a resistance might have resulted from the combination of a long-term exposure of African population to Old World diseases also familiar to Europeans and an array of tropical diseases endemic to Africa. As such, the expansion of the slave trade in early colonial America might throw light on the changing epidemiological situation in the Americas, resulting, in part, from the possible expansion across the Atlantic of pathogens originating in tropical Africa as much as from Eurasia.

Notes

1 This chapter would not have seen the light of the day without the generosity and gentle pressure of Lori Jones. Monica Green cleared an important path in the history of global health. Without her path breaking contributions to the field, her liberal sharing of material, and her encouragement, I doubt I would have attempted this chapter. Finally, some ideas discussed in this chapter emerged from inspiring conversations with Geoffroy de Saulieu, David Sebag, members of the Ife-Sungbo Archaeological Projects and of "Hiatus", an informal group of scholars exploring the impact of past pandemics on the African past.

2 Colbert had commissioned the drawings in the framework of his long-planned offensive against the United Provinces of the Netherlands.

3 Cape Lopez is located in modern Gabon. Lübelfing travelled in the late 1590s, Brun in the 1610s.

4 On diagnosis and the concept of disease in early modern Europe, see, for instance, Stein (2006). The identification and classification of diseases was radically distinct from modern practice.

5 The disease takes different forms depending on the specific parasitic flatworm involved; it is endemic to most of Atlantic Africa, from Senegambia to Angola (WHO 2016). Today, schistosomiasis disables more than it kills although long-term lethal complications exist. Microscopic haematuria is also a possible symptom of other tropical diseases transmitted by mosquitoes, including yellow fever (Monath and Barrett 2003, 346), dengue (Sriwijitralai and Wiwanitkit 2016), and malaria (George 2009) but could not have been noticed in the seventeenth century since microscopes were not part of the naval surgeon's toolkit (King 2018).

6 This textbook was first published in 1995 and is currently in its third edition (2017). In the first edition, Iliffe spoke of "innumerable insect vectors [that] made its disease environment exceptionally rich and diverse, far more than tropical America's" (Illife 1995, 10). This questionable comparison with America was removed from later revised editions.

7 For a longer discussion of this topic, please see Guillaume Linte's chapter 6 in this volume, especially pages 114–17.

8 It is worth noting that early modern Europeans might not have been able to distinguish between syphilis and other conditions such as Buruli ulcers or yaws.

9 The expression "other natural disease," in the original Dutch "andere natuerlycke cranckheden," can be understood as including all diseases except the six he had mentioned earlier. The use of the term "natural" suggests that he did not include diseases that could have a supernatural cause related to magical practices or witchcraft. He might have consciously or unconsciously borrowed this idea from the way Africans conceptualized disease (see below).

10 African history is replete with examples of such practices. See, for instance, Ogundiran (2020).
11 Here, I use the English translation modified according to the comments made by Albert Van Dantzig (1975–78) in his comparison of the English and Dutch versions.
12 To my knowledge, smallpox was not mentioned on the Gold Coast earlier in the seventeenth century, but Bosman suggests it was present from the late 1680s. Smallpox was a new imported disease in the Gulf of Guinea by the late seventeenth century. This probably explains Bosman's comment. It remained a threat throughout the eighteenth century (Alden and Miller 1987, 196, 205, 208). If Europeans posted on the Gold Coast primarily drank from the rainwater reservoirs built in forts and castles, they were less exposed to Guinea worms than Africans who drank from streams and wells potentially polluted by the larvae of *Dracunculus medinensis*.
13 On the dynamic nature of medicine in African history, see also Janzen (2011).
14 My translation of the original text, which reads "Pour les blessures ils ont une herbe dont le marc & le jus exprimé dessus fait des cures si inoüies, qu'ils se mettent peu en peine d'une blessure profonde de cinq doigts."
15 This category resembles Murdock's "theories of supernatural causation," although with a focus on human agency. Murdock subdivided his own category into mystical causation, animistic causation, and magical causation (1980, 17–27). Only the last of these had humans as core players.
16 For smallpox and a "human-caused" disease in Dahomey, see Quinn (1968).
17 In Nigeria, for instance, we can trace the bitter-sweet legacy of landscape epidemiology from the 1902–28 British campaign to eradicate mosquitos in Lagos, retraced by Jimoh Oluwasegun (2017), to the environmental Akalism of the 2010s, so pertinently captured by John Manton at Ibadan (Manton 2013).
18 The kingdom is also known as Matapa or Mutapa.
19 In a report dated 1921, Swynnerton suggested that such burning practices had been carried out for a least a century, if not longer.
20 The date of the epidemic is unknown, but likely was in the late eighteenth or early nineteenth century.
21 I was not able to identify the specific scientific name of this tree. On the burial of pre-modern smallpox victims in Dahomey, see Quinn (1968, 160).
22 Duffy antigens on red blood cells can be used as a receptor for *plasmodium vivax* malaria parasites. People without these antigens were subjected to a positive evolutionary selection pressure because they had better survival odds.
23 For a historiographical panorama of the Great Dying, see Green 2021, note 2.

References

Archival Sources

Central Regional Archives, Cape Coast, Ghana

Printed Sources

Acuna-Soto, Rodofo, David W. Stahle, Matthew D. Therrell, Richard D. Griffin, and Malcolm K. Cleaveland. 2004. "When Half of the Population Died: The Epidemic of Hemorrhagic Fevers of 1576 in Mexico." *FEMS Microbiology Letters* 240, no. 1: 1–5.
Akyeampong, Emmanuel. 2006. "Disease in West African History." In *Themes in West Africa's History*, edited by Emmanyel Akyeampong, 33–51. Oxford, Athens and Accra: James Currey, Ohio University Press, and Woeli Publishing Services.

Alden, Dauril, and Joseph C. Miller. 1987. "Out of Africa: The Slave Trade and the Transmission of Smallpox to Brazil, 1560–1831." *The Journal of Interdisciplinary History* 18, no. 2: 195–224.

Bayon, Germain, Bernard Dennielou, Joël Etoubleau, Emmanuel Ponzevera, Samuel Toucanne, and Sylvain Bermell. 2012. "Intensifying Weathering and Land Use in Iron Age Central Africa." *Science* 335, no. 6073: 1219–1222.

Bayon, Germain, Enno Schefuß, Lydie Dupont, Alberto V. Borges, Bernard Dennielou, Thibault Lambert, Gesine Mollenhauer, Laurence Monin, Emmanuel Ponzevera, Charlotte Skonieczny, and Luc André. 2019. "The Roles of Climate and Human Land-use in the Late Holocene Rainforest Crisis of Central Africa." *Earth and Planetary Science Letters* 505: 30–41.

Bianucci, Raffaella, Grazia Mattutino, Rudy Lallo, Philippe Charlier, Hélène Jouin-Spriet, Alberto Peluso, Thomas Higham, Carlo Torre, and Emma Rabino Massa. 2008. "Immunological Evidence of *Plasmodium falciparum* Infection in an Egyptian Child Mummy from the Early Dynastic Period." *Journal of Archaeological Science* 35, no. 7: 1880–1885.

Bosman, William. 1705. *A New and Accurate Description of the Coast of Guinea, Divided into the Gold, the Slave and Ivory Coasts*. London: James Knapton and Dan. Midwinter.

Boualam, Mahmoud, Bruno Pradines, Michel Drancourt, and Rémi Barbieri. 2021. "Malaria in Europe: A Historical Perspective." *Frontiers in Medicine*, 8: 691095.

Cagle, Hugh. 2018. *Assembling the Tropics. Science and Medicine in Portugal's Empire, 1450–1700*. Cambridge and New York: Cambridge University Press.

Chachage, C. 2020. "Social Distancing and 'Flatten the Curve': Africa Can Do It." *Corona Times*. https://www.coronatimes.net/social-distancing-africa-can-do-it/

Chouin, Gérard. 2001. "Seen, Said, or Deduced? Travel Accounts, Historical Criticism, and Discourse Theory: Towards an 'Archeology' of Dialogue in Seventeenth-Century Guinea." *History in Africa* 28: 53–70.

Chouin, Gérard. 2009. *Forests of Power and Memory: An Archaeology of Sacred Groves in the Eguafo Polity, Southern Ghana (c. 500–1900 AD)*. Unpublished PhD Dissertation, Syracuse University.

Chouin, Gérard. 2011. *Colbert et la Guinée: Le voyage en Guinée de Louis de Hally et Louis Ancelin de Gémozac (1670–1671)*. Saint-Maur-Des-Fossés: Éditions Sépia.

Chouin, Gérard. 2018. "Reflections on Plague in African History (14th–19th c.)." *Afriques* 9. http://journals.openedition.org/afriques/2228

Chouin, Gérard and Christopher Decorse. 2010. "Prelude to the Atlantic trade: New Perspectives on Southern Ghana's Pre-Atlantic History (800–1500)." *The Journal of African History* 51, no. 2: 123–45.

Chouin, Gérard and Olanrewaju Lasisi. 2019. "Crisis and Transformation in the Bight of Benin at the Dawn of the Atlantic Trade." In *Power, Political Economy, and Historical Landscapes of the Modern World Interdisciplinary Perspectives*, edited by Christopher DeCorse, 285–306. Albany, NY: SUNY Press.

Cooper, Frederick. 2011. "Nexus of Science and Colonialism." *Science* 333: 1577–1578.

Cunningham, Andrew. 2002. "Identifying Disease in the Past: Cutting the Gordian Knot." *Asclepio* 54, no. 1: 13–34.

Curtin, Philip D. 1961. "'The White Man's Grave': Image and Reality, 1780–1850." *Journal of British Studies* 1, no. 1: 94–110.

Curtin, Philip D. 1990. "The End of the 'White Man's Grave'? Nineteenth-century Mortality in West Africa." *The Journal of Interdisciplinary History* 21, no. 1: 63–88.

Delaunay, Karine. 1994. *Voyages à la Côte de l'Or (1500–1750). Etude historiographique des relations de voyage sur le littoral ivoirien et ghanéen.* Paris: Afera éditions.

De Marees, Pieter. 1602. *Beschrijvinghe ende historische verhael vant gout koninckrijck van Guinea.* Amsterdam: C. Claesz.

De Marees, Pieter. 1987. *Description and Historical Account of the Gold Kingdom of Guinea (1602).* Translated and edited by Albert Van Dantzig and Adam Jones. London: British Academy.

Depetris-Chauvin, Emilio, and David N. Weil. 2018. "Malaria and Early African Development: Evidence from the Sickle Cell Trait." *The Economic Journal* 128, no. 610: 1207–1234.

Derat, Marie-Laure. 2018. "Du lexique aux talismans : occurrences de la peste dans la Corne de l'Afrique du XIIIe au XVe siècle." *Afriques* 9. http://journals.openedition.org/afriques/2090

De Rosny, Eric. 1981. *Les yeux de ma chèvre.* Paris: Plon.

De Saulieu, Geoffroy, Yannick Garcin, David Sebag, Pascal R. Nlend Nlend, David Zeitlyn, Pierre Deschamps, Guillemette Ménot, Pierpaolo Di Carlo, and Richard Oslisly. 2021. "Archaeological Evidence for Population Rise and Collapse between ~2500 and ~500 cal. yr BP in Western Central Africa." *Afrique: Archéologie & Arts* 17: 11–32.

Dobson, Mary J. 1997. *Contours of Death and Disease in Early Modern England.* Cambridge: Cambridge University Press.

Echenberg, Myron. *Africa in the Time of Cholera: A History of Pandemics from 1817 to the Present.* Cambridge: Cambridge University Press, 2011.

Ehret, Christopher. 2002. *The Civilizations of Africa: A History to 1800.* Charlottesville: University of Virginia Press.

Ehret, Christopher. 2016. *The Civilizations of Africa: A History to 1800.* 2nd ed. Charlottesville: University of Virginia Press.

Etougbétché, Jonas, Gualbert Houémènou, Henri-Joël Dossou, Sylvestre Badou, Philippe Gauthier, Issaka Youssao Abdou Karim, Violaine Nicolas, and Gauthier Dobigny. 2020. "Genetic Diversity and Origins of Invasive Black Rats (*Rattus rattus*) in Benin, West Africa." *Journal of Vertebrate Biology* 69, no. 2. https://doi.org/10.25225/jvb.20014

Fauvelle, François-Xavier, ed. 2018. *L'Afrique ancienne de l'Acacus au Zimbabwe: 20,000 ans avant notre ère – XVIIᵉ siècle.* Paris: Belin.

Fury, Cheryl. 2012. "Health and Health Care at Sea." In *The Social History of English Seamen, 1650–1815,* edited by Cheryl Fury, 193–228. Woodbridge: Boydell Press.

Gallagher, Daphne and Stephen Dueppen. 2019. "Recognizing Plague Epidemics in the Archaeological Record of West Africa." *Afriques* 9. http://journals.openedition.org/afriques/2198

Garcin, Yannick, Pierre Deschamps, Guillemette Ménot, Geoffroy de Saulieu, Enno Schefuß, David Sebag, Lydie M. Dupont, Richard Oslisly, Brian Brademann, Kevin G. Mbusnum, Jean-Michel Onana, Andrew A. Ako, Laura S. Epp, Rik Tjallingii, Manfred R. Strecker, Achim Brauer, and Dirk Sachse. 2018. "Early Anthropogenic Impact on Western Central African Rainforests 2,600 y ago." *Proceedings of the National Academy of Sciences* 115, no. 13: 3261–3266.

George, Charles. 2009. "Blackwater Fever: The Rise and Fall of an Exotic Disease." *Journal of Nephrology* 22, suppl. 14: 120–28.

Giresse, Pierre, Jean Maley, and Alex Chepstow-Lusty. 2020. "Understanding the 2500 yr BP Rainforest Crisis in West and Central Africa in the Framework of the Late Holocene: Pluridisciplinary Analysis and Multi-archive Reconstruction." *Global and Planetary Change* 192: 103257.

Green, Edward. 1999. *Indigenous Theories of Contagious Disease*. Oxford: AltaMira Press.

Green, Monica H. 2014. "Taking 'Pandemic' Seriously: Making the Black Death Global." *The Medieval Globe* 1: 27–61.

Green, Monica H. 2017. "The Globalisations of Disease." In *Human Dispersal and Species Movement: From Prehistory to the Present*, edited by Nicole Boivin, Rémy Crassard, and Michael D. Petraglia, 11–43. Cambridge: Cambridge University Press.

Green, Monica H. 2018. "Putting Africa on the Black Death Map: Narratives from Genetics and History." *Afriques* 9. http://journals.openedition.org/afriques/2125

Green, Monica H. 2021. "The Great Dying: The Epidemiological and Medical Implications of Old and New World Encounters in the Pre- and Post-Contact Eras." *IsisCB* Special Issue, edited by Stephen P. Weldon and Neeraja Sankaran (under review, submitted), https://isiscb.org/special-issue-on-pandemics/essay.html?essayID=25

Harms, Robert. 2018. *Africa in Global History*. New York and London: W. W. Norton.

Hedrick, Philip. 2011. "Population Genetics of Malaria Resistance in Humans." *Heredity* 107, no. 4: 283–304.

Iliffe, John. 1995. *Africans: The History of a Continent*. Cambridge: Cambridge University Press.

Iliffe, John. 2017. *Africans: The History of a Continent*. 3rd ed. Cambridge: Cambridge University Press.

Janzen, John. 1982. *Lemba, 1650–1930. A Drum of Affliction in Africa and the New World*. New York and London: Garland Publishing.

Janzen, John. 2011. "Towards a Historical Perspective on African Medicine and Health." *Curare: Zeitschrift für Medizinethonologie* 34, no. 4: 282–95.

Joffe, Helene. 2011. "Public Apprehension of Emerging Infectious Diseases: Are Changes Afoot?" *Public Understanding of Science* 20, no. 4: 446–60. doi:10.1177/0963662510391604.

Jones, Adam. 1983. *German Sources for West African History 1599–1669*. Wiesbaden: Steiner.

Jones, Jared. 2011. "Ebola, Emerging: The Limitations of Culturalist Discourses in Epidemiology." *Journal of Global Health*, 1, no 1:1–6.

Jones, Lori. 2016. "The Diseased Landscape: Medieval and Early Modern Plaguescapes." *Landscapes* 17, no. 2: 108–23.

Kariuki, Silvia N. and Thomas N. Williams. 2020. "Human Genetics and Malaria Resistance." *Human Genetics* 139: 801–11.

King, Nathaniel. 2018. "An Examination of Sanitation and Hygiena Habit Artifacts Found Aboard Vasa: Health, Sanitation, and Life at Sea in Seventeenth-Century Sweden." Unpublished Masters Thesis, East Carolina University.

Laudisoit, Anne. 2009. *Diversity, Ecology and Status of Potential Hosts and Vectors of the Plague Bacillus Yersinia Pestis: Contribution to Plague Epidemiology in an Endemic Plague Focus: the Lushoto District (Tanzania)*. 2009. Unpublished PhD Dissertation, University of Liège and University of Antwerp.

Laudisoit, Anne, Simon Neerinckx, Rhodes H. Makundi, Herwig Leirs, and Boris R. Krasnov. 2009. "Are Local Plague Endemicity and Ecological Characteristics of Vectors and Reservoirs Related? A Case Study in North-East Tanzania." *Current Zoology* 55, no. 3: 200–11.

Leach, Melissa. 2010. "Time to Put Ebola in Context." *Bulletin of the World Health Organization* 88, no. 7: 488–89.

Liu, Weimin, Yingying Li, Gerald H. Learn, Rebecca S. Rudicell, Joel D. Robertson, Brandon F. Keele, Jean-Bosco N. Ndjango, et al. 2010. "Origin of the Human Malaria Parasite *Plasmodium falciparum* in Gorillas." *Nature* 467, no. 7314: 420–425.

Liu, Weimin, Yingying Li, Katharina S. Shaw, Gerald H. Learn, Lindsey J. Plenderleith, Jordan A. Malenke, Sesh A. Sundararaman, et al. 2014. "African Origin of the Malaria Parasite *Plasmodium vivax*." *Nature Communications* 5, no. 1: 1–10.

Loy, Dorothy E., Weimin Liu, Yingying Li, Gerald H. Learn, Lindsey J. Plenderleith, Sesh A. Sundararaman, Paul M. Sharp, and Beatrice H. Hahn. 2017. "Out of Africa: Origins and Evolution of the Human Malaria Parasites *Plasmodium falciparum* and *Plasmodium vivax*." *International Journal for Parasitology* 47, no. 2–3: 87–97.

Loyer, Godefroy. 1935. *Relation du voyage du royaume d'Issiny, Côte d'or, païs de Guinée en Afrique (1714)*. Edited by Paul Roussier. Paris: Larose.

Mackenbach, Johan. 2020. *A History of Population Health: Rise and Fall of Disease in Europe*. Amsterdam: Brill Rodopi.

Makundi, Rhodes H., Apia W. Massawe, Benny Borremans, Anne Laudisoit, and Abdul Katakweba. 2015. "We are Connected: Flea–Host Association Networks in the Plague Outbreak Focus in the Rift Valley, Northern Tanzania." *Wildlife Research* 42, no. 2: 196–206.

Manton, John. 2013. "'Environmental Akalism' and the War on Filth: The Personification of Sanitation in Urban Nigeria." *Africa* 83, no. 4: 606–22.

Marr, John S. and James B. Kiracofe. 2000. "Was the Huey Cocoliztli a Haemorrhagic Fever?" *Medical History* 44, no. 3: 341–62.

Mavhunga, Chakanetsa. 2018. *The Mobile Workshop: The Tsetse Fly and African Knowledge Production*. Cambridge: The MIT Press.

Monath, Thomas and Alan Barrett. 2003. "Pathogenesis and Pathophysiology of Yellow Fever." *Advances in Virus Research* 60: 343–97.

Murdock, George. 1980. *Theories of Illness: A World Survey*. Pittsburgh: University of Pittsburgh Press.

Neerinckx, Simon B., Andrew T. Peterson, Hubert Gulinck, Jozef Deckers, and Herwig Leirs. 2008. "Geographic Distribution and Ecological Niche of Plague in Sub-Saharan Africa." *International Journal of Health Geographics* 7, no. 1: 1–12.

Newfield, Timothy P. 2017. "Malaria and Malaria-like Disease in the Early Middle Ages." *Early Medieval Europe* 25, no. 3: 251–300.

Norris, Robert. 1789. *Memoirs of the Reign of Bossa Ahádee, King of Dahomy, an Inland Country of Guiney. To Which Are Added, the Author's Journey to Abomey, the Capital; and a Short Account of the African Slave Trade*. London: W. Lowndes.

Noya, Oscar, Naftale Katz, Jean Pierre Pointier, André Theron, and Belkisyolé Alarcón de Noya. 2015. "Schistosomiasis in America." In *Neglected Tropical Diseases – Latin America and the Caribbean*, edited by Franco-Paredes, Carlos, and José Ignacio Santos-Preciado, 11–43. Vienna: Springer.

Ogundiran, Akinwumi. 2020. "Managing Epidemics in Ancestral Yorùbá Towns and Cities: "Sacred Groves" as Isolation Sites." *African Archaeological Review* 37, no. 3: 497–502.

Oluwasegun, Jimoh Mufutau. 2017. "The British Mosquito Eradication Campaign in Colonial Lagos, 1902–1950." *Canadian Journal of African Studies/Revue canadienne des études africaines* 51, no. 2: 217–36.

Packard, Randall. 2021. *The Making of a Tropical Disease: A Short History of Malaria.* 2nd ed. Baltimore, MD: Johns Hopkins University Press.

Pépin, Jacques. 2021. *The Origins of AIDS.* 2nd ed. Cambridge: Cambridge University Press.

Puckett, Emily E., Jane Park, Matthew Combs, Michael J. Blum, Juliet E. Bryant, Adalgisa Caccone, Federico Costa, Eva E. Deinum, Alexandra Esther, Chelsea G. Himsworth, Peter D. Keightley, Albert Ko, Åke Lundkvist, Lorraine M. McElhinney, Serge Morand, Judith Robins, James Russell, Tanja M. Strand, Olga Suarez, Lisa Yon, and Jason Munshi-South. 2016. "Global Population Divergence and Admixture of the Brown Rat (*Rattus norvegicus*)." *Proceedings of the Royal Society B: Biological Sciences* 283, no. 1841: 20161762.

Quinn, Frederick. 1968. "How Traditional Dahomian Society Interpreted Smallpox?" *Abbia: Revue Culturelle Camerounaise* 20: 151–66.

Roberts, Jonathan. 2011. "Medical Exchange on the Gold Coast During the Seventeenth and Eighteenth Centuries." *Canadian Journal of African Studies/La Revue canadienne des études africaines* 45, no. 3: 480–523.

Rømer, Ludwig Ferdinand. 2000 (1760). *A Reliable Account of the Coast of Guinea (1760).* Translated and edited by Selena Axelrod Winsnes. Oxford: Oxford University Press.

Sebag, David, Laurent Brémond, Kathrin Jeffery, Makaya M'Vouboum, François Nguetsop, Richard Oslisly, Johan Ozwald, and Geoffroy de Saulieu. 2016. "Le rôle des bas-fonds dans l'évolution des paysages du parc national de la Lopé." In *Pour une écologie historique en Afrique centrale*, edited by Geoffroy de Saulieu, Martin Elouga, and Sonké Bonaventure, pp. 141–53. Yaoundé: AUF-IRD.

Shillington, Kevin. 2019. *History of Africa.* 4th ed. London: Palgrave Macmillan and Red Globe Press.

Siena, Kevin, ed. 2005. *Sins of the Flesh: Responding to Sexual Disease in Early Modern Europe.* Toronto: Centre for Reformation and Renaissance Studies.

Sriwijitralai, Won and Viroj Wiwanitkit. 2016. "Hematuria among Dengue Patients: A Note on Observation." *Indian Journal of Urology* 32, no. 3: 251.

Skotnes-Brown, Jules. 2019. "From the White Man's Grave to the White Man's Home? Experiencing 'Tropical Africa' at the 1924–25 British Empire Exhibition." *Science Museum Group Journal* 11. http://dx.doi.org/10.15180/191101.

Smythe, Kathleen. 2015. *Africa's Past, Our Future.* Bloomington: Indiana University Press.

Steckel, Richard. 2010. "The Little Ice Age and Health: Europe from the Early Middle Ages to the Nineteenth Century." Seminar Paper, University of Toronto. https://www.economics.utoronto.ca/index.php/index/research/downloadseminarpaper/3106

Steckel, Richard, Clark Spencer, Charlotte Roberts, and Joerg Baten, eds. 2019. *The Backbone of Europe: Health, Diet, Work, and Violence over two Millennia.* Cambridge: Cambridge University Press.

Stein, Claudia. 2006. "The Meaning of Signs: Diagnosing the French Pox in Early Modern Augsburg." *Bulletin of the History of Medicine* 80, no. 4: 617–48.

Thornton, John. 2012. *A Cultural History of the Atlantic World, 1250–1820.* Cambridge: Cambridge University Press.

Tilley, Helen. 2011. *Africa As a Living Laboratory: Empire, Development, and the Problem of Scientific Knowledge, 1870–1950.* Chicago, IL: University of Chicago Press.

Vågene, Åshild J., Alexander Herbig, Michael G. Campana, Nelly M. Robles García, Christina Warinner, Susanna Sabin, Maria A. Spyrou, et al. 2018. "*Salmonella enterica* Genomes From Victims of a Major Sixteenth-Century Epidemic in Mexico." *Nature Ecology & Evolution* 2, no. 3: 520–528.

Van Dantzig, Albert. 1975. "English Bosman and Dutch Bosman: A Comparison of Texts." *History in Africa* 2: 185–216.

Van Dantzig, Albert. 1976. "English Bosman and Dutch Bosman: A Comparison of Texts, II." *History in Africa* 3: 91–126.

Van Dantzig, Albert. 1978. "English Bosman and Dutch Bosman: A Comparison of Texts, IV." *History in Africa* 5: 225–56.

Wagoner, Phillip. 2003. "Precolonial Intellectuals and the Production of Colonial Knowledge." *Comparative Studies in Society and History* 45, no. 4: 783–814.

Watt, James, E. J. Freeman, and William F. Bynum. 1981. *Starving Sailors: The Influence of Nutrition upon Naval and Maritime History*. London: National Maritime Museum.

Wear, Andrew. 2008. "Place, Health and Disease: The *Airs, Waters, Places* tradition in Early Modern England and North America." *Journal of Medieval and Early Modern Studies* 38: 443–65.

Webb, James. 2006. "Ecology & Culture in West Africa." In *Themes in West Africa's History*, edited by Emmanuel Akyeampong, 33–51. Oxford, Athens and Accra: James Currey, Ohio University Press, and Woeli Publishing Services.

Webb, James. 2009. *Humanity's Burden: A Global History of Malaria*. New York: Cambridge University Press.

Webel, Mari. 2019. *The Politics of Disease Control: Sleeping Sickness in Eastern Africa, 1890–1920*. Athens: Ohio University Press.

Webster, Bonnie, Vaughan Southgate, and Timothy Littlewood. 2006. "A Revision of the Interrelationships of *Schistosoma* Including the Recently Described *Schistosoma guineensis*." *International Journal for Parasitology* 36, no. 8: 947–55.

Weil, David. 2014. "The Impact of Malaria on African Development over the Longue Durée." In *Africa's Development in Historical Perspective*, edited by Emmanuel Akyeampong, Robert Bates, Nathan Nunn, and James Robinson, 89–130. New York: Cambridge University Press.

WHO. 2016. *Schistosomiasis*. Accessed 12 March, 2020. https://www.who. int/news-room/fact-sheets/detail/schistosomiasis

Wilkinson, Annie and Melissa Leach. 2015. "Briefing: Ebola – Myths, Realities, and Structural Violence." *African Affairs* 114, no. 454: 136–48.

Yasuoka, Junko and Richard Levins. 2007. "Impact of Deforestation and Agricultural Development on *Anopheline* Ecology and Malaria Epidemiology." *The American Journal of Tropical Medicine and Hygiene* 76, no. 3: 450–60.

Ziegler, Michelle. 2016. "Landscapes of Disease." *Landscapes* 17, no. 2: 99–107.

8 The Rise and Fall of a Historical Plague Reservoir

The Case of Ottoman Anatolia

Nükhet Varlık

Introduction

The Black Death pandemic of the mid-fourteenth century swept across a sizeable portion of Afro-Eurasia, stretching from Central Asia to the Middle East, Europe, and North Africa, and likely beyond.[1] Thanks to recent historical, archaeological, and palaeogenetics research, we are now in a better position to piece together the temporal and spatial extent of this catastrophic event (Benedictow 2021, 2004; Chouin 2018; Green 2020, 2014). Given its geographic location at the intersection of southeast Europe, the Black Sea, and Middle East and North Africa (MENA), Anatolia (in modern day Turkey) was not immune to the pandemic. Historical evidence at hand helps us to establish a basic chronology and trajectory of plague's spread in that region (Schamiloglu 2004; Varlık 2015, 99–107).

The Black Death was a pandemic of plague – a bacterial infection caused by *Yersinia pestis* – that caused high levels of mortality (conventionally estimated as 40–60%, but most recently argued to be around 65% for Europe (Benedictow 2021, 869–76)). It, thus, fostered significant social, demographic, and economic transformations everywhere it affected. The fourteenth century was, indeed, a perfect storm for much of Eurasia: climatic instability and fluctuations, human and animal plagues, famine, wars, rebellions, and demographic reshuffling are all hallmarks of this era (Campbell 2016; Green 2018; Newfield 2009; Slavin 2012). As it did elsewhere, plague came to Anatolia and its surroundings on the heels of political, social, and environmental crises, adding yet another harsh blow onto its impoverished population. In the words of Şeyyad Hamza, a fourteenth-century Anatolian mystic poet who lost several children to plague, the Black Death was like a "wind of death": whomever it touched "fell down to the soil," much like dead leaves falling on the ground in the autumn (Akar 1987, 3).

However catastrophic it might have been, though, the Black Death was only a brief episode in the history of what is now called the Second Plague Pandemic. Plague outbreaks occurred repeatedly across Afro-Eurasia, beginning in the thirteenth century before the Black Death itself (Fancy and Green 2021; Green 2020). Likewise, the disease continued to break out in

DOI: 10.4324/9780429055478-12

different parts of Afro-Eurasia across several centuries after the Black Death – until the early eighteenth century in northern and western Europe, the late eighteenth century in Russian lands, and the late nineteenth century in the Middle East – before gradually retreating from these regions. Since it hosted the infection for the longest time (a full 600 years between 1347 and 1947), studying Anatolia's experience of plague promises to afford critical insights into the long-term rhythms, expansion, and contraction of the disease during the Second Pandemic (Varlık 2020a).

Plague's long history in Anatolia and its surroundings underscores the fact that Ottoman rule over the region overlapped almost squarely with the time-frame of the Second Pandemic. The plague outbreaks that kept recurring over six centuries were virtually contemporaneous with Ottoman power (c. 1300–1922). In other words, plague was a constant presence in Anatolia during the entire period of Ottoman rule – and even in its aftermath. Although existing scholarship has yet to acknowledge plague as one of the main historical agents of the era, any demographic and environmental study of Ottoman Anatolia must recognise plague's recurring presence and its cumulative impact. More importantly, for the purposes of this chapter, the fact that the infection lingered in this area longer than anywhere else in the historical record invites a host of questions. Why did the Second Pandemic continue in this region longer than elsewhere? How do we explain this long-term persistence? What were the social, economic, and, perhaps most importantly, environmental conditions that supported plague's persistence and later its disappearance from this region? Before addressing these questions, it is helpful to discuss the mechanisms of plague's persistence and extinction more generally.

Plague Persistence and Extinction

Plague is not an extinct disease. On the contrary, it is still active in some parts of the world, where it is enzootic (i.e., present in animal populations) and has the ability to "spill over" to human populations. Upon being introduced to a new environment, if the pathogen that causes plague – *Y. pestis* – finds a rodent population in which to sustain itself, it tends to form reservoirs (plague foci) that remain in the wild and are not a direct threat to humans. Only those individuals who come into close contact with infected or dead plague carriers (rodents or other mammals) and/or their ectoparasites (e.g., fleas, lice) are at risk. In such cases, the infection may be carried to human settlements and cause sporadic outbreaks that may remain undocumented in historical sources. When the infection is communicated from wild rodents to commensal rodents (i.e., species that "eat at the same table" as humans, mainly rats) that live in close proximity to human populations, localized outbreaks can occur (Gage and Kosoy 2005). Even when there is no contact with infected human settlements (no trade or travel), outbreaks with an animal origin can re-emerge, sometimes after many years of absence, for reasons that are not fully understood.

In recent years, a growing number of scholars from both the sciences and the humanities have started to pay closer attention to plague's long-term persistence (Carmichael 2014; Foley et al. 2007; Schmid et al. 2012; Slavin 2021; Wimsatt and Biggins 2009). These studies were further supported by new palaeogenetics findings suggesting that *Y. pestis* had a deep history in Eurasia, with outbreaks occurring since the Late Neolithic Bronze Age (Rasmussen et al. 2015; Spyrou et al. 2018; Valtueña et al. 2017). There is now a growing, albeit controversial, body of evidence about the environmental mechanisms that sustained *Y. pestis* infections over many centuries. The most heated debate revolves around the prolonged recurrences of plague in Europe during the Second Pandemic and largely involves two opposing hypotheses: namely, what will be referred to here as the "re-introductions hypothesis" and the "persistence hypothesis."

Some scholars insist that the prolonged presence of plague in Europe should be attributed to a series of introductions and re-introductions from outside the region, through trade and other forms of human-induced mobilities (Bramanti et al. 2021; Guellil 2018; Morozova et al. 2020; Namouchi et al. 2018; Schmid et al. 2015). According to this "re-introductions hypothesis," no local reservoirs were established in Western Europe that could sustain long-term persistence of the disease and hence European plagues had their origins elsewhere – anywhere from Eastern Europe to Central Asia (I discuss the historical background of such views that locate the origins of European plagues in the "Orient" in Varlık 2017 and 2020b). In other words, these scholars attribute the persistence of plague in Europe to repeated re-introductions of the pathogen from a non-European origin.

Given the imprecise nature of the point of origin in this line of argumentation, different views have been offered about the exact means by which the disease was transmitted to and spread within Europe. Some scholars emphasize climate fluctuations and their effects on disease-hosting rodents in Central Asia, arguing that each recurrent plague outbreak in Europe was associated with an individual "spill over" event in Central Asia and treated as a separate re-importation (Schmid et al. 2015). Some have identified the Ottoman Empire as the source of European plagues (Guellil 2018). Yet others emphasize the role of camels and human ectoparasites such as lice in plague's spread (Barbieri 2019; Dean et al. 2018). Recent historical scholarship has demonstrated that post–Black Death outbreaks were long imagined by contemporaries to have followed the same mechanisms as the Black Death itself, that is, introduced from a point of origin outside of Europe (see Lori Jones's chapter in this volume and Jones 2022). One wonders if these historical imaginations have influenced some of today's scientists.

At the opposite end of this debate are scholars who reject the idea of re-importations and suggest instead that the strains of *Y. pestis* that were introduced to Europe during the Black Death lingered in (or in the vicinity of) Europe to cause successive outbreaks over centuries. In a pioneering article, historian Ann Carmichael (2014) first proposed this "persistence hypothesis," arguing that the European Alps served as a potential plague reservoir and that the Alpine marmot served as a local rodent host from which European cities around the Mediterranean received repeated outbreaks of plague.

Recent studies confirm this historical claim, on the basis of evidence gathered by extracting and analysing ancient DNA (aDNA) fragments from human skeletal remains. For example, genetic evidence recovered from the victims of the Plague of Provence (1720–22) indicates that the bacterium that killed them descended directly from the lineage of *Y. pestis* involved in the Black Death. According to this research, "the strains responsible for the Black Death left descendants that persisted for several centuries in an as yet unidentified host reservoir population, accumulated genetic variation, and eventually contributed to the Great Plague of Marseille" (Bos et al. 2016, e12994). This finding supports the hypothesis that the infection was kept alive in (now extinct) plague reservoirs in or around western Europe and that it did repeatedly re-emerge even in the absence of new re-introductions from outside. This argument is also supported by historical research that indicates the absence of major plague outbreaks in the eastern Mediterranean region whence it is claimed to have been introduced (Varlık 2020b).

Other palaeogenetics studies from across Europe soon confirmed plague's persistence (Feldman et al. 2016; Seifert et al. 2016). These studies all agreed that upon the initial introduction of *Y. pestis* to Europe, different lineages of the bacterium emerged *within* Europe and then continued to circulate in and, importantly, *out of it* for centuries. This suggests, in turn, that there must have been plague reservoirs in Europe that supported the infection. Thus, there seems to be a newly emerging consensus about a single introduction of the pathogen to Europe (and probably to the larger Mediterranean world) during the Black Death and its persistence thereafter (Spyrou et al. 2016). This hypothesis is not only in line with our modern knowledge of *Y. pestis* ecology but also follows the broad outlines of the complicated histories of the emergence and distribution of Second Pandemic *Y. pestis* lineages more broadly (Fancy and Green 2021; Green 2020). Given the limited number of available *Y. pestis* aDNA genomes (especially outside of Europe), this consensus begs for more careful and historically grounded explanations about the social, epidemiological, and environmental conditions that made long-term persistence possible.

By the same token, the question of plague's "disappearance" from Europe at the end of the Second Pandemic has been equally controversial. Historians, public health officials, and medical authors who wrote about this issue during the nineteenth and twentieth centuries have produced a substantial scholarship. While some scholars have argued that plague's withdrawal was due to administrative actions, such as the implementation of quarantines and *cordons sanitaires*, others have emphasized the role of changes in urban planning, housing structures, and hygiene practices in European societies (Blažina-Tomić & Blažina 2015; Crawshaw 2012; Eckert 2000; Panzac 1985; Slack 1981). In an attempt to go beyond an anthropocentric (i.e., human) perspective, still others have suggested that the increased use of arsenic eradicated plague-bearing rats, that brown rats replaced black rats, or that rats themselves became immune to the infection (Appleby 1980; Konkola 1992). More recent contributions to this question came from palaeogenetics, which suggest that *Y. pestis* experienced gene deletion and decreased virulence in the late stages of the Second Pandemic (Spyrou et al. 2019). Currently, there is no consensus on this complex question, yet the recent debates on persistence, especially the persistence hypothesis, can offer insights for studying plague's retreat.

Plague's withdrawal from a region, much like its persistence, is governed by complex social, epidemiological, and environmental processes. Studying plague's withdrawal makes it necessary to shift our historical gaze away from contagion narratives – deeply rooted in Eurocentric, urban perspectives – to a dynamic multi-protagonist plague model that is closely associated with the rise and fall of historical plague reservoirs in the environment. The epidemiological fluctuations of the disease can be best studied in conjunction with changes in these plague reservoirs. How do such reservoirs expand or contract over time? What are the larger climatic, environmental, and human-induced changes that affect them? How do rodent colonies respond to such outside changes, and how do these responses affect their ability to sustain and transmit the infection?[2]

At this point, it may be helpful to underscore the privileged place that Europe holds in plague scholarship and how much Eurocentric views have distorted historical assumptions. Recent scientific and historical debates have focused almost exclusively on Europe, leading to false assumptions that certain phenomena were peculiar to the geographical, social, and environmental conditions of Europe. However, plague's persistence and extinction were hardly phenomena specific to Europe. The post-Black Death Mediterranean world was a rather unified epidemiological zone with an impressive array of micro-ecologies; some of the prominent characteristics of environments conducive to plague's persistence were common across the region. At first glance, one can pinpoint the major ports and hubs of infection, as well as principal trajectories of its circulation, both over the Mediterranean littoral (along the shoreline) and across its hinterland. Yet, a global outlook might be more helpful to understand patterns of plague.

Historical plague ports across the globe, especially those that gave rise to long-term persistence, seem to exhibit similar climatic features, typically characterized by warm wet winters and hot dry summers. These *mediterraneanoid* climate zones, located not only across the Mediterranean basin but also in California and Chile, effectively sustained the plague upon its introduction (Carmichael 2014, 181). Most Mediterranean ports received the infection during the First (c. 541–mid-eighth century) and the Second Pandemic, while California and Chile received it during the more globalized Third Pandemic (c. 1894–1950s); plague still exists in an enzootic state in the western United States and parts of South America, occasionally causing human cases. Given the conduciveness of this "Mediterranean environment" to the dissemination and persistence of the disease (but also its withdrawal in the long term), the

European experience needs to be better contextualized. Plague's persistence in and retreat from Europe was inevitably intertwined with near-immediate proxies – one of which, as I argue here, was Ottoman Anatolia. Hence, it is to Ottoman Anatolia and its plague experience that we now turn our attention.

Plague in Ottoman Anatolia

Anatolia had a long history of plague during the Second Pandemic – a sustained presence spanning six centuries. Repeated outbreaks continuously affected the region from the mid-fourteenth until the mid-twentieth century (Panzac 1985; Varlık 2015). This long history can hardly be explained by re-introductions of the infection each time from outside, which makes it imperative to study the mechanisms of plague's persistence and extinction in this environment. Moreover, the history of plague in Anatolia is closely entwined with the history of the rise and fall of the Ottoman Empire and needs to be studied in conjunction with it, as I discuss below.

Following the Black Death, plague affected only certain regions across Anatolia, circulating along its main trade and military routes. It eventually died down each time, only to reappear every 10–15 years. This pattern of recurrence continued more or less until the mid-fifteenth century when major anthropocentric transformations and their ecological ramifications changed plague epidemiology dramatically. Beginning in the second half of the fifteenth century, outbreaks started to reach previously untouched areas (smaller towns and villages in inner Anatolia, further away from main routes), and the intervals between epidemic episodes steadily diminished. The dissemination and frequency of plague outbreaks escalated to such an extent over the following century that there appears to be a recorded incidence of plague in one part of Anatolia or another almost every single year in the sixteenth century. Punishing epidemics continued into the seventeenth century with no sign of slowing down until the next century. Even though plague continued to break out in the nineteenth century and into the twentieth century, there seems to have been a gradual decline in epidemic activity, which begs further examination (Panzac 1985; Varlık 2015, 292).

I have argued elsewhere that the reasons for this epidemiological divergence need to be sought in the expansion of the Ottoman Empire and its imperial policies, which caused major ecological transformations in the Anatolian landscape, fauna, and flora (Varlık 2015). In short, to build and govern a centralized empire, the Ottoman administration managed, mobilized, and reshuffled the flow of its "natural" resources, including crops, livestock, people, and minerals, in entirely unprecedented ways. Anatolia was the main supplier of timber, livestock and beasts of burden, various animal products (such as silk, wool, and leather), and a variety of crops, silver, copper, and salt to the empire's capital, Istanbul (Constantinople) – a megacity whose population dwarfed any other in Afro-Eurasia, west of China – and to local and faraway industries and imperial projects (Mikhail 2012; White 2011).

Anatolia was also a hub where major maritime and overland trade networks converged. Roads crisscrossing the peninsula facilitated the constant flow of goods, which the Ottoman administration carefully fostered to secure tax revenues. The empire's policies of extraction and circulation of resources brought its diverse ecological zones into interaction with each other and intensified the mobilities of exchange among both humans and non-human agents, the sum of which resulted in the increased circulation of plague. Over the long-term, however, the empire's economic policies and the ecological strain it placed on Anatolia's resources resulted in a series of changes that may have led inadvertently to the extinction of plague from this region.

Studying the long-term persistence and withdrawal of plague in Anatolia in conjunction with the Ottoman Empire's imperial policies that altered the region's ecology allows us to question the ways in which late medieval and early modern societies interacted with nature, managed natural resources, and were, in turn, affected by the ecological consequences of their policies and interventions. To explore the complex ecology of plague in the Anatolian highlands and lowlands, it is crucial to stress the dynamic nature of plague reservoirs. This allows us to develop insights not only about the persistence of the infection but also of its gradual disappearance.

Anatolia is home to diverse microecologies and microclimates. The coastal strips of western and southern Anatolia are characterized by a warm Mediterranean climate: cool, rainy winters and hot and moderately dry summers. The immediate hinterland of the Mediterranean littoral is a semi-arid zone. The Black Sea coast enjoys a temperate oceanic climate that is wet, humid, and cooler; this area receives more precipitation, with its eastern parts receiving rainfall year around. The interior of the peninsula is characterized by a continental climate and low rainfall. Within these main zones, however, there also are multiple microclimatic zones that are starkly different one from the other.

The present-day temperature and humidity conditions for most of the peninsula seem to suggest that climatic conditions favourable to supporting epidemic activity can be found in some part of Anatolia almost year around. Needless to say, past climate fluctuations, and in particular the climate anomalies of the fourteenth century and the global cooling conditions of the Little Ice Age, need to be taken into consideration when studying the region's historical environmental conditions (Parker 2013; Tabak 2008; White 2012, 2011). They also may be contextualized more broadly, with respect to both time and space (Campbell 2016, 2010; Haldon 2014; Telelis 2008, 2005; Xoplaki et al. 2016).

A critical component of Anatolia's ecological diversity is its elevation. An ongoing digital study that assessed how mountainous the central Ottoman provinces were found that mountains covered 74% of the total area (Yaycıoğlu 2022). The Anatolian plateau itself comprised a major proportion of this percentage. This striking finding merits consideration, as it underscores the unusually mountainous condition of Ottoman topography. Mountains cover only 24% of the earth's entire land surface, yet here we are looking at a region that is home to three times that average. In fact, the same study established that the Ottoman Empire was "historically the most mountainous polity" when compared to other early modern and modern empires.[3]

The topography of Anatolia, characterized by mountains, thus needs to be recognized as a leading historical actor and an integral part of plague's complex ecology. The presence of mountains added significantly to the availability of microclimates and microecologies, which, in turn, contributed to the biological diversity of Anatolia: its flora, its fauna, and its pathogens. These are all critical considerations when studying plague's persistence and extinction.

One of the main mountain systems that defined Anatolia, the Taurus, divides the Mediterranean littoral from its hinterland. It is considered to be part of the Alpine-Himalayan belt of Eurasia, stretching from the Himalayas to the Atlantic and including the Alps and the Pyrenees. This mountain system and its surrounding basins contributed to Anatolia's complex topography and nurtured a rich biodiversity, especially in the pre-modern era (Çolak & Rotherham 2006; McNeill 1992; Michaux et al. 2004; Şekercioğlu et al. 2011; Yılmaz 1997). Within this wide range of biological diversity, the Taurus mountain system makes for a particularly great case study. Recent research shows that plague risk increases at higher elevations and where there is higher rodent biodiversity (Carlson et al. 2021). Given the specific ecological conditions conducive to plague, it was likely to house a conglomerate of plague hotspots (micro-foci). Especially the southern hills of this mountain range facing the Mediterranean and the northern hills facing the Black Sea seem to be ideal sites to study for their potential to harbour plague reservoirs.

These hills receive a substantial amount of rainfall (mostly in winter, spring, and autumn), which is generally believed to increase the volume of vegetation, and thus possibly help sustain large rodent populations (as well as their ectoparasites). The "Trophic Cascade Hypothesis" maintains that increased rainfall supports the growth of additional vegetation to feed rodents and can lead to the survival of an increased number of fleas in rodent burrows, possibly leading to epizootic conditions in natural reservoirs (Gage 2008; Parmenter et al. 1999, 814–21; Zell 2004, 16–26). Drawing from this model, it should be possible to examine whether the south-facing hills of the Taurus Mountains possessed conditions favourable to sustaining natural plague reservoirs. Presumably, if the large quantity of rainfall supported an adequate level of vegetation, it could also sustain a large rodent population and their ectoparasites. The climatic conditions of the hills facing the Mediterranean likely remained temperate even in winter, as the permanent snow line at approximately 3,500 m only applies to the highest peaks (Onur 1962). Even though we do not know exactly what species of (rodent) reservoir hosts and fleas were involved, it should be possible to test this hypothesis on the basis of historical evidence at hand. If plague persisted among the enzootic rodents and their fleas, one would expect to see early spring outbreaks; in fact, this seems to be supported by historical sources (Varlık 2015).

There are other reasons to look to the highlands as potential plague reservoirs. From the point of view of biogeography, mountain ecologies are considered similar to island ecologies (Hadjikyriacou 2011, 12–15; MacArthur and Wilson 1967). Paying attention to this type of insular biogeography is especially important for studying rodent and vector species and their distribution. The mechanisms that govern the introduction of new species and the growth or extinction of their population is likely similar in mountain ecologies and island ecologies alike. For example, zooarchaeological evidence documents the spectacular expansion of black rats (*Rattus rattus*) in the Mediterranean islands (Ruffino and Vidal 2010), while other studies show that plague is sustained in the highlands of Madagascar (above 800 m) where flea vectors (*Xenopsylla cheopis* and *Synopsyllus fonquerniei*) are more abundant (Andrianaivoarimanana et al. 2013; Vogler et al. 2011).

This is not to suggest that the Taurus mountain range is the only possible location that could have hosted plague reservoirs in Anatolia, and we can expand our gaze to different parts of ecologically diverse Anatolia. At this point, it may be helpful to consider a recent study from North Africa that has shown *Y. pestis*'s salt tolerance and its ability to persist in high saline environments (Malek et al. 2017); this opens additional possibilities for exploring Anatolia's hinterland.

Lake Tuz (Salt Lake) in inner Anatolia is the peninsula's largest hypersaline lake (over 30% salinity), and the microecology in the region around it may have historically served as plague reservoirs. That it continues to support a rich (albeit declining) biodiversity, with a large number of endemic species of plants and animals, may be indicative of its ability to host plague in the past. For example, Lake Tuz is still home to greater flamingos (*Phoenicopterus roseus*) in addition to a large number of birds and mammal species. Another potential implication of this region for Ottoman Anatolia is that the salt trade may have served as a potential conduit for the dissemination of plague, at least regionally. In addition to Lake Tuz, a number of other salt mines and salt beds in Ottoman Anatolia served the demands of local consumption and were heavily regulated by the Ottoman administration (İnalcık and Quataert 1994, 58–64).

Mountains, high saline environments, and many other ecological contexts: Ottoman Anatolia was home to a number of rodent species that could have contributed to the maintenance and amplification of plague. In the absence of systematic collection and inventorying of pre-modern zooarchaeological evidence, however, it is difficult to identify what species of rodents lived in the region at the time. Animal bones found in digs are documented in individual, oftentimes unpublished excavation reports or maintained in scattered museum collections; no knowledge system yet brings them together. Without a systematic inventory of historical rodent taxonomy in Ottoman Anatolia, we turn instead to studies from the Byzantine era (330–1453) that confirm the presence of *Rattus rattus* species (Kroll 2012). For the Ottoman era, information about rodents is mostly anecdotal, at times buried in narrative sources that need to be painstakingly teased out (Çelik 2022; Varlık 2014a, 207–13; 2015, 19–28).

Expanding the inquiry beyond rodents and small mammals may, however, offer additional insight about the rich fauna of Ottoman Anatolia. In addition to various documentary and narrative sources, treatises of veterinary medicine, hunting manuals, and practical works prepared for the maintenance of horses, dogs, and falconry (mostly for elite consumption) are helpful. Along with textual evidence, works of visual art representing animals in royal hunting scenes or the use of their fur can also be used fruitfully. Although illustrations of animals were produced to elicit certain emotional responses in their audience, and thus are not to be taken as realistic documents (Ben-Ami 2016, 31–41; Faroqhi 2010; Mikhail 2013), they nevertheless are a rich testament to the diversity of fauna – especially wildlife – that existed in Ottoman Anatolia.

Scattered descriptions in historical sources occasionally make it possible to identify rodents that are now extinct (or nearly extinct) in today's Anatolia. One such striking example may have been implicated in plague's history. The sixteenth-century German traveller Hans Dernschwam left a detailed description of one such animal he saw in northwest Anatolia. From his account, one can conclude that this was an animal species he had never encountered before, neither in his native homeland nor during his extensive travels in the Balkans and Anatolia. He wrote:

> It is slightly larger than a mouse, smaller than a vole, with delicate and well-proportioned limbs. It looked like a hare. Its head, mouth, and ears were well-balanced; its back was rather long and elegant. It had a very long tail. The tail was like a lion's tail with a little ball on its end. It held up its tail in the air. This way it looked like an African monkey.
>
> (Dernschwam 1987, 307–08).

This depiction brings to mind the jerboa (see Figures 8.1 and 8.2), a known plague carrier. It is difficult to identify exactly what species of jerboa Dernschwam saw based on this description alone. The great jerboa (*Allactaga major*) no longer exists in modern Anatolia, and the Euphrates jerboa (*Allactaga euphratica*) can be found marginally only in southeastern Turkey (Arslan et al. 2012). Fossil records indicate, however, that the great jerboa migrated to west and northwest Anatolia from its Central Asian steppe reservoir via the Balkans during the Late Pleistocene. Similarly, the Euphrates jerboa (also known as the Southwest Asian jerboa) inhabited much of inner Anatolia, Mesopotamia, and the area up to the Caspian Sea during the Late Pleistocene (Griffiths et al. 2013, 138).

Jerboa populations declined in Anatolia over time although we do not know exactly when this took place. If this sixteenth-century reference was,

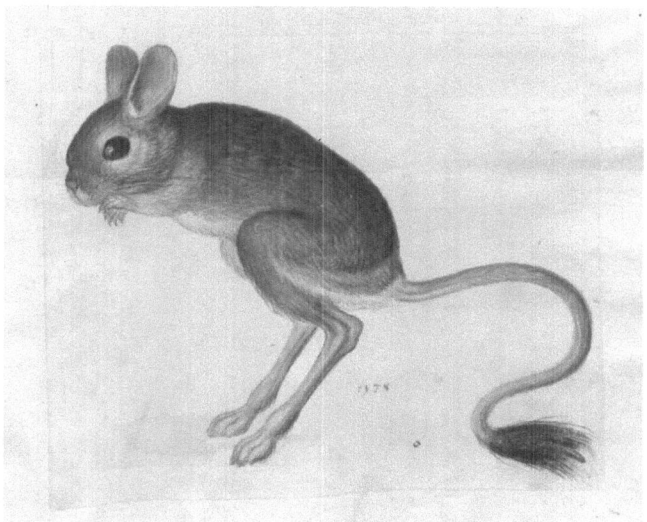

Figure 8.1 Image of a jerboa. Sketch possibly by Joris Hoefnagel or by or after Jacopo Ligozzi, c. 1578. In *Naturstudien Rudolfs II*. Österreichisches National Bibliothek, Cod. Min. 42, fol. 18, Public Domain.

indeed, to a type of jerboa, the decline in its population can reasonably be dated to a more recent era, as they were still being sketched and described in the eighteenth and nineteenth centuries, as the figures shown here attest. The jerboa population in modern-day Anatolia seems to be nearly depleted; even so, recent sightings in different parts of Turkey have been captured on camera and shared in the media.[4] These occasional sightings suggest the possible historical distribution of this species across central and eastern Anatolia. Even though there is no definitive scientific evidence to prove the existence of jerboas in Ottoman Anatolia, it is nevertheless interesting to reflect on the relationship between their extinction and the disappearance of plague – more on that below.

Other sixteenth-century European observers also noted this curious-looking animal, though sometimes misidentifying it as a small hare. Thanks to correspondence between Francesco I de' Medici, Grand Duke of Tuscany, and the Bolognese naturalist Ulisse Aldrovandi (d. 1605), and the former's commissioning of drawings by Jacopo Ligozzi, we can identify jerboas and even speculate about their origins. Francesco sent various European princes exotic goods, plants, and animals from the New World to secure political ties, including a series of shipments with jerboas to Archduke Ferdinand II of Austria in 1581. Francesco described the jerboa as "an animal from the Indies that they call a hare in that country" (Markey 2016, 52, 176 n38). Jerboas are not native to the New World, however, so they must have been brought

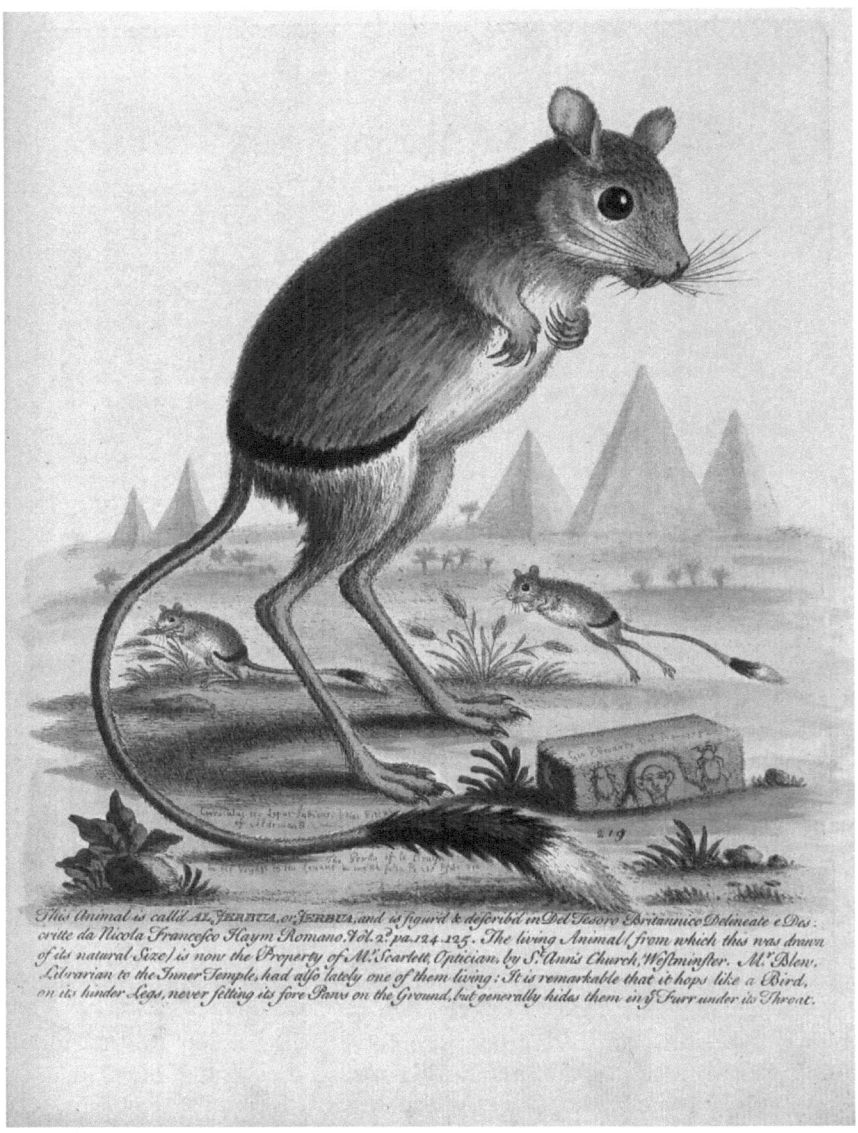

Figure 8.2 Image of a jerboa with pyramids in the background, showing the "Orientialist" perception of these rodents. Etching by George Edwards, 1752. Wellcome Collection, Public Domain Mark.

from somewhere else. Although their range across Afro-Eurasia is quite large, there is some evidence that might indicate its origin as Ottoman Anatolia: most of the items in Francesco's shipments were collected from the New World, but they occasionally included mineral, plants, and animals procured from elsewhere, including Anatolia (Markey 2016, 50).

The port of Livorno where Francesco conducted his business had strong ties to Ottoman trade networks and it is plausible to think of Anatolia or its surroundings as the jerboas' point of origin (Markey 2016, 50, 52, 177 n59). Sixteenth-century Ottoman imperial decrees forbade hunting wildlife with firearms, and we do not have much evidence regarding the smuggling of live wildlife for the same period (Yaycıoğlu 2022). Francesco's reference to jerboas as hares reminds us that they are referred to as "Arab hare" (*Arap tavşanı*) in Turkish, a vernacular term that may have circulated alongside terms such as "desert rat" (*çöl sıçanı*), used by the seventeenth-century Ottoman traveller Evliya Çelebi (Varlık 2015, 25 n23).

Later Ottoman sources refer to other species of rodents that are also known as plague carriers. For example, among the wild rodents of eighteenth-century Aleppo, the English physician Alexander Russell mentioned the short-tailed field mouse, dormouse, hamster, water rat, and jerboa (Russell and Russell 1794, 2:180–2). In the late nineteenth and early twentieth centuries, French epidemiologist Marcel Baltazard established that the Persian jird (*Meriones persicus*) was an active plague carrier in the mountainous regions between Anatolia and Iran (Baltazard et al. 1952). A nineteenth-century English traveller described marmot-like ground-burrowing rodents in Ilgın (in modern Konya) in central Anatolia, as follows:

> The plain swarmed with a species of burrowing animal about the size of a squirrel, which I had also seen in other parts of Asia Minor; but whether a species of marmotte, jerboa, lemming, or hamster, I could not ascertain... Their colour is a light yellowish brown, and they abound in the southern provinces of Russia, where the variety or species is known by the name of 'Rat des steppes'.
> (Hamilton 1842, 2:189; see also Panzac 1985, 123).

This rodent species may be identified as the white-throated woodrat (*Neotoma albigula*), which no longer survives in this part of the world (Wrobel 2006, 339). Unfortunately, given the general decline in Anatolia's biodiversity over recent centuries, the current distribution of rodent species in this region does not allow us to confidently map out species that lived there historically.

Something remains to be said about the relationship between, on the one hand, human interventions on the landscape and the decline in biological diversity in the region in general – the extinction of some rodent and vector species in particular – and the disappearance of plague in Anatolia, on the other. To this end, it is important to consider the effects of deforestation, changes in patterns of land use and agriculture, and hunting and the fur trade as well as any other major changes that affected populations of rodent species (Schwartz et al. 2006) and thus the persistence of plague.[5] Similarly, since the size of a reservoir affects how long plague can persist (Schmid et al. 2012), the building of roads or other types of disruptions to the environment that divides existing hotspots and reduces their size also influences their ability to sustain plague long-term.

The Highlands, the Lowlands, and Plague Dissemination

How were the Anatolian highlands connected to the lowlands in the late medieval and early modern eras? What types of links existed between them? These connections often may be too difficult to trace on the basis of documentary evidence alone. However, they are important to picture in the larger set of connections that comprised the origin and background of rural plague outbreaks. In such cases, it might be more helpful to look for evidence of plague in a cluster of villages or towns, rather than tracing isolated outbreaks. Sometimes, such cluster cases appear in the available archival sources from different parts of Anatolia, pointing to the need for further research.[6]

Trade offered one type of connection between Anatolia's highlands and lowlands. Local markets likely served this purpose. Even though the size, frequency, and distance between local markets in rural Anatolia varied immensely across the peninsula and over the centuries of Ottoman rule, archival documents allow us to pursue these connections. We know, for example, that some early modern Anatolian local markets served several villages. Many of those grew in the sixteenth century; some developed into small or mid-size towns, and others evolved into larger urban centres (Faroqhi 1984; Jennings 1976). A close study of local markets can help trace local or regional trade (although probably less so for long-distance trade). Furthermore, the circulation of certain commodities has been intimately connected to the spread of plague. For example, shipments of grains seem almost always to have been accompanied by plague, given rats' attraction to grains and of fleas to the grain debris. Similarly, the trade in meat, hides, and other animal products also attracted rats (Audoin-Rouzeau 2003; McCormick 2003). Other items, such as woollen textiles, furs, and salt were likely instrumental in spreading plague as well. For example, Russian furs became increasingly popular in Anatolia starting in the late fifteenth century. Italian woollen cloth can also be taken into consideration because both fur and woollen cloth can harbour infected fleas for a very long time (Varlık 2015, 153–5).

Individuals who were involved in the handling, transport, storage, and sale of such goods were more likely exposed to greater risk of infection. As such, workers in grain warehouses and mills, bakers, and people who handled infected animals (e.g., butchers) and their hides as well as those working in slaughterhouses or tanneries risked infection. Some Ottoman sources document the infection of people belonging to those professions, making it possible to link their illness to contact with infected items that circulated within the local or regional trade networks (Varlık 2014b, 261–88).[7]

In addition to local markets, other connections between the Anatolian highlands and lowlands included vertical nomadic transhumance (seasonal movement of livestock). Especially in western and southern Anatolia, groups of pastoralist nomads continued their seasonal migrations between lowland winter encampments and highland summer pastures for many centuries. By virtue of their role in connecting the highlands and lowlands, these nomads are of particular interest for our purposes. It is true that epidemics thrive especially in urban settings where people live in close proximity to each other; epidemiological studies have shown this with great authority. Nevertheless, there is also evidence for the spread of epidemics outside of urban centres, to the countryside, and to areas where nomads had extensive contacts (Borsch 2005, 24–54; Conrad 1981, 465–69; Dols 1977, 154–69). Because they lived in close contact with livestock and other animals, nomads were at high risk of infection. Moreover, they may have been instrumental in spreading plague by bridging areas where the disease was enzootic to places where it could become epidemic. Evidence from nomads in modern North Africa, for example, shows nomads' higher risk both of contracting the infection – given their contact with rodents and their ectoparasites – and of propagating it (Bitam et al. 2010; Néfissa and Moulin 2010). By the same token, the role of nomadic peoples in transmitting plague has also been brought into focus in historical studies of the disease (Buell 2012, 130–2). Finally, research from Madagascar reveals new insights about the transmission of enzootic plague from the highlands – where plague is sustained because of the abundance of flea vectors (Andrianaivoarimanana et al. 2013; Vogler et al. 2011) – to lowlands that may have implications for understanding the involvement of nomads in the process. If *Y. pestis* finds a favourable environment in the highlands in which to preserve itself from one season to the next, the pathogen can be carried either by humans or their animals (or their ectoparasites) to the lowlands, where commensal rodents subsequently can sustain the infection.

It is possible to reconsider the role of pastoralist nomads bridging the disease ecologies of the Anatolian highlands and lowlands, especially in view of their seasonal movements and their close proximity to animals. Recent research demonstrates that Asia's highland Silk Roads networks (elevation between 750 m and 4,000 m) emerged from the mobility trajectories of nomadic pastoralists (Frachetti et al. 2017). This supports the idea that the mobility patterns of Anatolia's pastoralist nomads can guide our thinking about the connections between the highlands and the lowlands. Moreover, nomads interacted with settled societies in various ways. For example, they supplied raw materials for the textile and leather industries, such as wool, dyes, and hides. They also produced carpets, rugs, and other textile items on their own. They supplied transportation animals, such as donkeys, horses, and camels. They participated in harvests in western Anatolia as migrant workers and also served in various military undertakings of the Ottoman state (Kasaba 2009, 31–5). Each of these activities brought them into contact with the settled populations of towns and cities. Economic interactions likely took place on the outskirts of Ottoman towns, where businesses such as tanneries, soap factories, and slaughterhouses were located and where low-income families and day labourers resided. These businesses likely attracted a great number of commensal rodents, exposed labourers to potentially infected materials, and, thus, functioned as possible gateways of infection leading to larger urban outbreaks (Ayalon forthcoming; Ben Néfissa and Moulin 2010; Bitam et al. 2010; Borsch 2005, 24–54; Conrad 1981, 465–69; Dols 1977, 154–69). All of these links could amplify the exchange of infection between the highlands and the lowlands, facilitated by the mediation of nomads.

Considering the complex patterns of disease dissemination, it is also helpful to pay attention to the role of mammalian carnivores, feeding on rodents, as potential transitory hosts that transported infected fleas between different rodent populations – and perhaps also between highlands and lowlands. These include wolves, jackals, and hyenas, all of which are mentioned in Ottoman sources. In addition, migratory birds (e.g., white storks) may have served in the long-distance transportation of infected fleas, causing metastatic leaps between different micro-foci (Varlık 2014, 213–16).

Connections to the Larger Mediterranean World

An infection carried by a single individual could hardly turn into an epidemic. In most cases, it is safe to assume that plague circulated locally without turning into an epidemic, unless and until it was communicated to a larger urban area, especially a port city. A wave of infection that circulated in a cluster, however, would more likely be communicated to an adjacent cluster and, thus, find a larger circulation outlet. Regardless of its point of origin, plague mostly moved along roads, facilitated by both humans and commodities that may have served as vectors of the disease.

A network of roads developed across Ottoman Anatolia, especially rigorously in the sixteenth century, to facilitate the movement of merchants, armies, pilgrims, and others. In addition to overland roads, rivers offered possible connections, not only for the movement of people and goods but for spreading rodent populations as well (Varlık 2015, 120). Similarly, mountain passes and valleys played a critical role in connecting plague reservoirs to larger urban areas, by facilitating the movement of caravans. What made it possible for local economies to be integrated, thus also seems to have contributed to the establishment of connections between different plague ecologies, and thereby the dissemination of the disease.

The question of how Anatolian plague reservoirs were connected to the larger Mediterranean networks requires further research. Did the Anatolian micro-foci feed the infection to Europe's local proxies? Did the Anatolian reservoirs directly "export" the infection to Europe? Historical sources seldom allow us to establish such direct connections. Based on the available evidence, it is possible to argue that plague's circulation between different ecologies before the sixteenth century must have been relatively slow and intermittent, yet along complex and intersecting trajectories that did not necessarily move unidirectionally. Maritime dissemination of the infection was more direct, much faster, and impressively effective in connecting urban foci of port cities to each other. It is also much better documented. Historical sources suggest that through the fourteenth and fifteenth centuries the circulation of plague was almost entirely in the west-to-east direction (Varlık 2015). Starting in the sixteenth century, the maritime circulation of plague in the Mediterranean became much more complex.

In comparison, overland circulation is much more elusive and challenging to trace in historical records, especially when the historical gaze moves away from urban areas. It is nearly impossible to trace the complex patterns of plague circulation (both local and long distance) in rural, sparsely populated parts of inner Anatolia on the basis of historical sources alone. These questions invite interdisciplinary studies that involve deeper analysis of climatic, ecological, and genetics data. Suffice it to say that this chapter is simply an exploration of the available evidence from a new perspective and calls for further research.

Notes

1 Earlier versions of this chapter were presented at various conferences and invited lectures, including at The Skilliter Centre for Ottoman Studies, Newnham College, University of Cambridge; The Graduate Center, CUNY; International Congress on Medieval Studies (Kalamazoo); Climate Change and History Research Initiative, Princeton University; The Center for Medieval and Renaissance Studies at the University of Oklahoma; Harvard University; Yale University; Georgetown University; Washington University in St Louis, School of Medicine; Institute for Advanced Study-Princeton; Ohio State University; Binghamton University, SUNY; University of Pennsylvania; and the Orient-Institut Beirut. I would like to extend my warm thanks to Kate Fleet, Seçil Yılmaz, Beth Baron, John Haldon, Kathleen Crowther, Evan Hepler-Smith, Paola Bertucci, Judith Tucker, Robert Feibel, Nicola Di Cosmo, Jane Hathaway, Meg Leja, Harun Küçük, and Fatih Ermiş for their kind invitations and those in the audience in each of those lectures for their valuable feedback. In addition, I thank Monica Green for inspiring me to pursue the connection between declining rodent populations and the waning of plague in Anatolia; Ann Carmichael for inspiring me to think about the role of mountains and animals in plague persistence; and Monica Azzolini for drawing my attention to jerboas in Aldrovandi's collection. Specials thanks to Lori Jones – the editor *extraordinaire* – for being the best interlocutor for exchanging ideas about plague's long history, and a constant source of support, encouragement, and friendship.

2 Gérard Chouin asks some of the same questions as they pertain to Africa in his chapter in this volume.

3 Following standard parameters for mountains, the study accepted an elevation over 500 meters and a slope of at least 5% as a mountain. See https://mapoe.stanford.edu/projects/environment-topographies-and-infrastructure.

4 Jerboas were recently spotted in several central and eastern cities in Turkey (e.g. in Sivas in August 2019, in Ankara in July 2020, in Amasya in September 2020, and in Şırnak in January 2021).
5 For a discussion of "dilution effect" hypothesis, that is, biodiversity conservation tends to lead to a decrease in infectious disease transmission, see for example, McCauley et al. (2015) and Keesing et al. (2006). For connections between biodiversity and infectious disease, including criticism of the hypothesis, see Young et al. (2017).
6 For example, published court records from late fifteenth-century Bursa point to the cluster of deaths of novice janissary boys in the outlying villages of Bursa. The date of the documents suggests that these deaths occurred at about the same time in a cluster of nearby villages (Varlık 2015, 149 n81).
7 For the plague death of individuals handling, buying, and selling flour in sixteenth-century Aleppo, see Mühimme Defteri 6, 55/114 (29 Muharrem 972 H./6 September 1564), published in Yılmaz and Yılmaz (2006, 2: 51).

References

Akar, Metin. 1987. "Şeyyad Hamza Hakkında Yeni Bilgiler." *Türklük Araştırmaları Dergisi* 2: 1–14.

Andrianaivoarimanana, Voahangy, Katharina Kreppel, Nohal Elissa, Jean-Marc Duplantier, Elisabeth Carniel, Minoarisoa Rajerison, and Ronan Jambou. 2013. "Understanding the Persistence of Plague Foci in Madagascar." *PLoS Neglected Tropical Diseases* 7, no. 11: e2382.

Appleby, Andrew B. 1980. "The Disappearance of Plague: A Continuing Puzzle." *The Economic History Review* 33, no. 2: 161–73.

Arslan, Atilla, Tarkan Yorulmaz, Kubilay Toyran, İrfan Albayrak, and Jan Zima. 2012. "C-Banding and Ag-NOR Distribution Patterns in Euphrates Jerboa, *Allactaga euphratica* (Mammalia: Rodentia), from Turkey." *Mammalia* 76, no. 4: 435–39.

Audoin-Rouzeau, Frédérique. 2003. *Les chemins de la peste: Le rat, la puce et l'homme*. Rennes: Presses universitaires de Rennes.

Ayalon, Yaron. Forthcoming. "When Nomads Meet Urbanites: The Outskirts of Ottoman Cities as a Venue for the Spread of Epidemic Diseases." In *Plagues in Nomadic Contexts: Historical Impact, Medical Responses, and Cultural Adaptations in Ancient to Mediaeval Eurasia*, edited by Kurt Franz, Ortrun Riha and Charlotte Schubert. Leiden: Brill.

Baltazard, M., M. Bahmanyar, Ch. Mofidi, and B. Seydian. 1952. "Le foyer de peste du Kurdistan." *Bulletin of the World Health Organization* 5, no. 4: 441–72.

Barbieri, Rémi, M. Drancourt, and D. Raoult. 2019. "Plague, Camels, and Lice." *Proceedings of the National Academy of Sciences* 116, no. 16: 7620–7621.

Ben-Ami, Ido. 2016. "The Expression of Wonder Regarding Animals in Ottoman Thought During the Early Modern Period." *Animals and Society* 54: 31–41 [in Hebrew].

Ben Néfissa, Kmar and Anne Marie Moulin. 2010. "La peste nordafricaine et la théorie de Charles Nicolle sur les maladies infectieuses." *Gesnerus-Swiss Journal of the History of Medicine and Sciences* 67, no. 1: 30–56.

Benedictow, Ole J. 2004. *The Black Death, 1346–1353: The Complete History*. Woodbridge: Boydell Press.

Benedictow, Ole J. 2021. *The Complete History of the Black Death*. Woodbridge: Boydell Press.

Bitam, Idir, Saravanan Ayyadurai, Tahar Kernif, Mohammed Chetta, Nabil Boulaghman, Didier Raoult and Michel Drancourt. 2010. "New Rural Focus of Plague, Algeria." *Emerging Infectious Diseases* 16, no. 10: 1639–40.

Blažina-Tomić, Zlata and Vesna Blažina. 2015. *Expelling the Plague: The Health Office and the Implementation of Quarantine in Dubrovnik, 1377–1533*. Montreal: McGill-Queen's University Press.

Borsch, Stuart J. 2005. *The Black Death in Egypt and England: A Comparative Study*. Austin: University of Texas Press.

Bos, Kirsten I., Alexander Herbig, Jason Sahl, Nicholas Waglechner, Mathieu Fourment, Stephen A. Forrest, Jennifer Klunk, Verena J Schuenemann, Debi Poinar, Melanie Kuch, G. Brian Golding, Olivier Dutour, Paul Keim, David M. Wagner, Edward C. Holmes, Johannes Krause and Hendrik N. Poinar. 2016. "Eighteenth-Century *Yersinia pestis* Genomes Reveal the Long-Term Persistence of an Historical Plague Focus." *eLife* 5: e12994.

Bramanti, Barbara, Yarong Wu, Ruifu Yang, Yujun Cui and Nils Chr. Stenseth. 2021. "Assessing the Origins of the European Plagues following the Black Death: A Synthesis of Genomic, Historical, and Ecological Information." *Proceedings of the National Academy of Sciences* 118, no. 36: e2101940118.

Buell, Paul D. 2012. "Qubilai and the Rats." *Sudhoffs Archiv* 96, no. 2: 127–44.

Carmichael, Ann G. 2014. "Plague Persistence in Western Europe: A Hypothesis." *The Medieval Globe* 1: 157–91.

Campbell, Bruce M. S. 2010. "Physical Shocks, Biological Hazards, and Human Impacts: The Crisis of the Fourteenth Century Revisited." In *Le Interazioni Fra Economia E Ambiente Biologico nell'Europa Preindustriale. Secc. XIII–XVIII (Economic and Biological Interactions in Pre-Industrial Europe from the 13th to the 18th Centuries)*, edited by Simonetta Cavaciocchi, 13–32. Florence: Firenze University Press.

Campbell, Bruce M. S. 2016. *The Great Transition: Climate, Disease and Society in the Late Medieval World*. Cambridge: Cambridge University Press.

Carlson, Colin J., Sarah N. Bevins, and Boris V. Schmid. 2021. "Plague Risk in the Western United States Over Seven Decades of Environmental Change." *Global Change Biology*. https://doi.org/10.1111/gcb.15966

Çelik, Semih. 2022. "Humans in Animalscapes: Reconstructing Vermin-Human Interactions in Rural Anatolia (c. 1600–1850)." *Diyâr: Journal of Ottoman, Turkish and Middle Eastern Studies*, special issue on "Human-Animal Encounters."

Chouin, Gérard, ed. 2018. *Sillages de la peste noire en Afrique subsaharienne: une exploration critique du silence / Black Death and Its Aftermaths in Sub-Saharan Africa: A Critical Exploration of Silence. Afriques* 9. https://journals.openedition.org/afriques/2084?lang=en

Çolak, Alper H. and Ian D. Rotherham. 2006. "A Review of the Forest Vegetation of Turkey: Its Status Past and Present and Its Future Conservation." *Biology and Environment: Proceedings of the Royal Irish Academy* 106 B, no. 3: 343–54.

Conrad, Lawrence I. 1981. "The Plague in the Early Medieval Near East." Unpublished PhD dissertation, Princeton University.

Crawshaw, Jane L. Stevens. 2012. *Plague Hospitals: Public Health for the City in Early Modern Venice*. Farnham: Ashgate.

Dean, Katharine R., Fabienne Krauer, Lars Walløe, Ole Christian Lingjærde, Barbara Bramanti, Nils Chr. Stenseth, and Boris V. Schmid. 2018. "Human Ectoparasites and Spread of Plague in Europe." *Proceedings of the National Academy of Sciences* 115, no. 6: 1304–9.

Dols, Michael W. 1977. *The Black Death in the Middle East*. Princeton, NJ: Princeton University Press.

Dernschwam, Hans. 1987. *İstanbul ve Anadolu'ya Seyahat Günlüğü*, translated by Yaşar Önen. Ankara: Kültür ve Turizm Bakanlığı.

Eckert, Edward E. 2000. "The Retreat of the Plague from Central Europe, 1640–1720: A Geomedical Approach." *Bulletin of the History of Medicine* 74, no. 1: 1–28.

Fancy, Nahyan and Monica H. Green. 2021. "Plague and the Fall of Baghdad (1258)." *Medical History* 65, no. 2: 157–77.

Faroqhi, Suraiya. 1984. *Towns and Townsmen of Ottoman Anatolia: Trade, Crafts, and Food Production in an Urban Setting, 1520–1650*. Cambridge: Cambridge University Press.

Faroqhi, Suraiya. 2010. *Animals and People in the Ottoman Empire*. Istanbul: Eren.

Feldman, Michal, Michaela Harbeck, Marcel Keller, Maria A. Spyrou, Andreas Rott, Bernd Trautmann, Holger C. Scholz, Bernd Päffgen, Joris Peters, Michael McCormick, Kirsten Bos, Alexander Herbig, and Johannes Krause. 2016. "A High-Coverage *Yersinia pestis* Genome from a Sixth-Century Justinianic Plague Victim." *Molecular Biology and Evolution* 33, no. 11: 2911–2923.

Foley, Janet E., Jennifer Zipser, Bruno Chomel, Evan Girvetz, and Patrick Foley. 2007. "Modeling Plague Persistence in Host-Vector Communities in California." *Journal of Wildlife Diseases* 43, no. 3: 408–24.

Frachetti, Michael D., C. Evan Smith, Cynthia M. Traub, and Tim Williams. 2017. "Nomadic Ecology Shaped the Highland Geography of Asia's Silk Roads." *Nature* 543, no. 7644: 193–198.

Gage, Kenneth L. and Michael Y. Kosoy. 2005. "Natural History of Plague: Perspectives from More than a Century of Research." *Annual Review of Entomology* 50, no. 1: 505–528.

Gage, Kenneth L., Thomas R. Burkot, Rebecca J. Eisen, and Edward B. Hayes. 2008. "Climate and Vectorborne Diseases." *American Journal of Preventive Medicine* 35: 436–450.

Green, Monica H. 2020. "The Four Black Deaths." *American Historical Review* 125, no. 5: 1600–1631.

Green, Monica H. 2018. "Climate and Disease in Medieval Eurasia." *Oxford Research Encyclopedia of Asian History*, edited by David Ludden. New York: Oxford University Press.

Green, Monica H., ed. 2014. "Pandemic Disease in the Medieval World: Rethinking the Black Death." *The Medieval Globe* 1.

Griffiths, Huw I., Kryštufek, Boris, and Jane M. Reed. 2013. *Balkan Biodiversity: Pattern and Process in the European Hotspot*. London: Kluwer Academic.

Guellil, Meriam, Oliver Kersten, Amine Namouchi, Stefania Luciani, Isolina Marota, Caroline A. Arcini, Elisabeth Iregren, Robert A. Lindemann, Gunnar Warfvinge, Lela Bakanidze, Lia Bitadze, Mauro Rubini, Paola Zaio, Monica Zaio, Damiano Neri, N. C. Stenseth, and Barbara Bramanti. 2020. "A Genomic and Historical Synthesis of Plague in 18th Century Eurasia." *Proceedings of the National Academy of Sciences* 117, no. 45: 28328–28335.

Hadjikyriacou, Antonis. 2011. "Society and Economy on an Ottoman Island: Cyprus in the Eighteenth Century." Unpublished PhD dissertation SOAS, University of London.

Haldon, John, Neil Roberts, Adam Izdebski, Dominik Fleitmann, Michael McCormick, Marica Cassis, Owen Doonan, Warren Eastwood, Hugh Elton, Sabine Ladstätter, Sturt Manning, James Newhard, Kathleen Nicoll, Ioannes Telelis, and Elena Xoplaki. 2014. "The Climate and Environment of Byzantine Anatolia: Integrating Science, History, and Archaeology." *Journal of Interdisciplinary History* 45, no. 2: 113–61.

Hamilton, William John. 1842. *Researches in Asia Minor, Pontus and Armenia: With Some Account of Their Antiquities and Geology.* London: J. Murray.

İnalcık, Halil and Donald Quataert, eds. 1994. *An Economic and Social History of the Ottoman Empire, 1300–1914*, vol. 1: 1300–1600 by Halil İnalcık. Cambridge: Cambridge University Press.

Jennings, Ronald. 1976. "Urban Population in Anatolia in the Sixteenth Century: A Study of Kayseri, Karaman, Amasya, Trabzon, and Erzurum." *International Journal of Middle East Studies* 7, no. 1: 21–57.

Jones, Lori. 2022. *Patterns of Plague: Changing Ideas about Plague in England and France, 1348–1750.* Montreal: McGill-Queen's University Press.

Kasaba, Reşat. 2009. *A Moveable Empire: Ottoman Nomads, Migrants, and Refugees.* Seattle: University of Washington Press.

Keesing, F, R. D. Holt, and R. S. Ostfeld. 2006. "Effects of Species Diversity on Disease Risk." *Ecology Letters* 9, no. 4: 485–98.

Konkola, Kari. 1992. "More Than a Coincidence? The Arrival of Arsenic and the Disappearance of Plague in Early Modern Europe." *Journal of the History of Medicine and Allied Sciences* 47, no. 2: 186–209.

Kroll, Henriette. 2012. "Animals in the Byzantine Empire: An Overview of the Archaeozoological Evidence." *Archeologia Medievale* 39: 93–121.

MacArthur, Robert H. and Edward O. Wilson. 1967. *Theory of Island Biogeography (MPB-1).* Princeton, NJ: Princeton University Press.

Malek, Maliya Alia, Idir Bitam, Anthony Levasseur, Jérôme Terras, Jean Gaudart, Said Azza, Christophe Flaudrops, Catherine Robert, Didier Raoult, and Michel Drancourt. 2017. "*Yersinia pestis* Halotolerance Illuminates Plague Reservoirs." *Scientific Reports* 7: 40022.

Markey, Lia. 2016. *Imagining the Americas in Medici Florence.* University Park: Penn State University Press.

McCauley, Douglas J., Daniel J. Salkeld, Hillary S. Young, Rhodes Makundi, Rudolfo Dirzo, Ralph P. Eckerlin, Eric F. Lambin, Lynne Gaffikin, Michele Barry, and Kristofer M. Helgen. 2015. "Effects of Land Use on Plague (*Yersinia pestis*) Activity in Rodents in Tanzania." *The American Journal of Tropical Medicine and Hygiene* 92, no. 4: 776–83.

McCormick, Michael. 2003. "Rats, Communications, and Plague: Toward an Ecological History." *The Journal of Interdisciplinary History* 34, no. 1: 1–25.

McNeill, John Robert. 1992. *The Mountains of the Mediterranean World: An Environmental History.* Cambridge: Cambridge University Press.

Michaux, J. R., R. Libois, E. Paradis, and M.-G. Filipucci. 2004. "Phylogeographic History of the Yellow-Necked Fieldmouse (*Apodemus flavicollis*) in Europe and in the Near and Middle East." *Molecular Phylogenetics and Evolution* 32, no. 3: 788–98.

Mikhail, Alan. 2012. *Nature and Empire in Ottoman Egypt: An Environmental History.* Cambridge: Cambridge University Press

Mikhail, Alan. 2013. *The Animal in Ottoman Egypt.* Oxford: Oxford University Press.

Morozova, Irina, Artem Kasianov, Sergey Bruskin, Judith Neukamm, Martyna Molak, Elena Batieva, Aleksandra Pudło, Frank J. Rühli, and Verena J. Schuenemann. 2020. "New Ancient Eastern European *Yersinia pestis* Genomes Illuminate the Dispersal of Plague in Europe." *Philosophical Transactions of the Royal Society B*, 375: 20190569.

Namouchi, Amine, Meriam Guellil, Oliver Kersten, Stephanie Hänsch, Claudio Ottoni, Boris V. Schmid, Elsa Pacciani, Luisa Quaglia, Marco Vermunt, Egil L. Bauer, Michael Derrick, Anne Ø. Jensen, Sacha Kacki, Samuel K. Cohn Jr., Nils C. Stenseth, and Barbara Bramanti. 2018. "Integrative Approach Using *Yersinia pestis* Genomes to Revisit the Historical Landscape of Plague during the Medieval Period." *Proceedings of the National Academy of Sciences* 115, no. 50: E11790–E11797.

Newfield, Timothy P. 2009. "A Cattle Panzootic in Early Fourteenth-Century Europe." *Agricultural History Review* 57, no. 2: 155–90.

Onur, Ayhan. 1962. "Türkiyede Daimi Kar Sınırı Hakkında." *Ankara Üniversitesi Dil ve Tarih Coğrafya Fakültesi Dergisi* 20, nos. 1–2: 119–23.

Panzac, Daniel. 1985. *La peste dans l'empire ottoman, 1700–1850*. Louvain: Édition Peeters.

Parker, Geoffrey. 2013. *Global Crisis: War, Climate and Catastrophe in the Seventeenth Century*. New Haven, CT: Yale University Press.

Parmenter, R. R., E. P. Yadav, C. A. Parmenter, P. Ettestad, and K. L. Gage. 1999. "Incidence of Plague Associated with Increased Winter-Spring Precipitation in New Mexico." *The American Journal of Tropical Medicine and Hygiene* 61, no. 5: 814–21.

Rasmussen, Simon, Morten Erik Allentoft, Kasper Nielsen, Ludovic Orlando, Martin Sikora, Karl-Göran Sjögren, Anders Gorm Pedersen, Mikkel Schubert, Alex Van Dam, Christian Moliin Outzen Kapel, Henrik Bjørn Nielsen, Søren Brunak, Pavel Avetisyan, Andrey Epimakhov, Mikhail Viktorovich Khalyapin, Artak Gnuni, Aivar Kriiska, Irena Lasak, Mait Metspalu, Vyacheslav Moiseyev, Andrei Gromov, Dalia Pokutta, Lehti Saag Liivi Varul, Levon Yepiskoposyan, Thomas Sicheritz-Pontén, Robert A. Foley, Marta Mirazón Lahr, Rasmus Nielsen, Kristian Kristiansen, and Eske Willerslev. 2015. "Early Divergent Strains of *Yersinia pestis* in Eurasia 5,000 Years Ago." *Cell* 163, no. 3: 571–82.

Ruffino, Lise and Eric Vidal. 2010. "Early Colonization of Mediterranean Islands by *Rattus rattus*: A Review of Zooarcheological Data." *Biological Invasions* 12: 2389–2394.

Russell, Alexander and Patrick Russell. 1794. *The Natural History of Aleppo: Containing a Description of the City, and the Principal Natural Productions in Its Neighbourhood: Together with an Account of the Climate, Inhabitants, and Diseases, Particularly of the Plague*. 2 Volumes. London: Printed for G. G. and J. Robinson.

Schamiloglu, Uli. 2004. "The Rise of the Ottoman Empire: The Black Death in Medieval Anatolia and Its Impact on Turkish Civilization." In *Views from the Edge: Essays in Honor of Richard W. Bulliet*, edited by Neguin Yavari, Lawrence G. Potter, and Jean-Marc Ran Oppenheim, 255–79. New York: Columbia University Press.

Schmid, Boris V., M. Jesse, L. I. Wilschut, H. Viljugrein, and J. A. P. Heesterbeek. 2012. "Local Persistence and Extinction of Plague in a Metapopulation of Great Gerbil Burrows, Kazakhstan." *Epidemics* 4, no. 4: 211–18.

Schmid, Boris V., Ulf Büntgen, W. Ryan Easterday, Christian Ginzler, Lars Walløe, Barbara Bramanti, and Nils Ch. Stenseth. 2015. "Climate-Driven Introduction of the Black Death and Successive Plague Reintroductions into Europe." *Proceedings of the National Academy of Sciences* 112, no. 10: 3020–3025.

Schwartz, Mark W., Louis R. Iverson, Anantha M. Prasad, Stephen N. Matthews, and Raymond J. O'Connor. 2006. "Predicting Extinctions as a Result of Climate Change." *Ecology* 87, no. 7: 1611–1615.

Seifert, Lisa, Ingrid Wiechmann, Michaela Harbeck, Astrid Thomas, Gisela Grupe, Michaela Projahn, Holger C. Scholz, and Julia M. Riehm. 2016. "Genotyping *Yersinia pestis* in Historical Plague: Evidence for Long-Term Persistence of *Y. Pestis* in Europe from the 14th to the 17th Century." *PLoS ONE* 11, no. 1: e0145194.

Şekercioğlu, Çağan H., Sean Anderson, Erol Akçay, Raşit Bilgin, Özgün Emre Can, Gürkan Semiz, Çağatay Tavşanoğlu, Mehmet Baki Yokeşi, Anıl Soyumert, Kahraman İpekdal, İsmail K. Sağlam, Mustafa Yücel, and H. Nüzhet Dalfes. 2011. "Turkey's Globally Important Biodiversity in Crisis." *Biological Conservation* 144, no. 12: 2752–2769.

Slack, Paul. 1981. "The Disappearance of Plague: An Alternative View." *The Economic History Review* 34, no. 3: 469–76.

Slavin, Philip. 2012. "The Great Bovine Pestilence and Its Economic and Environmental Consequences in England and Wales, 1318–501." *The Economic History Review* 65, no. 4: 1239–66.

Slavin, Philip. 2021. "Out of the West: Formation of a Permanent Plague Reservoir in South-Central Germany (1349–1356) and Its Implications." *Past & Present* 252, no. 1: 3–51.

Spyrou, Maria A., Rezeda I. Tukhbatova, Michal Feldman, Joanna Drath, Sacha Kacki, Julia Beltrán de Heredia, Susanne Arnold, Airat G. Sitdikov, Dominique Castex, Joachim Wahl, Ilgizar R. Gazimzyanov, Danis K. Nurgaliev, Alexander Herbig, Kirsten I. Bos, and Johannes Krause. 2016. "Historical *Y. pestis* Genomes Reveal the European Black Death as the Source of Ancient and Modern Plague Pandemics." *Cell Host and Microbe* 19, no. 6: 874–81.

Spyrou, Maria A., Rezeda I. Tukhbatova, Chuan-Chao Wang, Aida Andrades Valtueña, Aditya K. Lankapalli, Vitaly V. Kondrashin, Victor A. Tsybin, Aleksandr Khokhlov, Denise Kühnert, Alexander Herbig, Kirsten I. Bos, and Johannes Krause. 2018. "Analysis of 3800-Year-Old *Yersinia pestis* Genomes Suggests Bronze Age Origin for Bubonic Plague." *Nature Communications* 9, no. 1: 1–10.

Spyrou, Maria A , Marcel Keller, Rezeda I. Tukhbatova, Christiana L. Scheib, Elizabeth A. Nelson, Aida Andrades Valtueña, Gunnar U. Neumann, Don Walker, Amelie Alterauge, Niamh Carty, Craig Cessford, Hermann Fetz, Michaël Gourvennec, Robert Hartle, Michael Henderson, Kristin von Heyking, Sarah A. Inskip, Sacha Kacki, Felix M. Key, Elizabeth L. Knox, Christian Later, Prishita Maheshwari-Aplin, Joris Peters, John E. Robb, Jürgen Schreiber, Toomas Kivisild, Dominique Castex, Sandra Lösch, Michaela Harbeck, Alexander Herbig, Kirsten I. Bos, and Johannes Krause. 2019. "Phylogeography of the Second Plague Pandemic Revealed through Analysis of Historical *Yersinia pestis* Genomes." *Nature Communications* 10, no. 4470.

Tabak, Faruk. 2008. *The Waning of the Mediterranean, 1550–1870: A Geohistorical Approach*. Baltimore, MD: Johns Hopkins University Press.

Telelis, Ioannis G. 2008. "Climatic Fluctuations in the Eastern Mediterranean and the Middle East, AD 300–1500 from Byzantine Documentary and Proxy Physical Paleoclimatic Evidence: A Comparison." *Jahrbuch der Österreichischen Byzantinistik* 58: 167–208.

Telelis, Ioannis G. 2005. "Historical-Climatological Information from the Time of the Byzantine Empire (4th–15th Centuries AD)." *History of Meteorology* 2: 41–50.

Valtueña, Aida Andrades, Alissa Mittnik, Felix M. Key, Wolfgang Haak, Raili All-mäe, Andrej Belinskij, Mantas Daubaras, Michal Feldman, Rimantas Jankauskas, Ivor Janković, Ken Massy, Mario Novak, Saskia Pfrengle, Sabine Reinhold, Mario Šlaus, Maria A. Spyrou, Anna Szécsényi-Nagy, Mari Tõrv, Svend Hansen, Kirsten I. Bos, Philipp W. Stockhammer, Alexander Herbig, and Johannes Krause. 2017. "The Stone Age Plague: 1000 Years of Persistence in Eurasia." *Current Biology* 27, no. 23: 3683–3691.

Varlık, Nükhet. 2014a. "New Science and Old Sources: Why the Ottoman Experience of Plague Matters." *The Medieval Globe* 1: 193–227.

Varlık, Nükhet. 2014b. "Plague, Conflict, and Negotiation: The Jewish Broadcloth Weavers of Salonica and the Ottoman Central Administration in the Late Sixteenth Century." *Jewish History* 28, nos. 3–4: 261–88.

Varlık, Nükhet. 2015. *Plague and Empire in the Early Modern Mediterranean World: The Ottoman Experience, 1347–1600.* Cambridge: Cambridge University Press.

Varlık, Nükhet. 2017. "'Oriental Plague' or Epidemiological Orientalism?: Revisiting the Plague Episteme of the Early Modern Mediterranean." In *Plague and Contagion in the Islamic Mediterranean*, edited by Nükhet Varlık, 57–87. Kalamazoo, MI: Arc Humanities Press.

Varlık, Nükhet. 2020a. "The Plague That Never Left: Restoring the Second Pandemic to Ottoman and Turkish History in the Time of COVID-19." *New Perspectives on Turkey* 63: 176–89.

Varlık, Nükhet. 2020b. "Rethinking the History of Plague in the Time of COVID-19." *Centaurus* 62, no. 2: 285–93.

Vogler, Amy J., Fabien Chan, David M. Wagner, Philippe Roumagnac, Judy Lee, Roxanne Nera, Mark Eppinger, Jacques Ravel, Lila Rahalison, Bruno W. Rasoamanana, Stephen M. Beckstrom-Sternberg, Mark Achtman, Suzanne Chanteau, and Paul Keim 2011. "Phylogeography and Molecular Epidemiology of *Yersinia pestis* in Madagascar." *PLoS Neglected Tropical Diseases* 5, no. 9: e1319.

White, Sam. 2011. *The Climate of Rebellion in the Early Modern Ottoman Empire.* Cambridge: Cambridge University Press.

White, Sam. 2012. "The Little Ice Age Crisis of the Ottoman Empire: A Conjuncture in Middle East Environmental History." In *Water on Sand: Environmental Histories of the Middle East and North Africa*, edited by Alan Mikhail, 71–90. Oxford: Oxford University Press.

Wimsatt, Jeffrey and Dean E. Biggins. 2009. "A Review of Plague Persistence with Special Emphasis on Fleas." *Journal of Vector Borne Diseases* 46, no. 2: 85–99.

Wrobel, Murray. 2006. *Elsevier's Dictionary of Mammals.* Amsterdam: Elsevier.

Xoplaki, Elena, Dominik Fleitmann, Juerg Luterbacher, Sebastian Wagner, John F. Haldon, Eduardo Zorita, Ioannis Telelis, Andrea Toreti, and Adam Izdebski. 2016. "The Medieval Climate Anomaly and Byzantium: A Review of the Evidence on Climatic Fluctuations, Economic Performance and Societal Change." *Quaternary Science Reviews*, Special Issue: Mediterranean Holocene Climate, Environment and Human Societies, 136: 229–52.

Yaycıoğlu, Ali. 2022. "Ottoman Montology: Hazardous Resourcefulness and Uneasy Symbiosis in a Mountain Empire." In *Crafting History: Essays on the Ottoman World and Beyond in Honor of Cemal Kafadar*, edited by Ali Yaycıoğlu, Ilham Khuri-Makdisi, and Rachel Goshgarian, 351–80. Brookline, MA: Academic Studies Press.

Yılmaz, K. Tuluhan. 1997. "Ecological Diversity of the Eastern Mediterranean Region of Turkey and Its Conservation." *Biodiversity and Conservation* 7, no. 1: 87–96.

Coşkun Yılmaz and Necdet Yılmaz, eds. 2006. *Osmanlılarda Sağlık*. 2 Volumes. Istanbul: Biofarma.

Young, Hillary S.. Chelsea L. Wood, A. Marm Kilpatrick, Kevin D. Lafferty, Charles L. Nunn and Jeffrey R. Vincent. 2017. "Conservation, Biodiversity and Infectious Disease: Scientific Evidence and Policy Implications." *Philosophical Transactions of the Royal Society B* 372, no. 1722.

Zell, Roland. 2004. "Global Climate Change and the Emergence/Re-emergence of Infectious Diseases." *International Journal of Medical Microbiology* 293, Suppl 37: 16–26.

9 Survival in the Context of Urbanization and Environmental Change in Medieval and Early Modern London, England

Sharon N. DeWitte

Introduction

Medieval and Early Modern Crises in England

Medieval and early modern populations in England experienced repeated, widespread, and severe famines and disease epidemics.[1] Famine is the widespread shortage of or restricted access to food. It may have natural causes, such as the underproduction of crops resulting from drought conditions or the destruction of crops by plant diseases. It also can be artificially produced by human actions (i.e., it can be anthropogenic), such as the withholding of or purposeful destruction of food during times of conflict (Sen 1981). Epidemics are sudden increases in the number of cases of a disease within a population relative to the typical baseline number of cases under normal circumstances. Famine and infectious disease epidemics are often synergistically connected: malnutrition can reduce the effectiveness of human immune responses (Scrimshaw 2003), and thus famine conditions can increase susceptibility to, and the severity of, various diseases. As a result, infectious diseases are the primary cause of death during famines (Mokyr and Ó Gráda 2002).

In England, there were back-to-back harvest failures in 1256–58; this led to a famine in 1258. The severity of this famine is estimated to have been on par with that of the later, and generally more well-known, Great Famine of 1315–17 (Campbell 2016). The Great Famine killed approximately 10%–15% of the population of England and Wales, and had effects across the European continent (Campbell 2016; Hoyle 2017; Jordan 1996; Keene 2011). This was soon followed by the Great Bovine Pestilence (1319–20), an epidemic among animals (epizootic) that killed approximately 62% of bovines (cows, bulls, oxen, etc.) in England and Wales (Slavin 2012). In addition to having an immediate negative effect on available food resources, the Great Bovine Pestilence resulted in long-term dairy and animal protein deprivations that lasted until the early 1330s (DeWitte and Slavin 2013; Slavin 2012). These early fourteenth-century famines were soon followed by (and may have played a role in the severity of) catastrophic plague epidemics. The Black Death arrived in southern England in 1348 and spread across the entire length of

DOI: 10.4324/9780429055478-13

the country within approximately eighteen months. An estimated 30%–60% of the human population died in its wake (DeWitte and Kowaleski 2017). Genetic analyses of people who died during the Black Death have confirmed the long-held assumption that they suffered through an outbreak of bubonic plague, which is caused by a bacterium, *Yersinia pestis*, that continues to cause disease and death in human populations today (Bos et al. 2011; Haensch et al. 2010). This same pathogen was the cause of recurrent epidemics in England and elsewhere across Afro-Eurasia during the multi-century Second Plague Pandemic (Spyrou et al. 2016). The last major outbreak of plague in England was the so-called Great Plague in 1665–66 that killed an estimated 20% of London's population. The disease did not completely disappear for another century or so (Cummins et al. 2016).

Recent scholarship has linked several of these crises – famine and epidemic disease – to changes in global climatic conditions. In the mid-thirteenth century, the end of about 200 years of sustained high solar irradiance resulted in unstable and unseasonable weather in England (and more broadly) that caused the back-to-back harvest failures. This, in turn, produced famine conditions in 1258 (Campbell 2017). In 1257, the Samalas volcano on Lombok Island (Indonesia) erupted and released such a large amount of volcanic sulphur into the stratosphere that it ranks as one of the most significant volcanic events in the last 7,000 years (Lavigne et al. 2013; Mutaqin and Lavigne 2021). The eruption produced significant climatic effects such as cooler temperatures, particularly in the Northern Hemisphere. These effects were most pronounced in 1258 and persisted for 4–5 years after the eruption (Stoffel et al. 2015). This cataclysm and its effects post-date the beginning of the harvest failures that led to the terrible famine in 1258 and, thus, cannot be solely to blame for it. However, the cooling of temperatures in Northern Europe that the volcanic eruption likely caused might have led to continued crop failures, thereby extending pre-existing famine conditions and pushing mortality rates to extraordinarily high levels (Campbell 2017; Guillet et al. 2017).

Scholars have also linked the subsequent fourteenth-century crises to dramatic climate changes associated with the end of the Medieval Climate Anomaly in the 1270s and the beginning of the Little Ice Age. The period from the late thirteenth through fourteenth centuries was characterized by highly erratic weather patterns. Severe summertime storms in the North Atlantic led, in some years, to poor harvests and widespread famines across parts of Europe (Brooke 2014; Büntgen et al. 2011). Climate conditions during the Little Ice Age (c. 1300–1800) were also unstable, and European populations during this long period experienced periodic harvest failures, dramatically cold winters, and other climate-induced stressors (Appleby 1980; Brooke 2014; Williams and Larsen 2017).

Analysis of famines in several European countries from 1250 to the present (Alfani and Ó Gráda 2018) reveals a high frequency of famines immediately prior to the fourteenth-century Black Death, but relatively few famines for about 200 years afterward. This decrease in the frequency of famines in the aftermath of the epidemic likely reflects the substantially decreased population sizes and, thus, reduced population pressures that resulted from the Black Death. In other words, the factors that affect the ability of the environment to support a population's survival, e.g., via food availability, actually improved after the Black Death because the population was smaller.

All of these medieval and early modern crises occurred at a time of dramatic social inequality and, in London, of increasing urbanization. Greater urbanization, in turn, might have exacerbated the negative effects of social inequality. There is abundant evidence of the health effects of wealth inequality in living and past populations. Heterogeneity (variation) exists even within socioeconomic status levels; that is, the costs and benefits associated with socioeconomic status are not necessarily uniformly experienced by all people of a particular status but may be mediated by factors such as gender, sexuality, social race, and immigrant status. Nonetheless, in general, studies in living populations have shown that people of higher status are more likely to have access to health-promoting factors, such as sufficient and nourishing food, health education, and medical care. These individuals are also less likely to, among other things, live in overcrowded and polluted conditions or be the victims of violent crimes (Chen and Miller 2012; Evans and Kantrowitz 2002). There is evidence that even in populations with high general levels of wealth, inequality has negative effects on overall population health. For example, Suk and colleagues (2009) found that in European countries, wealth inequality was related to the prevalence of tuberculosis in 2006. That is, the greater the wealth inequality in a country, the higher its rates of tuberculosis. Increasing social inequality throughout medieval England, combined with a long-term trend of population growth prior to the Black Death (though with brief episodes of decline produced by crises), meant that a large proportion of the population was living in or near poverty. Since food crises disproportionately increased mortality rates among lower socioeconomic status people in pre-industrial populations (Hayward et al. 2012), the growth in the proportion of the medieval population that was low status likely compounded the population-level negative effects of famine until the Black Death.

Urbanization (the process whereby an increasing proportion of a population moves from rural areas to cities) and urban growth (increases in the population size and the geographic area of cities) also can have deleterious effects on human health. There are certainly benefits to living in cities today, such as enhanced access to health and social services, and better infrastructure for sanitation and water treatment. Indeed, several studies have found that standards of living and health conditions, as indicated by risks of mortality and life expectancy, for example, are generally better in cities today compared to surrounding rural areas in many areas of the world (Harpham 2009; Storper and Scott 2016; Thu Le and Booth 2014; Vlahov et al. 2007; Young 2013). However, these general population-level trends mask a tremendous amount of heterogeneity that exists within cities (e.g., Ezeh et al. 2017; Jian et al.

2019), and many of these positive aspects of urban living are relatively new phenomena associated with modernization.

During the period addressed in this chapter, England experienced a general trend of increasing urbanization. By 1300, approximately one-eighth of the total population lived in urban areas. London was the largest city in England at the time. With an estimated population size between 40,000 and 100,000, it housed about 2% of the total population (Campbell 2016; Jordan 1996; Keene 1989). By 1700, an estimated 10% of the population of England lived in London (Keene 1989). For both medieval and early modern London, it is likely that many inhabitants were at some risk of suffering from the negative consequences of living in an urban environment. Walter and DeWitte (2017) found, for example, that adults (at least females) in medieval London faced higher risks of death compared to those living at the same time in a rural environment elsewhere in England. The possible negative effects associated with urban contexts included: overcrowded housing conditions that favoured the spread of diseases reliant upon direct human-to-human transmission, contaminated water sources resulting in the spread of faecal-oral route diseases, insufficient waste disposal leading to the accumulation of garbage and human and animal waste – which attracts and sustains rodent and insect populations that spread numerous diseases. City dwellers also had no ability to produce most of their own food sources, making them vulnerable to food shortages. Altogether, the interaction of shifting climatic conditions, urbanization, infectious disease epidemics, and famine during the medieval and early modern periods might have powerfully shaped patterns of health and demography of people living in urban areas. Not all inhabitants of the city experienced the effects of these conditions equally. Evidence from seventeenth-century historical documents suggests that in wealthy urban parishes, births outpaced deaths, leading to increases in the population of those parishes (at least in years without plague epidemics). In poor parishes, by contrast, deaths exceeded births (making these areas so-called "demographic sinks") (Cummins et al. 2016). These varying patterns suggest that poorer inhabitants of London suffered disproportionately from the deleterious conditions associated with urbanization.

The scale of mortality that occurred during plague epidemics and famines in medieval and early modern England was not unique. They are examples of crisis mortality, a dramatic but temporary increase in mortality rate above the baseline level resulting from a single extraordinary factor. It can be caused by a variety of events, such as disease epidemics, famines, floods, and warfare (Bengtsson and Gagnon 2011; Bouckaert 1989; Sawchuk et al. 2013). The periodic mortality crises that affected England are, according to some scholars such as Omran (1971), typical of pre-industrial agricultural populations. They appear to have dominated pre-industrial population dynamics prior to relatively recent demographic transitions that occurred earliest in northern Europe approximately 300 years ago (Gage 2005; Wood 1998). Crisis mortality persists as an important phenomenon in many living populations today, particularly in lower-income countries (Baro and Deubel 2006; Wisner 2004). Given that crisis mortality likely shaped the lives of the majority of people in a variety of contexts around the world since the adoption of agriculture approximately 10,000 years ago, it is crucial to clarify the effects that these crises have had on human health and survival if we are to truly understand the full scope of human experience for much of our recent history. Such information is also relevant to understanding the experiences of, and potentially improving conditions within, living populations that have not undergone industrialization and modernization and that are, therefore, vulnerable to some of the same environmental, climatological, and human-produced hazards that existed in the past.

Bioarchaeological Research on Medieval England

Bioarchaeology is the study of human skeletal remains excavated from archaeological sites. The human skeleton is made up of living tissue that changes over both the short-term and the life course. Changes to the skeleton occur in response to homeostatic mechanisms that keep our bodies in balance, hormones associated with growth and reproductive functions, the stressors we inflict upon ourselves, the diseases and disorders from which we suffer, the chemicals to which we are exposed through our diets and the broader environment, and the normal wear and tear that occurs as a consequence of aging. Macroscopic, histological (microscopic), and molecular analyses of the skeleton provide information about biological sex (though see details below about the limitations thereof), age-at-death, body size, habitual activity patterns, infectious and non-communicable diseases, traumatic injury, nutritional status, dietary composition, and migration. The human skeleton, however, reflects more than just biological and physical conditions: it also reveals much about the sociocultural factors and structures that affect us, including racism, sexism, and socioeconomic inequality. This embodiment – i.e., the process by which social forces shape and are recorded by our physical bodies (Krieger 2005, 1999) – means that human skeletal remains can provide evidence of biosocial lives long after people have died and reveal a wider range of human experiences in the past than is possible using historical documents. Indeed, human skeletal remains provide the only source of information for many people who lived in the past and the environments in which they lived.

Previous bioarchaeological research focusing on human skeletons excavated from medieval cemeteries in London and dated to 1000–1540 revealed evidence of important changes in demography and health before and after the Black Death (DeWitte 2018, 2015). Prior to the Black Death, the population, in general, experienced declines in survivorship (i.e., people were not living as long) in the thirteenth century compared to the eleventh and twelfth centuries. At the same time, their bones exhibit increases in the frequencies of skeletal pathologies indicative of malnutrition, infectious disease, and other harmful conditions. Together, these findings indicate that there were declines in human health in the thirteenth century. It is possible that this downward trend in health explains, at least in part, why so many people died during the Black Death. That is, poor health for a large number of people in the time period right before the Black Death might have made the epidemic deadlier than it would have been if the population had been experiencing better health conditions. These studies also found that there were improvements in survivorship and changes in the frequency of several skeletal pathological conditions that suggest that health improved, in general, following the Black Death in the period from 1350 to 1540 (DeWitte 2018, 2014a, 2014b). These changes might reflect a short-term harvesting effect; i.e., the Black Death killed a large proportion of unhealthy people, leaving a population that consisted of relatively healthy people. Alternatively, they might suggest a longer-term selective effect, that is, the Black Death might have acted as a force of natural selection and, thus, favoured or disfavoured genetic variations associated with disease susceptibility or immune competence. This could have had effects across multiple generations. Finally, these changes might reflect improvements in the standards of living that followed the epidemic.

These findings raise the following questions: Were the improvements in health produced by improvements in the environment, especially in urban living conditions, that are described in contemporary written records (see details below)? Did the apparent improvements in health enjoyed by survivors of the epidemic last for only a generation or two after the epidemic? Were improvements in health the result of more fundamental changes to human biology or genetic composition (particularly in regions of the genome associated with disease susceptibility or immune competence) and therefore much more long-lasting? Further, were there any differences in survival between the sexes across the medieval and early modern periods? There are, in many living and past populations, important differences between the sexes with respect to immune competence, access to resources, and other factors that influence health and survival. There is also certainly evidence from the medieval period of sex differences in risks of death (DeWitte and Yaussy 2020; Walter and DeWitte 2017; Yaussy et al. 2016). This chapter expands on preliminary findings (DeWitte 2017) and uses data from human skeletal remains dated to the medieval and early modern periods in London to address these questions.

Materials and Methods

This chapter synthesizes previous bioarchaeological research and new (previously unpublished) analyses of temporal trends in survivorship at the time of these crises using a combined sample of 1431 adult skeletons from several medieval and early modern London cemeteries. Excavation of these human skeletal remains was licensed by the Ministry of Justice of England. All of the research reported here was done in full compliance with the ethical guidelines regarding the treatment of human remains established by the Church of England and English Heritage (which specifically pertain to remains from Christian burial grounds dating to the seventh to nineteenth centuries) and by professional anthropological associations (regarding research on human skeletal remains in general). Specifically, the human skeletal remains were treated with dignity and respect, and the research was not done in opposition to the wishes of living family or community members.

Skeletal Samples

The human skeletal remains used for this study come from the following London cemeteries: St. Nicholas Shambles (*c.* eleventh to twelfth centuries), Guildhall Yard (*c.* 1050–1230), St. Mary Graces (*c.* 1350–1538), St. Mary Spital (*c.* 1120–1540), and the New Churchyard (*c.* 1569–1739) (Bowsher et al. 2007; Connell et al. 2012; Grainger and Phillpotts 2011; Schofield 1997; White and Dyson 1988). All of the individuals included in this study were assigned, based on stratigraphy (i.e., the relative position of an object within layers of soil in the cemetery) or radiometric dating (based on the amount of radioactive carbon-14 present in a sample), to one of five time periods: 1000–1200 (n = 285), 1200–1250 (n = 302), 1350–1540 (n = 351), 1569–1670 (n = 308), and 1670–1739 (n = 182). While there are burials in St. Mary Spital that date to the period between 1250 and 1350, it is not possible to distinguish burials in that period associated with normal causes of death from those associated with the Black Death or other crises. Since the focus of this study is on patterns of mortality under normal conditions, these burials were excluded from analysis.

These samples include a mix of people of all ages and sexes, individuals of lower and higher socioeconomic status, laity, and monks and other members of the religious community. In order to ensure that the results of the analyses reported here reflect normal urban mortality patterns as closely as possible, the samples exclude burials from St. Mary Graces that are associated with a plague epidemic in 1361 (Bos et al. 2016; Gilchrist and Sloane 2005), mass burials from St. Mary Spital that are putative famine or plague burials (Connell et al. 2012), and mass burials from the New Churchyard that were likely seventeenth-century plague burials (Hartle et al. 2017).

Estimation of Age and Sex

The individuals included in this study were excavated from medieval Christian cemeteries, but none were retrieved from burials with grave markers nor are there any existing associated burial records that allow for their sex or ages at the time of death to be determined. Therefore, it was necessary to estimate each individual's age and (in the case of adults) sex from various skeletal features.

Ages for adults (i.e., those people who had completed skeletal growth) were estimated, based on features of the pelvis and skull that change with age, using an approach called transition analysis that was developed to overcome some of the limitations associated with conventional methods (Boldsen et al. 2002). In particular, transition analysis avoids a problem called "age mimicry" whereby conventionally estimated ages are biased toward the age distribution of the known–age-at-death samples that are used to develop age-estimation methods. This problem with conventional methods undermines confidence that estimated age-at-death patterns are truly revealing anything real about a past population. Conventional methods also lump all older (appearing) people into a single open-ended age category (e.g., 45+), which obscures potentially interesting variation that might occur at those older ages. In contrast, transition analysis allows age estimation for all ages, even the oldest ages, and thus enables the examination of patterns that occur among the elderly in a way not possible with conventional methods.

Ages for non–adult individuals (i.e., individuals who had not yet completed skeletal growth) were estimated based on the developmental stages of the bones (i.e., epiphyseal fusion), and dental development and eruption (Buikstra and Ubelaker 1994; Gustafson and Koch 1974; Moorrees et al. 1969; Scheuer et al. 1980; Scheuer and Black 2000; Smith 1991). For this study, non-adults were included only for estimation of the fertility proxy (a measure that reflects the numbers of offspring produced in a population), as described below, and were not included in estimates of adult survivorship. In order to compare the results of this study with those obtained by previous studies, Kaplan–Meier survival analysis (see below) was performed only on adults 15 years of age and above.

Sex was estimated, only for adults, based on features of the skull and pelvis that have been shown to appear more often in one sex than in the other. For this study, sex was estimated using the standards described in Buikstra and Ubelaker (1994) for multiple sexually dimorphic features of the skull and pelvis. The use of multiple skeletal indicators of sex improves the accuracy of sex estimation (Meindl et al. 1985; Rogers 2005; Walker 2008; Williams and Rogers 2006). However, because estimates of sex based on features of the pelvis have been shown to be more accurate than those based on features of the skull (Meindl et al. 1985; Walrath et al. 2004), for individuals in this study for which the skull and pelvis indicated different sexes, the pelvic scores were used in favour of those for the skull. Individuals for whom a sex estimation was not possible (i.e., those of indeterminate sex) were excluded from analysis. The possible presence of misclassified individuals within the samples used for this study would tend to underestimate the true differences between the sexes in temporal patterns of survivorship, assuming such differences exist.[2]

Estimation of Variation in Survival

As alluded to above, population-level estimates of life expectancy (how long on average people can expect to live in a particular context) can provide a general measure of the health of that population. In populations with high standards of living (as measured by such things as access to and rates of use of medical care, educational attainment, nutritional status, and per capital expenditure per household) and good health, people tend to suffer lower risks of mortality and live longer, on average, compared to people living in populations with lower standards of living and poorer general health. One way to assess longevity (i.e., long life) as a measure of health in past and present populations is the application of Kaplan–Meier survival analysis. This allows one to use data on age-at-death to estimate the proportion of the population that survives (or survived) to each age. This approach does not require the estimation of parameters (i.e., it is non-parametric), which makes it suitable for the small sample sizes that are typical of bioarchaeological research (parametric models, in contrast, require relatively large samples sizes). For this study, Kaplan–Meier survival analysis was used to assess temporal trends in survivorship for adults 15 years or older; comparisons were made across the five time periods detailed above and patterns were assessed separately for males and females to discern whether sex affected survival outcomes.

Fertility proxy (D_{30+}/D_{5+}): The use of skeletal samples from past populations to estimate demographic patterns and, by inference, the health of those populations is not a straightforward endeavour. Because most cemeteries are used for multiple generations, all the people in a skeletal sample who died at a particular age were not necessarily born at the same time. Imagine, for example, a cemetery used from 1900 to 2000. People buried in that cemetery who died at the age of thirty could have been born any time between 1870 and 1970. Even though they all died at the same age, their life experiences would have been very different depending on their years of birth. Some of those people would have lived their entire lives prior to the discovery of antibiotics, others experienced the 1918–1919 influenza pandemic, and still others lived through the Great Depression or, conversely, were born during times of economic growth. There is a tremendous amount of variation in experiences that might not be obvious or that is perhaps totally undetectable from aggregate patterns in a cemetery sample.

One problem, in particular, that must be considered when using age-at-death in skeletal samples to infer survival, and thus health, is the effect that changes in fertility rates over time can have on demographic patterns. Research has shown that changes in fertility (the number of offspring born into a population) can alter age-at-death distributions even if age-specific mortality remains unchanged over the same period. In fact, changes in fertility have a stronger effect on age-at-death distributions than do changes in mortality of the same magnitude (Milner et al. 1989; Paine 1989; Sattenspiel and Harpending 1983). For example, if fertility increases over time while age-specific mortality remains constant, an increasing number of infants will face those mortality risks each year and, thus, an increasing number will die annually and be buried in a cemetery. This, in turn, would skew the age-at-death distribution toward younger ages. The resulting skeletal sample might be incorrectly interpreted as reflecting an increase in mortality at younger ages and perhaps declines in health over time, even though risks of mortality have not actually changed at all. Given the possible effects of changes in fertility over the period from 1000 to 1739, this study controls for changes in fertility by calculating the number of the individuals above the age of thirty divided by the number of individuals above the age of five years, i.e., D_{30+}/D_{5+}, for each time period. Buikstra et al. (1986) found that there is a strong (negative) relationship between D_{30+}/D_{5+} and birth rate, such that the higher the number, the lower the birth rate and vice versa. This study estimated 95% comparison intervals for D_{30+}/D_{5+} values for each time period to determine whether birth rates differed significantly across those periods. The lack of overlap in the 95% comparison intervals suggests a real difference.

Results

Survivorship

The results of Kaplan–Meier survival analyses for each sex (mean survival times and their corresponding 95% confidence intervals) are shown in Table 9.1. As detailed above, these analyses include only individuals 15 years of age or older. The results reveal significant variation in mean survival time across the five time periods ($p < 0.001$). The highest survivorship for both sexes is seen in the period from *c*. 1000 to 1200 and from *c*. 1350 to 1540. Survivorship for both sexes drops from this high level in the period from *c*. 1569 to 1670. For males, survivorship improves thereafter *c*. 1670–1739. Although female survivorship also improves from 1670 to 1739, it does not do so to the same extent as it does for males. Note that for both sexes, the 95% confidence intervals for 1569–1670 and for 1670–1739 overlap. Thus, it is possible that survivorship did not actually change substantially over the period from 1569 to 1739 or that sex differences were not as marked as they appear at face value.

Table 9.1 Kaplan–Meier survival analysis results. Mean survival time and corresponding confidence intervals are shown in years

	Time Period	Mean Survival Time	95% CI
Females	**1000–1200**	40.96	34.48 – 44.44
	1200–1250	32.99	30.40 – 35.59
	1350–1540	38.23	35.22 – 41.23
	1569–1670	31.98	29.12 – 34.83
	1670–1739	33.29	29.80 – 36.78
Males	**1000–1200**	41.65	37.56 – 45.73
	1200–1250	33.14	30.53 – 35.75
	1350–1540	42.80	39.80 – 45.62
	1569–1670	34.27	31.61 – 36.94
	1670–1739	38.33	35.11 – 41.56

Table 9.2 D_{30+}/D_{5+} values and their 95% comparison intervals for each of the time periods

Time Period	D_{30+}/D_{5+}	95% CI
1000–1200	0.51	0.41 – 0.60
1200–1250	0.43	0.34 – 0.52
1350–1540	0.51	0.43 – 0.60
1569–1670	0.35	0.27 – 0.44
1670–1739	0.55	0.44 – 0.67

Fertility Proxy

The fertility proxies, i.e., the D_{30+}/D_{5+} values and their 95% comparison intervals, are shown in Table 9.2. Although there is variation in the numerical estimates over time, the 95% comparison intervals for the D_{30+}/D_{5+} values from all periods overlap. These results, therefore, indicate a lack of significant differences in birth rates among the periods.

Discussion

As previous studies have shown (DeWitte 2018, 2015), these results suggest that survivorship for both sexes and – by inference – health declined prior to the Black Death and improved in its aftermath during the medieval period. However, the new findings for the early modern period (1569–1739) reported here might indicate that improvements in survivorship and – again by inference – health were relatively short-lived for both sexes in the aftermath of the Black Death.

The Black Death might have shaped population patterns by altering exogenous factors (i.e., those factors external to an individual's physical body) that had immediate, but not long-lasting, effects on health and demography rather than shaping human genetics or biology in ways that had discernable effects over several centuries or longer. In particular, demography and health might have changed just after the Black Death because of improvements in standards of living resulting from the massive depopulation caused by the epidemic. After the Black Death, a severe shortage of labourers in England (as elsewhere) generally resulted in labourers' wages and payments in kind (such as extra food provisions) improving dramatically, while prices for food, goods, and housing fell (Bailey 1996; Campbell 2016; Dyer 1989). These changes led to improvements in the quality of peoples' diets, in general, and decrease in social inequities in diet after the Black Death. This, in turn, likely improved general levels of health, as good nutritional status can have positive effects on immune competence and other physiological systems related to health. Numerous studies in living populations have revealed evidence in support of the developmental origins of health and disease (DOHaD) hypothesis (also known as the Barker, foetal programming, and foetal origins hypotheses) that exposure to malnutrition *in utero* and early childhood can increase the risk of non-communicable diseases, such as cardiovascular disease, later in life (Barker 1990; Thayer and Kuzawa 2014; Worthman and Kuzara 2005). Similar underlying mechanisms might have linked early-life exposure to stress and adult health in the past. As mentioned above, Alfani and Ó Gráda (2018) found that across the entire period from 1250 to 2017, the 200 years following the Black Death were characterized by the lowest frequencies of famines. They also find evidence that, in the past, overpopulation was a crucial factor in the production of famine, rather than warfare, purposeful attempts to withhold food, or other similar human actions. Thus, for several generations after the Black Death in England, people appear to have experienced relatively few famines (because of epidemic-induced reduced population sizes) and also better diet in general; both of these factors could have promoted better health conditions with respect to both infectious and non-communicable diseases through the mid-sixteenth century.

However, the estimated general declines in survivorship beginning in 1569, shown in this study, might indicate that the apparent gains in health and survival observed in London after the Black Death might have been lost as the population and available resources achieved a new equilibrium following the epidemic. Following the Black Death, the population of England was slow to recover to its pre-epidemic size, and sustained recovery was not achieved until the sixteenth century (Bailey 1996). Population growth in the sixteenth century and thereafter would have produced the population pressure that Alfani and Ó Gráda cite as the predominant cause of pre-modern famine. With the unstable and periodically unfavourable climate conditions of the Little Ice Age, subsistence crises increased in frequency in the 1500s after a 200-year "hiatus." Alfani and Ó Gráda (2018) found that from 1250 to 2017, the frequency of famines in Europe was highest between 1550 and 1719. During that period, England, in particular, experienced famines in 1555–1557, 1585–1587, 1594–1598, 1622–1623, and 1698, with the last serious famine arguably occurring in 1622–1623 (Alfani and Ó Gráda 2018). These famines, as well as an increasing number of people vulnerable to the short- and long-term effects thereof, might have resulted in deteriorating health, in general, as reflected by declines in estimated survivorship shown here. The estimated improvement in survivorship (at least for males) in the period from *c.* 1670 to 1739 might reflect a reduction in the severity and frequency of famines in eighteenth-century England. It is worth noting, however, that there were elevated grain prices, food riots, and a spike in mortality levels in England in 1728–1729; although this was not described by contemporaries as a famine *per se*, it was nonetheless England's last subsistence crisis (Alfani and Ó Gráda 2018; Appleby 1980) and had a "scarring" effect. That is, it increased the risk of death and decreased life expectancy across the lifespan for people born in those years (Klemp and Weisdorf 2012).

Alternatively, rather than truly reflecting trends in health for the population of London, or England more broadly, the apparent decline in survivorship from 1569 onward might be an artefact of the socioeconomic composition of the people buried in the New Churchyard compared to the other cemeteries used here. The New Churchyard cemetery, which is the sole source of data for the period from 1569 to 1739 in this study, contains mostly lower-status burials (Hartle et al. 2017). In contrast, the other burial grounds (*c.* 1000–1540) contain a mixture of higher- and lower-status individuals that might be less heavily biased toward low status. It is possible that in the period 1569–1739 there were substantial differences in survivorship between high-and low-status people in London, as has been estimated (at least among children) for skeletal samples dated to the eighteenth and nineteenth centuries (DeWitte et al. 2016). There is abundant evidence from living populations of associations between socioeconomic status and health, including findings in a variety of contexts that people of low status suffer higher risks of mortality and reduced life expectancy compared to high-status individuals (Cavigelli and Chaudhry 2012; Phelan et al. 2010; Robertson et al. 2013). How far back in time these status differentials in health existed is, however, not fully understood and is, thus, the subject of debate. Some scholars argue that substantial health gradients or disparities by wealth are a relatively recent by-product of the Industrial Revolution (see, e.g., Antonovsky 1967), while others contend they likely existed any time wealth inequalities existed (see, e.g., Marmot 2005). If health disparities are generally a consequence of inequality, and not strictly associated with industrialization, the patterns observed in the period from 1569 to 1739 in this study might reflect the conditions among urban London's poor inhabitants rather than general declines in survivorship, and thus health, in the broader population.

If the upward trend in male survivorship from 1670 to 1739 is real, it might reflect gendered differences in access to resources or exposures to stressors at this time that benefitted males and negatively affected (or at the very least failed to benefit) females. Females are innately better equipped to resist and survive infectious and non-communicable diseases and other physiological stressors for a variety of reasons, including the general immune-boosting effects of oestrogen (levels of which are typically much higher in females) and the immune compromising effects of testosterone (levels of which tend to be higher in males) (Klein and Roberts 2010; Zarulli et al. 2018). However, during the medieval and early modern periods, cultural preferences for male heirs and discrimination against women in male-dominated English society may have meant that males had access to better care, food, and other resources throughout their lives compared to females (Bardsley 1999; Green 1994). Such cultural buffering of males, at the expense of females, could have outweighed inherent female biological advantages and, therefore, resulted in sex differences in improvements in health and, thus, survivorship from 1670 onward. Further, as Walter and DeWitte discuss (2017), the predominant occupations of young females in London might have exposed them to certain diseases at greater rates than was true for males: female servants charged with food preparation, for example, might have experienced higher risks of exposure to diseases transmitted by animals.

This apparent trend in male survivorship might also be an artefact of sex-specific effects of selective mortality during the seventeenth-century plague epidemics, each of which killed approximately 20% of the population of London (*c.* 1603, 1625, 1636, and 1665; see Cummins et al. 2016). A similar mechanism has been suggested elsewhere, with respect to the Black Death, to explain sex differences in risks of mortality *c.* 1350–1540 (DeWitte and Yaussy 2020; Yaussy et al. 2016). In general, selective mortality refers to the process by which only certain individuals, typically those that are the most frail, die at a particular age. Mortality, thus, is generally non-random, but rather is selective with respect to health condition or physiological function. Previous analyses have revealed evidence that the Black Death killed more frail males than frail females (perhaps because of inherent female biological buffering). This would mean that in the aftermath of the Black Death, the males who survived the epidemic might have been, on average, healthier (less frail) than female survivors (DeWitte 2010). If similar patterns of selective mortality occurred during seventeenth-century plague epidemics in London, the cumulative effects could have preserved greater heterogeneity in frailty among females but resulted in lower average frailty among males, as reflected by increases in average survivorship for males, but not females *c.* 1670–1739.

Lastly, it is possible that the apparent increase in male survivorship during this period occurred because of sex differences in rates of migration or in the health status of immigrants to the city in the early modern period. Rural to urban migration was common in England throughout the medieval period, and both women and men (particularly young adults) were drawn to London because of the greater economic opportunities available there compared to their rural homes (Bailey 1996; Childs 2006; Kowaleski 1988). Some studies of modern populations have found that successful migrants are, at least temporarily, healthier on average than people in both their source and receiving populations (e.g., Anson 2004; Lu 2008). A similar effect of "migrant selectivity" (also referred to as the healthy migrant effect) might have operated in pre-modern England. However, it is also possible that at least some adult migrants to London might have been vulnerable to diseases endemic in London that they were not exposed to in rural areas during childhood and, thus, died from these diseases at greater rates than people who were raised in London (Alirol et al. 2011). If, as some historical evidence indicates for the medieval period (Kowaleski 1988), young adult migrants to early modern London were predominantly female, there might have been a larger pool of vulnerable females who died from infectious diseases during adolescence and young adulthood in the city compared to males. This, in turn, might have resulted in survivorship differences between the sexes from 1569 to 1739. Evaluating which of these alternative scenarios is most plausible requires further study with additional lines of evidence.

Future Work

My current project (in collaboration with stable isotope experts Julia Beaumont and Janet Montgomery) seeks to discern which underlying mechanisms might have produced the demographic patterns summarized in this chapter. This new project will integrate isotopic, demographic, and pathological data to examine trends in diet and sex and socioeconomic status differences thereof in the medieval period in an attempt to determine whether improvements in health after the Black Death were the result primarily (or exclusively) of dietary changes or migration. Specifically, we will explore how variation in diet changed in England following the Black Death and whether improvements in diet (as described in historical documents) were equally enjoyed by everyone, regardless of age, sex, and socioeconomic status. Importantly, we will also assess whether improvements in diet, if discernible from the stable isotopic data, contributed to substantial improvements in health. Our project also uses stable isotopic data to assess trends in migration and the health status of migrants in London across the medieval period. Ultimately, our goal is to evaluate whether improvements in survivorship after the Black Death might reflect the influx of healthy migrants following the epidemic and whether there is any evidence of gendered variation thereof.

The findings summarized in this chapter demonstrate the dramatic effects that the environment – and specifically the interaction of natural forces (e.g., climatic conditions and disease epidemics) and anthropogenic factors (e.g., urbanization and socioeconomic disparities) – had on human health in past populations. As is often true of scientific research, the results presented here raise additional questions, in this case, specifically about the intersection of urbanization, climate change, and socioeconomic and gender disparities in health. Thus, these findings highlight the need for interdisciplinary perspectives and multiple lines of evidence to improve our understanding of health and the environment in the past.

Notes

1 I am grateful to Jelena Bekvalac and Rebecca Redfern at the Museum of London Centre for Human Bioarchaeology, and Don Walker at Museum of London Archaeology (MOLA) for providing access to the human skeletal remains used in this study and for generously providing the physical facilities for this work. Funding to support the collection of data used in this work was provided by the National Science Foundation (BCS-1261682), The Wenner Gren Foundation (#8247), The American Association of Physical Anthropologists, and the University of South Carolina Office of the Provost.

2 I acknowledge that the approach I have taken views sex as a dichotomy, and thus ignores the variation in sex that is known to exist in human populations. I also note that sex (which is determined by biological factors such as genetics, hormones, and reproductive organs) is not the same as gender, which is a social construct that is assigned and performed and varies cross-culturally. Though in bioarchaeology we often view sex estimated from skeletal remains as a proxy for gender, this overly simplifies reality and ignores and erases the experiences of people who were, for example, non-binary with respect to sex, or gender fluid.

References

Alfani, Guido and Cormac Ó Gráda. 2018. "The Timing and Causes of Famines in Europe." *Nature Sustainability* 1: 283–88. https://doi.org/10.1038/s41893-018-0078-0

Alirol, Emilie, Laurent Getaz, Beat Stoll, François Chappuis, and Louis Loutan. 2011. "Urbanisation and Infectious Diseases in a Globalised World." *Lancet Infectious Diseases* 11. no. 2: 131–41. https://doi.org/10.1016/S1473-3099(10)70223-1

Anson, Jon. 2004. "The Migrant Mortality Advantage: A 70 Month Follow-up of the Brussels Population." *European Journal of Population/Revue européenne de Démographie* 20: 191–218. https://doi.org/10.1007/s10680-004-0883-1

Antonovsky, Aaron. 1967. "Social Class, Life Expectancy and Overall Mortality." *Milbank Memorial Fund Quarterly* 45, no. 2, Part 1: 31–73.

Appleby, Andrew B., 1980. "Epidemics and Famine in the Little Ice Age." *Journal of Interdisciplinary History* 10, no. 4: 643–63. https://doi.org/10.2307/203063

Bailey, Mark. 1996. "Demographic Decline in Late Medieval England: Some Thoughts on Recent Research." *Economic History Review* 49, no. 1: 1–19.

Bardsley, Sandy. 1999. "Women's Work Reconsidered: Gender and Wage Differentiation in Late Medieval England." *Past & Present* 165: 3–29.

Barker, D.J. 1990. "The Fetal and Infant Origins of Adult Disease." *British Medical Journal* 301: 1111.

Baro, Mamadou and Tara F. Deubel. 2006. "Persistent Hunger: Perspectives on Vulnerability, Famine, and Food Security in Sub-Saharan Africa." *Annual Review of Anthropology* 35: 521–38. https://doi.org/10.1146/annurev.anthro.35.081705.123224

Bengtsson, Tommy and Alain Gagnon. 2011. "Revisiting Mortality Crises of the Past: Introduction." *Genus* 67, no. 2: 1–7. https://doi.org/10.2307/genus.67.2.1

Boldsen, Jesper L., George R. Milner, Lyle W. Konigsberg, and James W. Wood. 2002. "Transition Analysis: A New Method for Estimating Age from Skeletons." In *Paleodemography: Age Distributions from Skeletal Samples*, edited by Robert D. Hoppa and James W. Vaupel, 73–106. Cambridge: Cambridge University Press.

Bos, Kirsten I., Verena J. Schuenemann, G. Brian Golding, Hernán A. Burbano, Nicholas Waglechner, Brian K. Coombes, Joseph B. McPhee, Sharon N. DeWitte, Matthias Meyer, Sarah Schmedes, James Wood, David J. D. Earn, D. Ann Herring, Peter Bauer, Hendrik N. Poinar, and Johannes Krause. 2011. "A Draft Genome of *Yersinia pestis* from Victims of the Black Death." *Nature* 478: 506–10.

Bos, Kirsten I., Alexander Herbig, Jason Sahl, Nicholas Waglechner, Mathieu Fourment, Stephen A. Forrest, Jennifer Klunk, Verena J. Schuenemann, Debi Poinar, Melanie Kuch, G. Brian Golding, Olivier Dutour, Paul Keim, David M. Wagner, Edward C. Holmes, Johannes Krause, and Hendrik N. Poinar. 2016. "Eighteenth-Century *Yersinia pestis* Genomes Reveal the Long-Term Persistence of an Historical Plague Focus." *eLife* 5: e12994. https://doi.org/10.7554/eLife.12994

Bouckaert, Andre. 1989. "Crisis Mortality: Extinction and Near-Extinction of Human Populations." In *Differential Mortality: Methodological Issues and Biosocial Factors*, edited by Lado Ruzicka, Guillaume Wunsch, and Penny Kane, 217–30. Oxford: Clarendon Press.

Bowsher, David, Tony Dyson, Nick Holder, and Isca Howell. 2007. *The London Guildhall: An Archaeological History of a Neighbourhood from Early Medieval to Modern Times*. 2 Volumes. London: Museum of London Archaeology Service.

Brooke, John L. 2014. *Climate Change and the Course of Global History*. New York: Cambridge University Press.

Buikstra, Jane E. and Douglas H. Ubelaker, eds. 1994. *Standards for Data Collection from Human Skeletal Remains: Proceedings of a Seminar at the Field Museum of Natural History* (Arkansas Archaeology Research Series 44). Fayetteville, AR: Arkansas Archeological Survey Press.

Büntgen, Ulf, Willy Tegel, Kurt Nicolussi, Michael McCormick, DavidFrank, Valerie Trouet, Jed. O. Kaplan, Franz Herzig, Karl-Uwe Heussner, Heinz Wanner, Jürg Luterbacher, and Jan Esper. 2011. "2500 Years of European Climate Variability and Human Susceptibility." *Science* 331: 578–82. https://doi.org/10.1126/science.1197175

Campbell, Bruce M. S. 2016. *The Great Transition: Climate, Disease and Society in the Late-Medieval World.* Cambridge: Cambridge University Press.

Campbell, Bruce M. S. 2017. "Global Climates, the 1257 Mega-Eruption of Samalas Volcano, Indonesia, and the English Food Crisis of 1258." *Transactions of the Royal Historical Society* 27: 87–121. https://doi.org/10.1017/S0080440117000056

Cavigelli, Sonia A. and Hashim S. Chaudhry. 2012. "Social Status, Glucocorticoids, Immune Function, and Health: Can Animal Studies Help Us Understand Human Socioeconomic-Status-Related Health Disparities?" *Hormones and Behavior* 62, no. 3: 295–313. https://doi.org/10.1016/j.yhbeh.2012.07.006

Chen, Edith and Gregory E. Miller. 2012. "Socioeconomic Status and Health: Mediating and Moderating Factors." *Annual Review of Clinical Psychology* 9: 723–49. https://doi.org/10.1146/annurev-clinpsy-050212-185634

Childs, Wendy R. 2006. "Moving Around." In *A Social History of England 1200–1500*, edited by Rosemary Horrox and W. Mark Ormrod, 260–75. Cambridge: Cambridge University Press.

Connell, Brian, Amy Gray Jones, Rebecca Redfern, and Don Walker. 2012. *A Bioarchaeological Study of Medieval Burials on the Site of St. Mary Spital: Excavations at Spitalfields Market, London E1: 1991–2007.* London: Museum of London Archaeology.

Cummins, Neil, Morgan Kelly, and Cormac Ó Gráda. 2016. "Living Standards and Plague in London, 1560–1665." *Economic History Review* 69, no. 1: 3–34.

DeWitte, Sharon N. 2010. "Sex Differentials in Frailty in Medieval England." *American Journal of Physical Anthropology* 143, no. 2: 285–97. https://doi.org/10.1002/ajpa.21316

DeWitte, Sharon N. 2014a. "Mortality Risk and Survival in the Aftermath of the Medieval Black Death." *PLoS ONE* 9, e96513. https://doi.org/10.1371/journal.pone.0096513

DeWitte, Sharon N. 2014b. "Health in Post-Black Death London (1350–1538): Age Patterns of Periosteal New Bone Formation in a Post-Epidemic Population." *American Journal of Physical Anthropology* 155, no. 2: 260–67. https://doi.org/10.1002/ajpa.22510

DeWitte, Sharon N. 2015. "Setting the Stage for Medieval Plague: Pre-Black Death Trends in Survival and Mortality." *American Journal of Physical Anthropology* 158, no. 3: 441–51. https://doi.org/10.1002/ajpa.22806

DeWitte, Sharon N. 2017. "Living Longer? Demographic Trends in London Using Transition Analysis." In *The New Churchyard: From Moorfields Marsh to Bethlem Burial Ground, Brokers Row and Liverpool Street*, edited by Hartle, Robert, Niamh Carty, Michael Henderson, Elizabeth L. Knox, and Don Walker, 113–14. London: Museum of London Archaeology.

DeWitte, Sharon N. 2018. "Stress, Sex, and Plague: Patterns of Developmental Stress and Survival in Pre- and Post-Black Death London." *American Journal of Human Biology* 30, no. 1: e23073. https://doi.org/10.1002/ajhb.23073

DeWitte, Sharon N. and Phil Slavin. 2013. "Between Famine and Death. Physiological Stress and Dairy Deficiency in England on the Eve of the Black Death (1315–50): New Evidence from Paleoepidemiology and Manorial Accounts." *Journal of Interdisciplinary History* 44, no. 1: 37–61.

DeWitte, Sharon N., Gail Hughes-Morey, Jelena Bekvalac, and Jordan Karsten. 2016. "Wealth, Health and Frailty in Industrial-Era London." *Annals of Human Biology* 43, no. 3: 241–54. https://doi.org/10.3109/03014460.2015.1020873

DeWitte, Sharon N. and Maryanne Kowaleski. 2017. "Black Death Bodies." *Fragments: Interdisciplinary Approaches to the Study of Ancient and Medieval Pasts* 6: 1–37.

DeWitte, Sharon N. and Samantha L. Yaussy. 2020. "Sex Differences in Adult Famine Mortality in Medieval London." *American Journal of Physical Anthropology* 171, no. 1: 164–69.

Dyer, Christopher 1989. *Standards of Living in the Later Middle Ages: Social Change in England, c. 1200–1500.* Cambridge: Cambridge University Press.

Evans, Gary W. and Elyse Kantrowitz. 2002. "Socioeconomic Status and Health: The Potential Role of Environmental Risk Exposure." *Annual Review of Public Health* 23. no. 1: 303–31. https://doi.org/10.1146/annurev.publhealth.23.112001.112349

Ezeh, Alex, Oyinlola Oyebode, David Satterthwaite, YenFu Chen, Robert Ndugwa, Jo Sartori, Blessing Mberu, G. J. Melendez-Torres, Tilahun Haregu, Samuel I. Watson, Waleska Caiaffa, Anthony Capon, and Richard J. Lilford. 2017. "The History, Geography, and Sociology of Slums and the Health Problems of People Who Live in Slums." *The Lancet* 389, no. 10068: 547–58. https://doi.org/10.1016/S0140-6736(16)31650-6

Gage, Timothy B. 2005. "Are Modern Environments Really Bad for Us?: Revisiting the Demographic and Epidemiologic Transitions." *American Journal of Physical Anthropology* 128, no. S41: 96–117. https://doi.org/10.1002/ajpa.20353

Gilchrist, Roberta and Barney Sloane. 2005. *Requiem: the Medieval Monastic Cemetery in Britain.* London: Museum of London Archaeology Service.

Grainger, Ian and Christopher Phillpotts. 2011. *The Cistercian Abbey of St Mary Graces, East Smithfield, London.* MoLA Monograph 44. London: Museum of London Archaeology.

Green, Monica H. 1994. "Documenting Medieval Women's Medical Practice." In *Practical Medicine from Salerno to the Black Death,* edited by Luis Garcia-Ballester, Roger French, Jon Arrizabalaga, and Andrew Cunningham, 322–52. Cambridge: Cambridge University Press.

Guillet, Sébastien, Christophe Corona, Markus Stoffel, Myriam Khodri, Franck Lavigne, Pablo Ortega, Nicolas Eckert, Pascal Dkengne Sielenou, Valérie Daux, Olga V. Churakova (Sidorova), Nicole Davi, Jean-Louis Edouard, Yong Zhang, Brian H. Luckman, Vladimir S. Myglan, Joël Guiot, Martin Beniston, Valérie Masson-Delmotte, and Clive Oppenheimer. 2017. "Climate Response to the Samalas Volcanic Eruption in 1257 Revealed by Proxy Records." *Nature Geoscience* 10, 123–28. https://doi.org/10.1038/ngeo2875

Haensch, Stephanie, Raffaella Bianucci, Michel Signoli, Minoarisoa Rajerison, Michael Schultz. Sacha Kacki, Marco Vermunt, Darlene A. Weston, Derek Hurst, Mark Achtman, Elisabeth Carniel, and Barbara Bramanti. 2010. "Distinct Clones of *Yersinia pestis* Caused the Black Death." *PLoS Pathogogy* 6, e1001134. https://doi.org/10.1371/journal.ppat.1001134

Harpham, Trudy. 2009. "Urban Health in Developing Countries: What Do We Know and Where Do We Go?" *Health & Place* 15, no. 1: 107–16. https://doi.org/10.1016/j.healthplace.2008.03.004

Hartle, Robert, Niamh Carty, Michael Henderson, Elizabeth L. Knox, and Don Walker, eds. 2017. *The New Churchyard: From Moorfields Marsh to Bethlem Burial Ground, Brokers Row and Liverpool Street*. London: Museum of London Archaeology.

Hayward, Adam D., Jari Holopainen, Jenni E. Pettay, and Virpi Lummaa. 2012. "Food and Fitness: Associations Between Crop Yields and Life-History Traits in a Longitudinally Monitored Pre-Industrial Human Population." *Proceedings of the Royal Society B: Biological Sciences* 279, no. 1745: 4165–4173. https://doi.org/10.1098/rspb.2012.1190

Hoyle, R., 2017. "Britain." In *Famine in European History*, edited by Guido Alfani and Cormac Ó Gráda, 141–65. Cambridge: Cambridge University Press.

Jian, Yun, Lucas Neas, Lynne C. Messer, Christine L. Gray, Jyotsna S. Jagai, Kristen M. Rappazzo, and Danelle T. Lobdell. 2019. "Divergent Trends in Life Expectancy Across the Rural-Urban Gradient and Association with Specific Racial Proportions in the Contiguous USA 2000–2005." *International Journal of Public Health* 64: 1367–1374. https://doi.org/10.1007/s00038-019-01274-5

Jordan, William C. 1996. *The Great Famine: Northern Europe in the Early Fourteenth Century*. Princeton, NJ: Princeton University Press.

Keene, Derek. 2011. "Crisis Management in London's Food Supply, 1250–1500." In *Commercial Activity, Markets and Entrepreneurs in the Middle Ages: Essays in Honour of Richard Britnell*, edited by Ben Dodds and Christian D. Liddy, 45–62. Woodbridge: Boydell and Brewer.

Klein, Sabra L. and Charlotte Roberts. 2010. *Sex Hormones and Immunity to Infection*. Heidelberg: Springer.

Klemp, Marc and Jacob Weisdorf. 2012. "The Lasting Damage to Mortality of Early-Life Adversity: Evidence from the English Famine of the Late 1720s." *European Review of Economic History* 16, 233–46.

Kowaleski, Maryanne, 1988. "The History of Urban Families in Medieval England." *Journal of Medieval History* 14, no. 1: 47–63. https://doi.org/10.1016/0304-4181(88)90016-4

Krieger, Nancy. 1999. "Embodying Inequality: A Review of Concepts, Measures, and Methods for Studying Health Consequences of Discrimination." *International Journal of Health Services* 29, no. 2: 295–352. https://doi.org/10.2190/M11W-VWXE-KQM9-G97Q

Krieger, Nancy. 2005. "Embodiment: A Conceptual Glossary for Epidemiology." *Journal of Epidemiology and Community Health* 59, no. 5: 350–55. https://doi.org/10.1136/jech.2004.024562

Lavigne, Franck, Jean-Philippe Degeai, Jean-Christophe Komorowski, Sébastien Guillet, Vincent Robert, Pierre Lahitte, Clive Oppenheimer, Markus Stoffel, Céline M. Vidal, Surono, Indyo Pratomo, Patrick Wassmer, Irka Hajdas, Danang Sri Hadmoko, and Edouard de Belizal. 2013. "Source of the Great A.D. 1257 Mystery Eruption Unveiled, Samalas Volcano, Rinjani Volcanic Complex, Indonesia." *Proceedings of the National Academy of Sciences* 110, no. 42: 16742–16747. https://doi.org/10.1073/pnas.1307520110

Lu, Yao. 2008. "Test of the 'Healthy Migrant Hypothesis': A Longitudinal Analysis of Health Selectivity of Internal Migration in Indonesia." *Social Science & Medicine 1982* 67, no. 8: 1331–1339. https://doi.org/10.1016/j.socscimed.2008.06.017

Marmot, Michael. 2005. *The Status Syndrome: How Social Standing Affects Our Health and Longevity.* New York: Holt Paperbacks.

Meindl, Richard S., C. Owen Lovejoy, Robert P. Mensforth, and Lydia Don Carlos. 1985. "Accuracy and Direction of Error in the Sexing of the Skeleton: Implications for Paleodemography." *American Journal of Physical Anthropology* 68, no. 1: 79–85. https://doi.org/10.1002/ajpa.1330680108

Milner, George R., Dorothy A. Humpf, and Henry C. Harpending. 1989. "Pattern Matching of Age-at-Death Distributions in Paleodemographic Analysis." *American Journal of Physical Anthropology* 80, no. 1: 49–58. https://doi.org/10.1002/ajpa.1330800107

Mokyr, Joel and Cormac Ó Gráda. 2002. "What Do People Die of During Famines: The Great Irish Famine in Comparative Perspective." *European Review of Economic History* 6, no. 3: 339–63. https://doi.org/10.1017/S1361491602000163

Mutaqin, Bachtiar W. and Franck Lavigne. 2021. "Oldest Description of a Caldera-forming Eruption in Southeast Asia Unveiled in Forgotten Written Sources." *GeoJournal* 86, no. 2: 557–566. https://doi.org/10.1007/s10708-019-10083-5

Omran, Abdel R. 1971. "The Epidemiologic Transition: A Theory of the Epidemiology of Population Change." *Milbank Memorial Fund Quarterly* 49, 509–38.

Paine, Richard R. 1989. "Model Life Table Fitting by Maximum Likelihood Estimation: A Procedure to Reconstruct Paleodemographic Characteristics From Skeletal Age Distributions." *American Journal of Physical Anthropology* 79, no. 1: 51–61. https://doi.org/10.1002/ajpa.1330790106

Phelan, Jo C., Bruce G. Link, and Parisa Tehranifar. 2010. "Social Conditions as Fundamental Causes of Health Inequalities: Theory, Evidence, and Policy Implications." *Journal of Health and Social Behavior* 51, no. 1 Suppl: S28–40. https://doi.org/10.1177/0022146510383498

Robertson, Tony, G. David Batty, Geoff Der, Candida Fenton, Paul G. Shiels, and Michaela Benzeval. 2013. "Is Socioeconomic Status Associated With Biological Aging as Measured by Telomere Length?" *Epidemiologic Reviews* 35, no. 1: 98–111. https://doi.org/10.1093/epirev/mxs001

Rogers, Tracy L. 2005. "Determining the Sex of Human Remains Through Cranial Morphology." *Journal of Forensic Sciences* 50, no. 3: 493–500.

Sattenspiel, Lisa, and Henry Harpending. 1983. "Stable Populations and Skeletal Age." *American Antiquity* 48, no. 3: 489–98.

Sawchuk, Lawrence A., Lianne Tripp, Sotirios Damouras, and Mark DeBono. 2013. "Situating Mortality: Quantifying Crisis Points and Periods of Stability." *American Journal of Physical Anthropology* 152, no. 4: 459–70. https://doi.org/10.1002/ajpa.22380

Schofield, John. 1997. "Excavations on the Site of St. Nicholas Shambles, Newgate Street, City of London, 1975–9." *Transactions of the London and Middlesex Archaeological Society* 48, 77–135.

Scrimshaw, Nevin S. 2003. "Historical Concepts of Interactions, Synergism and Antagonism Between Nutrition and Infection." *The Journal of Nutrition* 133, no. 1: 316S–21S.

Sen, Amartya. 1981. *Poverty and Famines: An Essay on Entitlement and Deprivation.* Oxford: Clarendon Press.

Slavin, Phil. 2012. "The Great Bovine Pestilence and its Economic and Environmental Consequences in England and Wales, 1318–50." *Economic History Review* 65, no. 4: 1239–1266. https://doi.org/10.1111/j.1468-0289.2011.00625.x

Spyrou, Maria A., Rezeda I. Tukhbatova, Michal Feldman, Joanna Drath, Sacha Kacki, Julia Beltrán de Heredia, Susanne Arnold, Airat G. Sitdikov, Dominique Castex, Joachim Wahl, Ilgizar R. Gazimzyanov, Danis K. Nurgaliev, Alexander Herbig, Kirsten I. Bos, Johannes Krause. 2016. "Historical *Y. pestis* Genomes Reveal the European Black Death as the Source of Ancient and Modern Plague Pandemics." *Cell Host & Microbe* 19, no. 6: 874–81. https://doi.org/10.1016/j.chom.2016.05.012

Stoffel, Markus, Myriam Khodri, Christophe Corona, Sébastien Guillet, Virginie Poulain, Slimane Bekki, Joël Guiot, Brian H. Luckman, Clive Oppenheimer, Nicolas Lebas, Martin Beniston, and Valérie Masson-Delmotte. 2015. "Estimates of Volcanic-Induced Cooling in the Northern Hemisphere Over the Past 1,500 Years." *Nature Geoscience* 8: 784–88. https://doi.org/10.1038/ngeo2526

Storper, Michael and Allen J. Scott. 2016. "Current Debates in Urban Theory: A Critical Assessment." *Urban Studies* 53, 1114–1136. https://doi.org/10.1177/0042098016634002

Suk, Jonathan E., Davide Manissero, Guido Büscher, and Jan C. Semenza. 2009. "Wealth Inequality and Tuberculosis Elimination in Europe." *Emerging Infectious Diseases* 15, no. 11: 1812–1814.

Thayer, Zaneta M., and Christopher W. Kuzawa. 2014. "Early Origins of Health Disparities: Material Deprivation Predicts Maternal Evening Cortisol in Pregnancy and Offspring Cortisol Reactivity in the First Few Weeks of Life." *American Journal of Human Biology* 26, no. 6: 723–30. https://doi.org/10.1002/ajhb.22532

Thu Le, Huong and Alison L. Booth. 2014. "Inequality in Vietnamese Urban–Rural Living Standards, 1993–2006." *Review of Income and Wealth* 60, no. 4: 862–86. https://doi.org/10.1111/roiw.12051

Vlahov, David, Nicholas Freudenberg, Fernando Proietti, Danielle Ompad, Andrew Quinn, Vijay Nandi, and Sandro Galea. 2007. "Urban as a Determinant of Health." *Journal of Urban Health* 84, no. 1: 16–26. https://doi.org/10.1007/s11524-007-9169-3

Walker, Phillip L. 2008. "Sexing Skulls Using Discriminant Function Analysis of Visually Assessed Traits." *American Journal of Physical Anthropology* 136, no. 1: 39–50. https://doi.org/10.1002/ajpa.20776

Walter, Brittany S. and Sharon N. DeWitte. 2017. "Urban and Rural Mortality and Survival in Medieval England." *Annals of Human Biology* 44, no. 4: 338–48.

White, William J. and Tony Dyson. 1988. *Skeletal Remains from the Cemetery of St Nicholas Shambles, City of London.* London: London and Middlesex Archaeological Society.

Williams, Brenda A. and Tracy L. Rogers. 2006. "Evaluating the Accuracy and Precision of Cranial Morphological Traits for Sex Determination." *Journal of Forensic Sciences* 51, no. 4: 729–35.

Williams, Leslie Lea and Clark Spencer Larsen. 2017. "Health and the Little Ice Age in Southeastern Germany and Alpine Austria: Synergies between Stress, Nutritional Deficiencies, and Disease." Bioarchaeology International 1, no. 3/4: 148–70. https://doi.org/10.5744/bi.2017.0012

Wisner, Ben, ed. 2004. *At Risk: Natural Hazards, People's Vulnerability and Disasters.* 2nd Edition. London: Routledge.

Wood, James W. 1998. "A Theory of Preindustrial Population Dynamics Demography, Economy, and Well-Being in Malthusian Systems." Current Anthropology 39, no. 1: 99–135. https://doi.org/10.1086/204700

Worthman, Carol M. and Jennifer Kuzara. 2005. "Life History and the Early Origins of Health Differentials." *American Journal of Human Biology* 17, no. 1: 95–112. https://doi.org/10.1002/ajhb.20096

Yaussy, Samantha L., Sharon N. DeWitte, and Rebecca C. Redfern. 2016. "Frailty and Famine: Patterns of Mortality and Physiological Stress Among Victims of Famine in Medieval London." *American Journal of Physical Anthropology* 160, no. 2: 272–83. https://doi.org/10.1002/ajpa.22954

Young, Alwyn. 2013. "Inequality, the Urban-Rural Gap, and Migration." *The Quarterly Journal of Economics* 128, no. 4: 1727–1785. https://doi.org/10.1093/qje/qjt025

Zarulli, Virginia, Julia A. Barthold Jones, Anna Oksuzyan, Rune Lindahl-Jacobsen, Kaare Christensen, and James W. Vaupel. 2018. "Women Live Longer Than Men Even During Severe Famines and Epidemics." *Proceedings of the National Academy of Sciences* 115, no. 4: E832–E840. https://doi.org/10.1073/pnas.1701535115

Index

Note: Page number followed by "n" refer to end notes.